Praise for *The Per*

"*The Personalized Autism Nutrition Plan* empowers parents with a flexible, science-backed approach to addressing their child's unique needs through diet and nutrition. With clear guidance, adaptable meal plans, and kid-friendly recipes, this book is a game changer for families seeking holistic ways to manage symptoms and support well-being."

—David Perlmutter, MD, FACN, #1 *New York Times* bestselling author of *Grain Brain* and *Drop Acid*

"Parents of neurodivergent kids, *The Personalized Autism Nutrition Plan* by Julie Matthews is your secret weapon! Julie breaks down how simple dietary shifts can improve your child's brain health and happiness. With 50 kid-approved recipes, easy meal plans, and clear explanations of the science behind it all, you'll feel empowered to support your child's well-being—without overwhelm."

—JJ Virgin, four-time *New York Times* bestselling author

"By following a few simple dietary suggestions, you can see a marked improvement in many chronic symptoms. You'll systematically pinpoint the best ingredients for your child's holistic health and discover new favorite recipes that you can return to again and again."

—Izabella Wentz, PharmD, *New York Times* bestselling author of *Hashimoto's Protocol*

"Whether you're the parent of a child with autism, ADHD, or anxiety, *The Personalized Autism Nutrition Plan* is the perfect kitchen companion to keep your child healthy and thriving. Even picky eaters will find something to enjoy."

—Terry Wahls, MD, FACP, author of *The Wahls Protocol*

"*The Personalized Autism Nutrition Plan* will empower parents of children with autism, ADHD, and related disorders, and remind them they are not alone on this journey. Julie Matthews ensures you are competent and confident on matters of your child's nutrition."

—Dr. Elana Roumell, ND, founder of Med School for Moms

"This is a great guide to both introductory diets and advanced diets and supplements based on research and many years of experience. Highly recommended."

—James B. Adams, PhD, professor at Arizona State University and director of Arizona State University's Autism/Asperger's Research Program

"In *The Personalized Autism Nutrition Plan*, Julie Matthews brilliantly combines clinical expertise with a genuine understanding of the unique needs of children on the spectrum. This guide not only empowers parents but also inspires a holistic approach to care that can transform lives."

—Kurt Woeller, DO, biomedical autism specialist and integrative medicine physician

"*The Personalized Autism Nutrition Plan* provides science-based nutritional knowledge and biochemical foundations for the parents of a child with autism, ADHD, or anxiety. What makes this book stand out is the deep dive on how to use therapeutic diets—including low-salicylate, low-glutamate, low-oxalate, low-histamine, low-amine, gluten- and grain-free, GAPS, Paleo, and low-FODMAP—using a personalized approach. By following Julie's dietary suggestions, you'll see dramatic improvements in many chronic symptoms."

—Trudy Scott, nutritionist and author of *The Antianxiety Food Solution*

"Julie Matthews has always been a leader in the nutritional care of our children with special needs and this book does not disappoint. She gives parents and practitioners easily digestible recipes for picky eaters, adjustable meal plans, and detailed, evidence-based, ideal foods and nutritional supplements for children with special needs. There is no such thing as junk food; it is either junk or food. Learning from the best, this book gives you all you need to understand, implement, and succeed in making a quality food and overall nutritional plan for your child.

—Nancy O'Hara, MD, MPH, FAAP, board-certified pediatrician

"*The Personalized Autism Nutrition Plan* is an empowering resource for all parents who want to help their children heal. It marries good science with a clear, actionable, and nourishing plan that all children can benefit from."

—Vicki Kobliner, MS, RDN

"There is no greater expert on effective therapeutic nutrition for autism than Julie Matthews. *The Personalized Autism Nutrition Plan* is a fantastic step-by-step, easy-to-follow resource, backed by scientific research and decades of clinical practice. This should be required reading for any parent or practitioner supporting a child with autism, ADHD, or other neurodevelopmental conditions."

—Beth Lambert, author of *A Compromised Generation* and founder and executive director of Documenting Hope

"Working out the right nutritious foods to feed your child can be a minefield, and Julie breaks this down so beautifully to make it easy for you. You'll learn how to become your child's nutritional detective with this wonderful book's help; your child will reap the benefits of better sleep, mood, and behavior. Don't wait to start your child's nutrition journey today with this brilliant book!"

—Lucinda Miller, author of *Brain Brilliance* and clinical lead of NatureDoc

"*The Personalized Autism Nutrition Plan* is your best solution to information overload. Julie Matthews's excellent book provides you with the knowledge and confidence to support your child toward optimal health."

—James Greenblatt, MD, functional psychiatrist and author of *Finally Focused*

"I have been serving children with autism for over a decade now. I only wish I had this remarkable book to share with my families earlier. It is not only comprehensive, more importantly it is super practical and easy to implement. The information in *The Personalized Autism Nutrition Plan* is outstanding and an absolute must-read for any family whose child is struggling with autism."

—Pejman Katiraei, DO, board-certified pediatrician
and cofounder of Wholistic Kids

"This is a very comprehensive and evidence-based book, which starts by outlining all the comorbidities that can accompany most cases of autism and related childhood developmental disorders, based on the latest research. With the nutritional guidance in this book, parents and caregivers are able to help many children ameliorate and even reverse many symptoms of autism."

—Rebecca Sherry Eshraghi, PhD, board-certified doctor of natural medicine

"Julie Matthews is a pioneer in personalized nutrition for children with autism, and it is a great gift that she's now sharing her copious experience and wisdom in a book. Her book offers valuable, evidence-based guidance that has worked successfully to help not just countless struggling kids but also their families. It's wonderful that now so many more people will have the insight and support Julie offers in this excellent reference."

—Maya Shetreat, MD, pediatric neurologist and author of *The Dirt Cure*

"The nutrition guidelines in this book have been been life-changing! Julie Matthews's newest book explains how diet and supplements can impact autism and behavioral symptoms. It's a practical guide backed by science that tells you exactly what you need to know so you can make the right changes to improve your child's health, and even your own!"

—Annika Rockwell, RDN

THE
PERSONALIZED
AUTISM
NUTRITION PLAN

Also by Julie S. Matthews, MS

*Nourishing Hope for Autism: Nutrition and Diet Guide
for Healing Our Children*

THE
PERSONALIZED
AUTISM
NUTRITION PLAN

Nourishing Hope for Kids with
ASD, ADHD, Anxiety, and
Neurodevelopmental Delays

JULIE S. MATTHEWS, MS

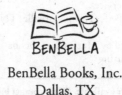

BenBella Books, Inc.
Dallas, TX

BioIndividual Nutrition® and Nourishing Hope® are registered trademarks of Julie Matthews. Nourishing Hope Food Pyramid™, Low SAG diet™, and V123™ are trademarks of Julie Matthews.

The Personalized Autism Nutrition Plan copyright © 2025 by Julie S. Matthews

BenBella Books, Inc.
8080 N. Central Expressway
Suite 1700
Dallas, TX 75206
benbellabooks.com
Send feedback to feedback@benbellabooks.com

BenBella is a federally registered trademark.

Printed in the United States of America
10 9 8 7 6 5 4 3 2 1

Library of Congress Control Number: 2024039029
ISBN 9781637746110 (trade paperback)
ISBN 9781637746127 (electronic)

Editing by Claire Schulz
Copyediting by Jessica Easto
Proofreading by Rebecca Maines and Lisa Story
Indexing by WordCo Indexing Services
Text design and composition by PerfecType, Nashville, TN
Cover design by Morgan Carr
Interior graphics support provided by María Clara Ochoa
Printed by Lake Book Manufacturing

To my Nourishing Hope mothers and families,
you have enriched my life and inspire me.

To my daughter, who has taught me so much and inspires
me to be a better person. I love you with all my heart.

CONTENTS

SECTION 2
The Nourishing Hope Essentials

SECTION 3
BioIndividual Nutrition and Therapeutic Diets

SECTION 4
Fifty Family-Friendly Recipes

FOREWORD

Aidan was a six-year-old boy who was struggling. He was anxious, agitated, and angry most of the time. He didn't feel right in his own body or brain. He couldn't stand loud sounds or certain sensations or food textures—not even the sound of his mother chewing or a hug or kiss from her, which he would promptly wipe away. He was diagnosed with attention deficit/hyperactivity disorder, oppositional defiant disorder, sensory processing disorder, and possible autism spectrum disorder. His mom was overwhelmed and knew that there was more that could help Aidan before they started medications, but she didn't know where to start. So we sat down and decided on one step to take first: swap out his Takis for Siete Fuego chips without the artificial dyes and monosodium glutamate; swap out the after-soccer Gatorade for unsweetened coconut water; and eliminate all artificial dyes, artificial flavors, preservatives, and emulsifiers from the foods he was eating.

Two weeks later, Mom sent me a note saying that Aidan was a different kid. He still had a long way to go, but he wasn't getting into fights at school, he was able to sit more calmly during circle time, he didn't fly into rages when the slightest thing went wrong, and—most important—he didn't wipe away her kisses and even started asking her for hugs. She was amazed by the change and grateful for the opportunity to connect.

This is the power of food as medicine. This is what I want every practitioner and parent to understand. The right foods have the power to heal, while the wrong foods can keep our children stuck in their current state of dis-ease (a term some practitioners use to describe when a body is out of its optimal state of wellness, or "ease").

But just what are the "right foods" for your child?

As an integrative pediatrician and pediatric functional medicine expert of more than twenty years, I know from firsthand experience that there is no one-size-fits-all approach when it comes to nutrition—especially for our children. Each child has their own unique story, family history, life circumstances, gut-brain connection, and epigenetic profile that requires a personalized approach to nutrition that is as unique as they are.

This is exactly why every parent and practitioner needs Julie's book, *The Personalized Autism Nutrition Plan: Nourishing Hope for Kids with ASD, ADHD, Anxiety, and Other Neurodevelopmental Delays.*

Julie is my go-to expert for all my nutrition and food-as-medicine questions and needs for my patients and my own family. I am honored to call Julie a colleague and, most important, a dear friend. Julie and I started our holistic careers at the same time. I still remember traveling up to San Francisco to meet in the little recording studio that she used for her radio show (yes—she had a radio show and was on the leading edge of the podcast movement!), marveling at how dedicated, passionate, and knowledgeable she was about everything nutrition and autism. Julie has been my sister in our common mission to revolutionize the future of children's health. Our paths have been intertwined in many ways; we had our baby girls the same year. And now, we have birthed our book babies just a year apart!

Julie's passion has led her around the world to speak as the leading expert in therapeutic diets and personalized nutrition for children with special needs and neurodevelopmental concerns. She is a published researcher with a degree in medical nutrition and has the superpower to translate complex science into practical, actionable steps for parents and clinicians. I am grateful to have learned so much from Julie over the years that has benefited my patients and my own family alike.

The Personalized Autism Nutrition Plan is the personalized nutrition bible that I wish I had when I was starting my practice twenty years ago, navigating my way through the research coming out that neurodiverse children might benefit from a gluten-free, casein-free diet, or a Feingold diet, or low oxalate, keto, low histamine, and on and on (if you don't know what these are, don't worry—Julie will walk you through them in this book). It was enough to make my head spin as a practitioner, much less a parent. But I was lucky: I had Julie's ear and phone number on speed dial. And now with her book, you get to as well—whether you're a parent of a child with neurodiversity who is struggling with symptoms that are impacting their ability to thrive or a practitioner who wants to know how to serve the children in their practice to help them thrive.

In this essential guidebook, you will learn:

- Why a personalized nutrition approach is so important to address the underlying factors and symptoms of children with autism or any neurodevelopmental concern
- The foundations of a nourishing diet for all children
- How to successfully address picky eating
- The specifics of different therapeutic diets (including low salicylate, low glutamate, low histamine, SCD, GAPS, Paleo, low oxalate, low FODMAP, and more) and how to create a personalized nutrition plan that's right *for your child*
- An evidence-based guide to supplements to support your child's microbiome, immune system, mood/behavior, attention/focus, mitochondria, and speech/language/communication
- Fifty recipes to help you get started and set yourself up for success on your child's personalized nutrition journey
- 375+ references to share with your family, friends, and practitioners who may need more evidence before they're ready to join you on your journey
- And so much more

This will be your nutrition resource for decades to come. In *The Personalized Autism Nutrition Plan*, Julie helps parents and practitioners cut through the nutrition noise and find solutions that *nourish hope* for your whole family!

Elisa Song, MD
Integrative Pediatrician and Pediatric Functional Medicine Expert
Author of the national bestseller *Healthy Kids, Happy Kids: An Integrative Pediatrician's Guide to Whole Child Resilience*

INTRODUCTION

At four years old, Matthew had very little language. His frequent feelings of frustration and anxiety led to a lot of tantrums. His sleep problems frequently woke up his older sister, who shared a bedroom with him, and kept his parents awake for hours at a time, causing a lot of stress and exhaustion for the family. His mother, Terri, was almost at the end of her rope, but his mother and father were determined to do everything they could to help Matthew sleep and relieve his emotional distress.

Fortunately, Terri learned of the improvements other families were getting with dietary intervention and realized changing Matthew's diet was something her family could try. She also worked with an integrative physician (a friend and colleague of mine, Dr. Kurt Woeller, who recommended me to her), who did laboratory testing to see what was happening in his body and gave him the nutrients and supplements he needed.

After starting a gluten-free and casein-free diet, Matthew had significant improvements in his behavior, mood, and sleep. Over several years, as his care team learned more and his needs changed, they combined additional therapeutic diets: removing food sensitivities and following a low oxalate diet, an anti-yeast diet, and a grain-free diet (all of which we will discuss in the book). His mother told me, "His symptoms of autism began to fade. It was incredible to see better cognition, language, and sleep, fewer tantrums, and more eye contact as we changed his diet, removing even the 'healthy' foods that did not work with his body. Less inflammation led to less meltdowns, food cravings, and negative behaviors. Even therapists and teachers were beginning to see the connection and got a glimpse of how powerful food is for mood and behavior."

Today Terri is one of my best friends, and I've been blessed to witness many of Matthew's milestones. At the time of this writing, Matthew is twenty years old, and his doctors no longer diagnose him with autism. He graduated from high school, became an Eagle Scout, and is now going to college. He is an aspiring author, and as I write this, he just won an award at his college for student of the year in writing and literacy. The change Matthew experienced is dramatic, and not everyone will undergo the same—but his story offers one example of change that is possible for children and adults with autism.

I have spent more than two decades working with children and adults with autism spectrum disorder (ASD) to improve their symptoms through diet and nutrition interventions. These interventions can change their lives and the lives of their loved ones. In my work, I've seen children gain language, converse with a parent for the first time, connect with their siblings, increase eye contact, sleep better, feel calmer, and have reduced abdominal pain. It's my life's work and my passion to help people with autism lead healthier, happier lives.

People ask me how I got interested in autism. When I was in school to become a certified nutrition consultant many years ago, I first studied attention deficit/hyperactivity disorder (ADHD). I interviewed a father, Michael Lang, who had expertise in the field and who had recovered his children from autism with dietary interventions. While I was supposed to be learning more about food for ADHD, he was so passionate about autism that we spent the entire time talking about diet and nutrition approaches for ASD. He shared with me the pain and challenges of these children and the tremendous help diet was—and the underlying science of why it worked. I had never heard such a thing, and I wondered, *Why was no one talking about this?* He told me how there were very few nutrition professionals in this field and how needed they were. I knew this was what I had to do in the world. I dove in headfirst and never looked back. My second-year school paper would eventually become my first book, *Nourishing Hope for Autism* (self-published in 2005), and inform the future of my work. I attended autism parent and medical conferences—many of which Michael also attended—to learn and eventually speak. (Michael since passed away of pancreatic cancer, but I think of him as my guide in this work and a guardian angel.)

Since those early days, I have gotten a master's degree in medical nutrition and published nutrition research. I've worked with thousands of clients and parents, trained doctors, and nutritionists, read thousands of scientific studies on autism, and presented at medical conferences around the world. I've developed a process of strategically using diet and nutrition to improve symptoms of autism. A fundamental principle of my approach is personalized nutrition, a methodology I call BioIndividual Nutrition, which I'll introduce in depth in later chapters. After decades fine-tuning this approach, I've achieved better results and integrated my best practices into a framework that is easy for parents to pick up and use successfully and get real results. I call my approach Nourishing Hope—also the name of my organization and website of resources. It's an individual healing journey to offer hope for a healthy, happy future. There's no real right or wrong in this process. No situation is too dire, and there is no shame. It's not about being perfect but rather getting started.

Some of my clients say they have "recovered" from autism, which means their doctor no longer diagnoses them with autism. I don't use the word *cured*. It doesn't accurately describe the experience. Not everyone will lose their diagnosis. However, this possibility opens the pathway to see the potential for improving autism. Recovery isn't the goal. The goal is improvement and relief of symptoms so that people with autism can live their best lives.

A Note on Terms

Since the official diagnosis is autism spectrum disorder, or ASD, this is the term we often use in the field. (Meanwhile, some people call autism "autism spectrum *condition*" because they do not see it as a disorder.) Throughout this book, I refer to it as autism spectrum disorder, ASD, and sometimes simply autism. I do not mean anything different by these various terms.

A Note on Neurodiversity

Before moving on, I want to address a valid concern that arises whenever people talk about treating autism. Some people maintain that autism is just neurodiversity and we should accept people with autism exactly as they are. Sometimes, they will bring up amazing stories of gifted autistic savants. Neurodiversity is wonderful. And of course, we *should* accept people as they are. But when I and other professionals in my field talk about improving autism, we are not talking about trying to "change" someone just to make them like their neurotypical peers. We are trying to relieve their suffering so their true neurodiverse gifts can shine. Most people with autism are not savants. As we will discuss in later chapters, the symptoms of autism can make life very difficult for people with ASD. Among my clients are people with severe gut pain or chronic diarrhea who wear diapers as teenagers. Many have anxiety so debilitating they can't leave the house. They may have no speech at all or can't effectively communicate with their loved ones. They may be highly distraught when their routine changes, or they may try to elope from the house (and sadly, some don't make it back). This is more than an issue of neurodiversity. These are individuals who are hurting and want help. You can both love and accept your child exactly as they are *and* want a better life for them. This book can help.

HOW TO EXPLORE THIS BOOK AND THE NOURISHING HOPE PROGRAM

In this book, you will learn the principles behind nutrition and diet interventions and the Nourishing Hope process to apply them to address your child's unique needs and see real results. The process is from my Nourishing

Hope program called Nourishing Hope for Healing Kids. The steps are laid out in a specific order to deliver the best results easily and quickly. The process works for beginners who have not done any dietary or nutritional intervention and those who have tried everything without the results they are seeking. This program will help you create a personalized autism nutrition plan for your child.

Section 1 of the book explains core concepts of autism as a whole-body disorder, the important underlying factors to know, and how it all connects to diet and nutrition.

Section 2 lays out the first half of the Nourishing Hope process, which includes eating healthy, ditching junk food and toxins, incorporating supplements, addressing picky eating, and starting a gluten-free, casein-free, soy-free diet. This part ends with the critical step of taking care of yourself. These are the Nourishing Hope Essentials, solid principles that most families will be able to follow and benefit from. This half of the program is built on the most common, widely beneficial strategies. Most people end up implementing most of the steps and strategies in this part (families who are already using nutritional interventions for ASD may be using them now). These are great for both families new to nutrition and eating healthfully and experienced families that want to get back to the basics and re-evaluate where to go from here.

Section 3 walks you through the second half of Nourishing Hope involving bioindividual nutrition and therapeutic diets, in which you'll refine *your* child's *personalized autism nutrition plan*. These next steps cover the most common and beneficial therapeutic diets. For this part of the program, I suggest you read through all the therapeutic diets, then determine which you would like to try out. It is not intended for *everyone* to do *everything* in section 3. Which diet(s) you choose will depend on your child's unique needs. This part of the book is a great place for people who have tried everything, are stuck at a plateau and need further support, or are ready to personalize their nutrition plan further. If you're new and you find you are still working on getting a solid foundation going in the first half, don't feel you have to proceed to this part right away. It will be waiting here for you when you are ready! Finally, I'll share some of my best tips for working with your health care provider.

And the recipe section of this book provides you with some tried-and-true recipes to get you started making nutritious, diet-compliant meals.

What If Your Child Doesn't Have an Autism Diagnosis?

You don't need an autism diagnosis to benefit from this program. The principles in this book address underlying factors that cause symptoms, regardless of the diagnosis. Many of the underlying conditions that contribute to autism are also factors in other neurological conditions. The diet and nutrition principles in this book help provide the body and brain what they need and remove what is causing challenges. As such, this program is good for many neurological conditions, such as ADHD, Tourette's syndrome, Down syndrome, learning delays, anxiety, aggression, and defiant disorders.

Additionally, an individual with autism may have several of these conditions, so it's not just autism symptoms or the condition of ASD that may improve. You might find these principles helpful for a variety of neurological and physical symptoms. Gastrointestinal conditions and poor sleep, also common in autism, often improve with these dietary approaches.

What If You Are Reading This Book for Yourself?

If you are an adult with ASD reading this book for yourself, welcome! While I wrote this book with kids in mind because families are the majority of my clients, the information and suggestions in this book are not only for children. They work for adults, too. In our randomized controlled trial of individuals with ASD, we found there was no correlation between age and improvements from nutritional intervention.[1] In other words, adults showed improvements along with children. And my experience with Nourishing Hope families finds the same. So, while I am often addressing parents and caregivers and referring to children in this book, know that I'm speaking to you, too.

WISHING YOU A HOPEFUL JOURNEY

Think of this program as a road map and you as a driver on a journey. Each step is like a streetlight illuminating aspects of your diet and nutrition journey. In some cases, you will get to the streetlight and out of your car, stay awhile, trying out the nutrition information, then move on your way. In other cases, particularly in the second half, the step is meant to enlighten you (like a light on the road) to a certain dietary or nutritional intervention to consider. In this case, you might just pull over, read the information, and keep moving. I created the program to go in an order that I've found to be most helpful, so most people will drive along following the road map step-by-step. However, this program is meant to be flexible. Some people who have been implementing a diet for a while may zoom past some steps quickly. Others, who are longtime veterans to diet and nutrition, may take a shortcut, bypassing steps to get to what they'd like to explore more. If something isn't right for you—skip it. Come back to it later. Discuss it with your health care provider; this book isn't meant to replace that relationship but enhance it. You can implement some of these nutrition strategies (such as eating more vegetables) on your own, you'll want to research other concepts further, and you'll ask your doctor about other concepts.

Over the years, I've met people who falsely believed autism could not be improved at all. Or those who don't believe ASD can be improved with nutrition. Or those who believe their child's symptoms are too severe for diet to help and that I and other workers in this field are giving false hope. Or those who think a special diet is too difficult to follow. To them I say: There is science supporting this approach, and it is worth it. There are only upsides. This is why I have dedicated my life to studying and sharing this approach. This program is based on my two decades of work with children with autism and other conditions like ADHD, learning delays, anxiety,

Tourette's syndrome, and even Down syndrome. Thousands of families have used the principles in this book and/or the steps in this program to help their children. And these principles are what I have used to train practitioners all over the world to better serve their patients and clients. And now I'm so excited to share it with you, whether you are a beginner to nutrition or diet veteran. Above all, my goal is to help parents and families feel empowered and inspired to try diet and nutrition interventions so that their children can thrive and live to their fullest potential.

SECTION 1

Core
Concepts

WHAT CAUSES AUTISM?

Underlying Factors and How Food Can Help

W hen people find out I specialize in autism spectrum disorder, the most common question I get is, "What causes autism?" That's a million-dollar question—literally. Millions if not billions of dollars have been spent over decades to find one cause of autism (and a cure), but no single cause has been found. We know it's not purely genetic because, when ASD is diagnosed among identical twins, sometimes only one twin has it.[1] And it's not purely environmental because not everyone with a particular exposure will get autism.

But while we can't predict exactly who will get autism, we know it is increasingly common. When I was in elementary school in the 1970s, researchers estimated 1 in 10,000 children had autism. When I began my nutrition career in the early 2000s, ASD was estimated to affect 1 in 150 children in the United States, and rates have continued to rise steadily: 1 in 54 in 2016 and 1 in 44 in 2018.[2] At the time of this writing, 1 in 36 children are diagnosed with ASD.[3] This is a steep rise. While many people will suggest that the increased rates are simply a matter of more awareness and better diagnosis, a Danish study showed that while 60 percent of the increased prevalence of ASD may be attributed to better diagnostic and reporting practices, the remaining 40 percent could not be attributed to these changes and something more is causing the rise in autism.[4]

In fact, there are multiple underlying causes and contributing factors, which are different for each person, making each individual with autism different and the condition diverse. The technical term for this is *heterogeneous condition*. The symptoms can be quite different from person to person as well. (It is considered a spectrum disorder because there is wide variation in the presentation of the condition from person to person.) This makes autism a complex condition for parents trying to understand it, practitioners working to treat it, and researchers attempting to study it. But this is not to say that ASD is a complete anomaly; most chronic diseases are caused by an interplay of genes and environment. Autism is no different. The good news is that nutrition is the key to unraveling the complexities of this interplay and addressing symptoms.

But, before we get there, let's take a step back to understand what we know about autism. Understanding autism is fundamental to addressing it in a thoughtful, comprehensive way.

AUTISM IS A WHOLE-BODY DISORDER

If you've talked to a doctor about your child's autism, you'll know that few medical treatment options are available. Diagnosing physicians often recommend speech and behavioral therapy (this is the common experience among my clients). And while these are supportive therapies, they are not medical treatments for improving autism. They address neither the underlying medical conditions that cause symptoms nor conditions that often accompany ASD, such as seizures and gastrointestinal disorders.

Among doctors and parents alike, ASD is commonly misunderstood as an exclusively psychiatric (brain) disorder. Autism is identified by the American Psychiatric Association's *Diagnostic and Statistical Manual of Mental Disorders* (DSM-5) as a developmental disorder with impairments in communication and social interaction, and repetitive behaviors. And it *is* studied with psychiatric and brain conditions.

However, we must understand autism as a whole-body disorder. The brain is affected, but the brain is not an island unto itself. It is part of the body, and what's going on in the rest of the body affects the brain. For instance, our brain's nutrient status is only as good as the nutrient levels in the body. If the body is deficient, in most cases, the brain will be also. Or the deficiencies will cause other biochemical problems that negatively affect the brain. Additionally, we only have one immune system, so conditions such as inflammation that become systemic in the body will affect the brain.

Dr. Martha Herbert, a prominent pediatric neurologist and associate professor at Harvard Medical School who sees autism as a whole-body disorder, wrote that we should consider autism a "disorder that affects the brain,"[5] which I think is a more useful way to understand it. As she explains, instead of a brain-based condition, it's more accurate to think of it as a disorder that affects multiple systems of the body and in turn affects the brain.

Researchers and clinicians are also finding that there are subtypes within autism, and these subtypes can make it more difficult to see clear results in studies. For example, some children mainly have gastrointestinal issues, others immune system dysfunction or mitochondrial dysfunction. It may seem obvious, but treatments intended to address one underlying cause will work for only the children (or research participants) who have that issue. This can make research results mixed from study to study. This is because research typically uses general populations. So, with subtypes existing, the diet or nutrient will work best for certain people, and the results may appear watered down when looking at its effect in a general autism population. This doesn't mean that the diet or nutrient doesn't work. In fact, it likely means that for those that it works for, it works even better than studies show. The key is to figure out what underlying factors affect the individual and which diet and nutrition interventions address those factors.

By understanding the underlying factors that contribute to autism, we can not only evolve future medical treatments and nutrition interventions but also help those with ASD today.

Let's examine those underlying factors, some of which might be affecting you or your child. However, don't be discouraged if it feels too technical for you right now. Feel free to skip ahead, as there is plenty you can do to help your child without understanding the biological underpinnings of the condition. It will be here later if you reach a point that you want to come back to it. And don't feel you have to figure it all out yourself. Any information you absorb will help you seek out answers from health experts because you will know who to go to and how to ask the right questions. With that, let's jump into it.

UNDERLYING FACTORS

Autism has many underlying causes and contributing factors, which includes a combination of genetic variants and impaired bodily systems that manifest differently from person to person. Researchers explain that these factors "act synergistically" to affect the child's system and cause autism spectrum disorder.[6] These factors include:

- Food reactions and nutrient deficiencies
- Gastrointestinal issues and microbiome imbalances
- Immune system dysfunction and inflammation
- Mitochondrial dysfunction
- Impaired detoxification
- Endocrine/metabolic issues
- Genetics (nutrigenetics and nutrigenomics)
- Issues of methylation and other important biochemical pathways

Food Reactions and Nutrient Deficiencies

Let's start with how food reactions and nutrient deficiencies can impact autism. In the subsequent sections on underlying factors, we'll also discuss the role of food and nutrient deficiencies and these bodily systems specifically—so parts of this chapter may begin to feel repetitious!—but here, we'll set the framework of food and nutrients and how food and nutrients play a direct role.

Certain foods can cause or exacerbate symptoms of autism directly. For example, artificial food additives in foods can cause hyperactivity—this is why we remove them in step 1 of the program. Additionally, certain food proteins poorly broken down by improper digestion can form compounds that directly affect the brain. That said, it is important to note that food is a contributor to, rather than the cause of, autism. I am not suggesting that food causes autism. It is an important area to address to improve the underlying factors affecting the individual, but eating a particular food or foods is not the *sole cause* of autism.

Removing foods that inhibit or damage the body's cells and systems can reverse many ASD-related problems and symptoms. And introducing the right foods can help the body and brain work better. This can improve how your child feels, thinks, and behaves.

Nutrient deficiencies are another contributing factor. We need nutrients for the body and brain to function. Deficiencies can cause or exacerbate the biochemical imbalances in autism.

While getting proper nutrition can help, nutrient deficiencies are not always due to insufficient intake. They can be the result of a system or biochemical pathway that is not functioning optimally. So, for instance, even if your child eats enough meat, they may still be deficient in protein or B_{12} because their body isn't digesting or absorbing the nutrient properly. Also, many nutrients are made or converted to their active forms in the body, and genetic variants involved in those processes can cause deficiencies. Nutrient deficiencies can also stem from inflammation and oxidative stress, because the nutrients we do have end up being used to resolve those issues instead of other biochemical processes. Poor gastrointestinal function and gut microbial imbalance can also cause nutrient deficiencies.

And of course, deficiencies can be caused by consuming a poor diet low in nutrients. The standard American or western diet, which is filled with sugar, starches, and very few vegetables, often does not provide enough nutrients for children's growth and development. And children with autism are likely to have picky eating habits, which further contribute to poor nutrition. (We tackle picky eating in step 4.)

You might notice that these underlying factors and nutritional aspects can create a vicious cycle. The underlying factors can cause reactions to foods and deficiencies, and the foods and deficiencies can fuel the underlying factors. While this can make the vicious cycle complex, it also means that when we address diet and nutrition, we can break the cycle! This is great news. We can have a profound effect through the food we eat and nutrition we get. The next sections will look at these relationships and how diet and nutrition can impact the other underlying factors.

Gastrointestinal Issues and Microbiome

The gastrointestinal (GI) tract, also known as the digestive system, is critical for health. It's also a key player in autism: up to 70 percent of children with autism have gastrointestinal symptoms.[7] Gastrointestinal problems are significantly more prevalent in children with autism than their siblings without autism, and the severity of autism has been associated with gastrointestinal symptoms in multiple studies.[8] The top two symptoms of ASD-related GI problems are constipation and diarrhea.[9]

The gut and brain are connected. The gut is often called the second brain because of its connection to and influence on brain function. Neurotransmitters such as serotonin are prevalent in the gut. And we know traumatic injury to the brain can negatively impact the gut, and impairments in the gut can create damage or dysfunction in the brain, showing that this connection is a two-way street.[10]

Since the digestive system breaks down the food we eat and ensures vitamins, minerals, and other nutrients get absorbed, our gastrointestinal system is closely intertwined with the nutrition factors we discussed previously. For example, our digestive system ensures the proteins in our food get broken down and absorbed as amino acids. It digests starches and sugars into single-molecule sugars to get absorbed and digests fat for proper absorption. We need these nutrients for our cells, body systems (including our gastrointestinal system), and brain. Proper gastrointestinal function in children is important for health, growth, and repair, as well as cognition, mood, and behavior.

In addition to allowing nutrients into the bloodstream, the intestinal barrier also keeps toxins and problematic substances out. When the proteins in foods are not broken down properly and the intestinal barrier is too permeable (a condition known as leaky gut), long protein chains are absorbed into the blood in a form that doesn't belong there. The body sees these protein chains as invaders, and they can create immune system reactions and inflammation.

An important part of gut health is the microbes, or the gut microbiome. The gut microbiome, the milieu of bacteria and other microbes both good and bad that occupy the gastrointestinal tract, is essential for a healthy digestive system, body, and mind. Beneficial bacteria in our gut aid digestion; regulate bowel movements; reduce inflammation; manufacture B vitamins, including folate, B_6, B_{12}, and more; aid in the absorption of minerals; produce short-chain fatty acids for a healthy gut and brain; and perform many more important functions for our health.

The gut microbiome can affect the brain, positively or negatively, depending on the microbes present.

Researchers have found children with autism have different gut bacteria than neurotypical children.[11] Lower levels of *Bifidobacterium* and higher levels of *Lactobacillus* are found in children with autism. In this study led by my mentor, Dr. James B. Adams, children with autism had lower levels of short-chain fatty acids—substances produced by bacteria that our intestinal cells use as fuel, promoting intestinal health. And this study found a strong correlation between gastrointestinal symptoms and the severity of autism.[12]

Gut pathogens increase the inflammatory response locally in the GI tract and systemically. An imbalance in gut microbes, known as dysbiosis, can also cause other health problems such as obesity, insulin resistance, decreased energy availability, and leaky gut and can negatively affect the brain. Pathogens such as bacteria (especially *Clostridia*) and yeast (*Candida*) in the gut can release toxins that can cause mood problems—and are suspected to contribute to the decreased digestive and brain health of people with autism and have been associated with increased autism symptom severity.[13] You can read more on *Clostridia* and *Candida* in "Beyond Diet and Nutrition."

In ASD, disturbances in the gut microbiome and dysbiosis can lead to inflammation, oxidative stress, leaky gut, immune dysfunction, metabolic dysregulation, and changes to gene expression.[14] This microbiome disruption may in part be due to increased antibiotic use in ASD in early childhood; this antibiotic use has been associated with significant increased risk of GI diagnosis.[15] Conversely, improving the microbiome can have profound effects.

Two groundbreaking studies show how powerful a healthy microbiome is in ASD. In one study, fecal microbiota from healthy individuals was given to eighteen children with ASD via microbiota transfer therapy. While this may cause some of us to feel squeamish, the results were amazing. The children had an 80 percent reduction in their gastrointestinal symptoms, improvements in their bacterial diversity and abundance, and significant improvements in their ASD behavioral symptoms that continued past the eight weeks of the study.[16] Two years later, a follow-up study was done, and researchers found that most of the participants' GI improvements remained and that the ASD symptoms continued to improve significantly years after the therapy had ended. In fact, before the microbiota transfer therapy, fifteen of the eighteen children rated as having severe ASD according to the Childhood Autism Rating Scale (CARS), while two years later, only three children were still considered severe, seven were rated mild to moderate, and eight were below the level of an ASD diagnosis score![17]

Because the gut and brain are so intricately connected and negatively affected in autism, healing the gut is a key priority. Fortunately, diet and nutrition intervention can be very beneficial here. Food and the gut, and food and the microbiome, have two-way relationships: Food reactions can contribute to gut issues, and underlying conditions in the gut affect the ability to tolerate certain foods. Moreover, foods we eat can also help or harm our microbiome, and the microbiome can influence the foods we do and don't tolerate.

This is where therapeutic diets come in. Therapeutic diets are designed to remove problematic substances and focus on those that are tolerated and can help the healing process. Some therapeutic diets are even designed with the specific purpose of positively affecting the gut microbiome.[18] Research shows that autism, as well as mental health conditions such as ADHD, anxiety, and depression, can be improved with therapeutic diets because of their influence on the microbiome.[19] Researchers who study this subject also state that therapeutic diets should be personalized according to the microbiome and other underlying factors,[20] something you will learn to do in this program.

No single diet works for all GI issues. It is important to consider many different dietary strategies when creating a personalized nutrition plan. You'll notice that many of the therapeutic diets in this book address gut healing in different ways. We will get into much more detail on these diets in later chapters, and you'll find a summary of how diet supports gut healing and the microbiome in step 11.

Immune System Dysfunction and Inflammation

Inflammation is a normal and healthy process of the immune system. We need a certain amount of inflammation to fight infections and heal wounds. Normally, our bodies turn inflammation on and off as needed. It is when the immune system is not in balance and cannot turn off the inflammatory process that we have a problem.

This chronic inflammation can negatively affect the brain. Inflammation in utero and early childhood can cause neurodevelopmental conditions including ASD, epilepsy, and cognitive impairment.[21] In part, inflammation can cause the intestinal and blood-brain barriers to become overly permeable to toxins that can cause damage to the brain in ASD.[22]

Although strong local inflammatory conditions, such as in the gut, are common in autism, systemic inflammation (inflammation throughout the body) is also an issue and can affect multiple organs,[23] including the brain.[24] In fact, research consistently finds strong associations between inflammation and ASD.[25]

Immune system dysregulation in autism contributes to this inflammation, as well as to allergies, autoimmune reactions, increased oxidative stress, decreased antioxidant function, and decreased ability to fight infections.[26] Immune system dysfunction is implicated as a cause of autism and its continuation.[27]

What causes this inflammation? Inflammation can be caused by infections, gut microbes, toxins, imbalanced blood sugar, and mast cell activation. (Mast cells are a part of the immune system and release histamine, which causes inflammation and has neurotoxic effects. Mast cell activation in autism may contribute to brain inflammation and may be a causative factor in ASD.)[28] Inflammation can be caused by anything that triggers an immune response. Foods can be a big cause of inflammation. Beyond certain inflammatory foods and dietary proteins that cause inflammation in ASD,[29] our overall diet, the food additives we consume, and the chemicals in our cookware and food storage containers can all cause inflammation as well. Conversely, other foods, such as fatty fish and antioxidant-rich fruits, can be beneficial for the immune system but need to be personalized to the individual. (As you'll learn in later chapters, a food that's great for one person may cause reactions in another.) Think of oxidative stress as a fire in our body that causes inflammation, and our consumption of antioxidants as the strategy to put the fire out. Reducing inflammation through the foods children eat and substances they avoid is important and can make a significant difference. Additionally, nutritional supplements can reduce inflammation and improve immune function.

Higher histamine, allergies, immune system hyperactivity, and autoimmunity in autism can cause more reactions to foods. Therapeutic diets can be helpful. We discuss specific strategies for reducing inflammation through therapeutic diets and nutritional supplementation later in the book, particularly in steps 7, 8, 10, and 12.

Mitochondrial Dysfunction

Mitochondria are the powerhouse of the cell, providing all the energy our body and brain cells need. To make energy, our mitochondria are involved in cellular metabolism (burning fuel for energy). In this process, the mitochondria also produce free radicals, which need to be neutralized by antioxidants. Without sufficient antioxidants, free radicals can cause oxidative stress and damage. When there is oxidative stress and decreased antioxidant function, as is the case in ASD, mitochondria can be damaged, causing impaired mitochondrial function and damage to neurons in the brain.[30] Additionally, poor mitochondrial function can lead to further inflammation. Given all this, it's perhaps not surprising that the prevalence of mitochondrial dysfunction in autism is high—as many as four out of five kids with ASD may have it (though the rate varies from study to study).[31]

Since every cell relies on mitochondria, poor mitochondrial function can lead to challenges in virtually any or every organ system, including the brain, gastrointestinal tract, immune system, liver, kidneys, lungs, and heart. This can make it challenging to recognize mitochondrial dysfunction because the trouble isn't limited to one system. And it means that mitochondrial dysfunction in children with autism can cause many challenges, including extreme fatigue. However, when you and your doctor realize this connection and notice multiple systems are dysfunctional, you can recognize that poor mitochondria function may be involved and get the help you need.

Fortunately, there are things that can improve mitochondrial function, including (you guessed it!) diet and nutrition interventions. There are nutrients and antioxidants that are important for mitochondrial function and support, as well as diets that can be beneficial: those that avoid anything that might cause inflammation (as discussed previously), those that cut oxalates (discussed in step 10), and the ketogenic diet (step 11).

Impaired Detoxification

Detoxification is our body's way of neutralizing and/or clearing out chemicals and toxins that, if not dealt with, can damage the brain (physically and cognitively), gut, mitochondria, immune system, and most cells and organs. To clear out these toxins, our liver relies on antioxidants that it gets from our diet and that our body makes, such as glutathione, as well as other vitamins and minerals.

Children with ASD tend to have low levels of glutathione, which is often called the master antioxidant.[32] Glutathione detoxifies chemicals, heavy metals, and other toxins. A study of fifty-two boys with ASD found they had higher levels of lead and mercury than controls, along with lower glutathione activity and vitamin E levels—all of which are strongly linked to social and cognitive impairment.[33]

Additionally, other impaired systems in children with ASD can add to detoxification challenges: Excess inflammation, imbalanced microbiome, and mitochondrial dysfunction cause important antioxidants and detoxifying nutrients to be insufficient (either not made or all used up). Unfortunately, as is a common theme in this chapter, these associations go two ways: The conditions themselves can cause poor detoxification, and poor detoxification and higher toxin levels can exacerbate the conditions.

So what's the role of food in detoxification? Nutrients such as antioxidants and sulfur in food help detoxify. Additionally, nutritional supplements that boost our detoxification system can be beneficial. On the other hand, food additives and chemicals in pesticides and food storage containers have to be detoxified, adding to the burden on our system. Fortunately, this also means that there are things you can easily do to reduce your child's body burden of toxins and support their improved detoxification capacity. We will discuss these toxins in more detail, how you can avoid them in your food and environment, and safer alternatives in step 1.

Environmental Factors

While we're on the topic of toxins . . . there are other external factors that can contribute to symptoms, deplete nutrients, and affect our bodily systems. These include pathogens, stressors, and trauma. We'll take a look at these, and what you can do about them, in "Beyond Diet and Nutrition."

Endocrine/Metabolic Issues

Our endocrine system includes hormones, such as sex hormones, cortisol, insulin, and thyroid hormones. Hormones are chemical messengers, so our endocrine system makes sure our body systems are communicating and functioning properly: keeping puberty and fertility on track, turning the stress response on and off as needed, and supporting proper metabolic function. Metabolic function, or metabolism, includes making energy in our mitochondria. Hormones also regulate aspects of behavior and cognitive function, and endocrine system disruption is present in autism.[34]

Metabolic dysfunction in autism includes low-grade inflammation, increased oxidative stress and damage, decreased glucose oxidation, and increased fatty acid oxidation. These conditions are associated with insulin resistance (when cells in the body don't respond well to insulin—the hormone that regulates blood glucose). Insulin resistance has been found in children with autism, and the condition can negatively affect the brain.[35] While researchers are still studying whether insulin resistance is causative in ASD, reducing sugar and processed food that can have negative effects on blood glucose and long-term health has numerous benefits regardless.

Furthermore, dozens of genetic disorders of metabolism are associated with autism, including metabolic disorders of amino acids, organic acids, neurotransmitters, purine metabolism, folate transport, folate metabolism, cerebral folate deficiency, cholesterol production, copper metabolism, and iron excess.[36] In fact, there are so many that it's no wonder that some children are so severely affected, and I believe we will discover many subtypes of autism tied to these metabolic issues.

We've talked about diets and supplements that support mitochondrial function. And there are also personalized approaches that help metabolic function, including how much carbohydrate we tolerate and need. And genetic disorders of metabolism may have specific dietary and nutrient support. Since some of these are rarer than others and do not affect a large percentage of children with autism, a personalized nutrition approach is best.

Genetics (Nutrigenetics and Nutrigenomics)

Our genes make us who we are. They shape our nutritional status and health risks. While no single gene has been found to cause autism, dozens of genetic variants are associated with the condition. Many are single nucleotide polymorphisms (SNPs). These are not rare mutations but rather variants in genes that exist in more than 1 percent of the population, sometimes much more. These genes affect methylation, oxidative stress, inflammation, neurotransmitter levels, and other biochemical factors that impair brain function and development. Additionally, our microbiome has its own genome, so that is an additional factor outside our genes.

That said, our genes do not set our fate in stone. Our nutrition and lifestyle choices shape our lives and health, too, because they can affect which genes are expressed. (Our genes are regulated—turned on or off as needed—through gene expression; methylation, a process discussed in the next section, is involved with this.) In fact, genes and nutrition are a two-way street. Our genes affect our body's response to food and nutrients (the study of nutrigenetics), and the foods and nutrients we consume affect our gene expression, the process called epigenetics (the study of nutrigenomics).

The good news is that our diet, nutrients, toxins, and microbiome can affect our gene expression, and steps 1, 2, and 3 outline these strategies.

Issues of Methylation and Other Important Biochemical Pathways

Now that we have a working understanding of autism as a whole-body disorder, I will dig deeper into three important biochemical pathways that are disrupted in people with autism: methylation, transsulfuration, and sulfation. These pathways are linked, so when one isn't working right, the next will also be affected. They can influence our ability to process toxins, cause nutrient deficiencies, impact our ability to tolerate certain foods, and negatively impact organs and body systems. It's important to understand these systems because the biochemistry informs the diet and nutrient strategies we use to improve nutrition and symptoms.

Methylation

Let's start with methylation, the first pathway. Methylation is an important biochemical process that happens billions of times per second in every cell! Methylation is the process of passing a small molecule called a methyl group (CH_3, one carbon atom and three hydrogen atoms) to something (DNA, an enzyme, a hormone, or a neurotransmitter) to make something happen. For example, to turn off a gene, such as a cancer gene, a methyl group is added to DNA—a process called DNA methylation. DNA methylation silences gene expression and turns off the cancer gene.

Beyond gene expression, methylation is involved with processes such as:

- Neurotransmitter production, which affects mood and behavior
- Mitochondrial function, which is needed for energy
- Histamine metabolism, which affects allergy response
- Hormone metabolism such as healthy estrogen metabolism
- Insulating the nerves or myelin sheath in the brain

Diminished methylation capacity is associated with anxiety, depression, ADHD, impaired detoxification, allergy conditions, histamine intolerance, imbalanced hormones, inflammatory conditions, poor immune function, cancer, and heart disease.

The Science of Methylation

Our primary methyl donor is S-adenosylmethionine (SAM or SAMe). Think of a methyl group as the baton that one runner passes to another runner in a race. It gets transferred from "person" to "person," until it reaches SAM. SAM is the teammate that ultimately receives the baton to transfer (or donate) the methyl groups for all the uses of methylation described in the previous section.

How do we make SAM? It starts with folate in a process called the folate cycle. We will talk again about folate and MTHFR (methylenetetrahydrofolate reductase) in step 3, but for now the important part is that the enzyme MTHFR makes methylfolate (officially known as 5-methyltetrahydrofolate)—active folate that has a methyl group.

With the help of vitamin B_{12}, folate passes its methyl group to homocysteine, which becomes methionine through the enzyme methionine synthase (and the gene MTR), and ultimately SAM. After SAM donates its methyl group, it becomes S-adenosylhomocysteine (SAH), then homocysteine, and the cycles can start again. From here, homocysteine can pick up a new methyl group, then is recycled back to methionine (we call this cycle the methionine cycle or the methionine-homocysteine cycle).

Imagine the folate cycle and the methionine cycle as two gears in a machine. The two interact, the first influencing the second, passing methyl groups along for the process of methylation. Side note: This recycling process (from homocysteine to methionine) is important so there is a secondary process that uses trimethylglycine (TMG) instead of folate and B_{12}, but more on that in step 3.

METHYLATION, TRANSSULFURATION, AND SULFATION

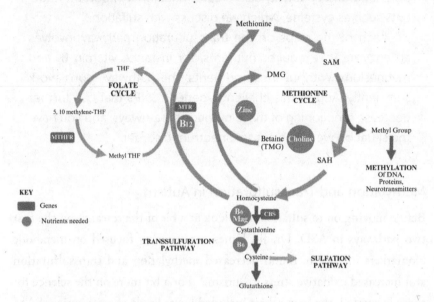

Transsulfuration

Transsulfuration is the next of these important biochemical pathways. This process produces glutathione, our master antioxidant. Therefore, this pathway is important for antioxidant function, inhibiting oxidation, and protecting the cells and mitochondria from damage. Glutathione is also important for detoxication and immune function. Diminished transsulfuration can contribute to inflammation, pain, digestive symptoms, difficulty fighting infections, decreased detoxification, and fatigue.

The Science of Transsulfuration

As shown in the pathway graphic above, the transsulfuration pathway requires adequate methylation to start. After SAM becomes homocysteine, it has two potential routes: (1) recycling back to methionine, as discussed, or (2) progressing down the transsulfuration pathway to create glutathione. Both are important. The transsulfuration pathway also creates additional important nutrients such as cysteine, which we discuss with sulfation.

Each of the steps on the transsulfuration pathway involves an enzyme that requires nutrients, for instance vitamin B_6 and magnesium. Without these nutrients, the pathways don't work sufficiently. Add to this challenge genetic SNPs that can further decrease functioning of these nutritional pathways, and you have the situation we see in autism spectrum disorder.

Methylation and Transsulfuration in Autism

Before moving on to sulfation, let's look at a bit of the research on the first two pathways in ASD. Dr. Jill James, a researcher focused on metabolic biomarkers in autism, found decreased methylation and transsulfuration and increased oxidative stress in autism.[37] For a bit more on the science for those interested, the biomarkers included lower levels of methionine, SAM (with higher SAH), homocysteine, cystathionine, cysteine, and total glutathione (though higher levels of oxidized glutathione—in other words, not the good stuff). To put it more simply, the children with ASD were low in all the good things they need for these biochemical pathways to function adequately and high in those that indicate dysfunction.

Impaired folate cycle, methylation, and transsulfuration biochemistry is so common in ASD that researchers were able to accurately identify children with autism and those without autism 96 to 97 percent of the time through these specific metabolite measurements.[38]

Sulfation

After methylation and transsulfuration comes sulfation. Sulfation is a mechanism that uses sulfate, a form of sulfur, for many biochemical processes, including detoxifying chemicals and certain natural food compounds (such as salicylates and amines, discussed in step 7), maintaining gut and brain barrier integrity, and aiding in digestion, neurodevelopment, immune function, and hormone regulation.[39]

The sulfate required for sulfation mostly comes from cysteine, which is created partway down the transsulfuration pathway. Poor sulfation can affect health, behavior, digestion, and food reactions. Children with autism have been found to have low sulfation and low levels of sulfate.[40] (Researchers have also discovered poor sulfation in many other chronic conditions, such as chronic fatigue syndrome, sensitivity to foods or other chemicals, IBS or chronic diarrhea, depression, migraines, and hyperactivity.)[41]

The Role of Diet and Nutrition in These Biochemical Pathways

Methylation, transsulfuration, and sulfation can all be improved by supplying the nutrients needed for these pathways to function adequately. We'll cover these in steps 3 and 7. Understanding the genes that affect these pathways can further support your personalized nutrition approach and help you determine the forms and amounts of these nutrients to consume. But you don't have to do gene testing and understand your genes from day one. You can start with the simple steps, and over time you can work up to the more complex things. Remember, you don't have to do it all by yourself, either. You can get additional support from your health care team without being an expert in everything (more on this in "Beyond Diet and Nutrition").

Furthermore, addressing underlying factors that deplete these biochemical pathways helps reduce the burden on the system and provides improvement. Some food compounds (salicylates and amines) require sulfation to process, and so reducing them is often very beneficial; we'll cover these diets in step 7.

OTHER CONDITIONS PRESENT IN AUTISM

Beyond the underlying biochemical factors that make up this whole-body condition, there are also many comorbidities (additional diseases or conditions present) in autism. The following mental and physical conditions often accompany ASD:

- ADHD
- Anxiety

- Depression
- Learning disorders
- Gastrointestinal disorders
- Immune system dysregulation
- Mitochondrial dysfunction
- Sleep disturbances
- Seizures[42]

The presence of comorbidities is important for several reasons. Comorbidities can give us clues about underlying factors that can be causing these coexisting conditions and autism symptoms. For instance, if someone with autism has anxiety and depression, we might investigate their methylation capacity, or if they have anxiety and gastrointestinal issues, we might consider imbalances in the microbiome. Comorbidities can exacerbate the symptoms and challenges of autism. Addressing comorbidities through nutrition strategies gives us another way to improve a child's quality of life. And recognizing comorbidities provides an additional way for us to gauge improvement in ASD.

Let's take ADHD, one of the most common comorbidities, as an example. ADHD is present in 30.6 percent of children with autism, and an additional 24.7 percent exhibit some ADHD symptoms, though they're below the threshold for diagnosis.[43] This means more than half of children with autism have ADHD or some symptoms of it. This is important because these ADHD symptoms can add to the difficulty those with ASD have; a study of forty-nine children with autism found that, for those with ADHD, their ADHD symptoms exacerbated their autism by impairing executive control and adaptive behavior and reducing verbal working memory.[44] By using diet and nutrition strategies that address the ADHD symptoms directly, we can help children with autism improve their quality of life.

THE BOTTOM LINE

This chapter is science heavy, but you don't have to be a biochemist or deeply understand it all to benefit. The most important takeaway is that diet and nutrition strategies can address current biochemistry challenges, address comorbidities, minimize food reactions, and improve symptoms. These strategies are firmly within your control as a parent, and this means there is much you can do to help your child with autism thrive. Before we get to those steps, however, let's pause to understand some of my research, which is a pillar of the Nourishing Hope program.

THE SCIENCE BEHIND NOURISHING HOPE

The Therapeutic Diets and Supplements Best Supported by Research

Throughout this book, I summarize findings from research on how diet and nutrition can support your child with autism, help them feel better, and improve their symptoms. In this chapter, however, I'd like to present you with detailed findings from two studies I coauthored. This research underpins the choice of the specific therapeutic diets and supplements you may try throughout the Nourishing Hope program. Together, these different studies show that diet and nutrient intervention for ASD can provide tremendous improvement and that a personalized nutrition approach is best.

COMBINING SUPPLEMENTATION AND A GLUTEN-FREE, CASEIN-FREE, SOY-FREE DIET

After years of working with families, I had the opportunity to share my expertise as a coauthor of a study entitled "Comprehensive Nutritional and Dietary Intervention for Autism Spectrum Disorder—A Randomized, Controlled, 12-Month Trial," which was published in the peer-reviewed journal *Nutrients* in 2018. The lead researcher was James Adams, PhD, a well-known and prolific autism nutrition researcher and a mentor of mine.

Our study was a randomized controlled trial, a study design considered the gold standard in nutrition research. A total of 117 individuals, aged three to fifty-eight years, were enrolled in the study. More than half (sixty-seven) of the participants had autism spectrum disorder and were randomly assigned to a treatment group (thirty-seven participants) or a control group (thirty participants). The remaining fifty participants were neurotypical, and their baseline results were used for comparison to the ASD group before and after treatment. Our study measured the effects of six interventions added one at a time approximately monthly:

1. Vitamin/mineral supplementation
2. Essential fatty acid supplementation
3. Epsom salt baths
4. Carnitine supplementation
5. Digestive enzyme supplementation
6. Healthy gluten-free, casein-free, soy-free (GFCFSF) diet

These common diet and nutrient strategies have all been previously studied and/or used by clinicians and families with beneficial results. This was one of the first nutrition studies for ASD that *combined* multiple nutrition interventions.

The participants were followed over the course of a year. We found that dietary changes combined with nutritional supplements are safe and can help address underlying factors in autism, improve debilitating symptoms, and improve health, learning, and behavior. We also found that the interventions helped no matter the participants' age. The comprehensive diet and nutrition intervention provided significant benefits:

- Improved cognitive function: 6.7-point increase in nonverbal IQ, on average
- Improved developmental age: 4.5 times improvement, increased from four months in control group to eighteen months in treatment group, on average

- Decreased autism severity: 28 percent decrease in Autism Treatment Evaluation Checklist (ATEC) score, a measure of autism severity, compared to a 6 percent decrease in control group, on average
- Increased speech and language comprehension
- Reduced gastrointestinal symptoms
- Increased vitamin status
- Improved levels of carnitine, red blood cell minerals, and fatty acids
- Improvements in language, hyperactivity, anxiety, physical symptoms, and more based on the Parent Global Impressions (PGI) symptom rating scale

PARENT GLOBAL IMPRESSIONS

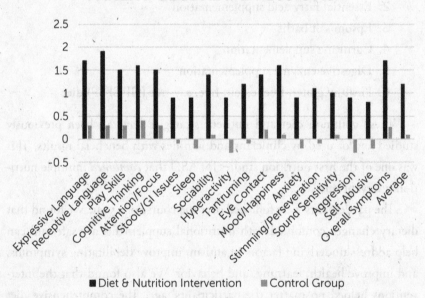

■ Diet & Nutrition Intervention ■ Control Group

Data from: James B. Adams et al., "Comprehensive Nutritional and Dietary Intervention for Autism Spectrum Disorder—A Randomized, Controlled 12-Month Trial," *Nutrients* 10, no. 3 (March 17, 2018): E369, https://doi.org/10.3390/nu10030369.

Several individual cases were so impressive they warrant mention here.

One seven-year-old boy had severe pica, a potentially very dangerous condition involving eating nonfood items. This boy had very low levels of vitamin B_{12}, vitamin C, beta-carotene, and several more B vitamins. Within one week of starting the healthy GFCFSF diet, his pica was fully resolved and remained that way throughout the study.

A twenty-seven-year-old man struggled with kidney stones and a severe inability to urinate, which required catheterization daily, leading to urinary tract and bladder infections. Because his health care team couldn't find a cause, it was assumed to be neurological. However, four days after eliminating dairy products on the healthy GFCFSF diet, he was able to urinate on his own. On two separate occasions in the following months, he ingested dairy (ice cream and cheese) and was again unable to urinate for several days after each incident. With a strict dairy-free diet, he no longer needed catheterization, so he stopped getting infections and his quality of life improved significantly.

A nine-year-old girl with severe autism had very low energy levels and strength. She could not get up from the floor on her own, climb stairs, get into the family van, or walk more than a quarter mile. Because of this she used a wheelchair when out in public. Her lab tests revealed that, at the start of the study, her carnitine levels were very low. Carnitine is a nutrient that helps with mitochondrial function to support energy levels. Her diet up until that point included no red meat or pork, which are the main sources of carnitine in our diet. Four months into the study, after starting carnitine supplements, her endurance and strength significantly improved. And by one year from the start of the study, she could get up and climb independently and walk up to two miles at a time, and she no longer required her wheelchair. At the end of the study, when her energy had returned, her carnitine levels tested above average.

It's interesting to note that not all children respond to carnitine; however, this supplement was life-changing for her—testament to the importance of personalizing nutrition!

ANALYZING 13 THERAPEUTIC DIETS AND THE PERSONALIZED APPROACH

The second study I coauthored with Dr. Adams was "The Ratings of the Effectiveness of 13 Therapeutics Diets for Autism Spectrum Disorder: Results of a National Survey," which was published in the *Journal of Personalized Medicine* in 2023. One of this study's strengths was its large sample size: 818 participants. We got our data from a large survey that asked about participants' experience with therapeutic diets, as well as supplements ("nutraceuticals") and psychiatric and seizure medications. For our study, we included data on diets that were followed by at least twenty survey responders.

"Which diets were the most beneficial and most popular?" you might ask. Here's how they stacked up, from highest to lowest rated (the number of participants following each is in parentheses):

1. Healthy diet (179 users)
2. Feingold diet* (74 users)
3. Food avoidance diet, based on IgG/IgE testing (54 users)
4. Low sugar diet (104 users)
5. Food avoidance diet, based on observation (82 users)
6. Gluten-free and casein-free diet (221 users)
7. Specific Carbohydrate Diet (37 users)
8. Ketogenic diet (21 users)
9. Corn-free diet (46 users)
10. Casein-free diet (134 users)
11. Paleo diet (21 users)
12. Soy-free diet (62 users)
13. Gluten-free diet (114 users)

Interestingly, some of the moderately popular or less common diets had some excellent overall benefit and/or symptom improvements. So, the "best" diet isn't necessarily the most popular. It's what works best for the individual's needs. (Note: This study didn't include all the diets I've found through my research and clinical experience to be beneficial. Some of the diets in the

---

* This is a low salicylate, additive-free diet.

Nourishing Hope program aren't on this list, either because they weren't included in the survey or they did not have enough responses to meet our threshold. Some diets missed being included by only a few responses!)

This study also rated the overall benefit of each diet and the adverse effects. All diets rated well, providing moderate to good benefit with very few adverse effects. You can see how the diets stack up in the following chart.

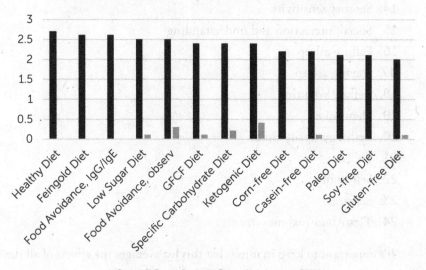

OVERALL BENEFIT AND ADVERSE EFFECT

■ Overall Benefit   ■ Overall Adverse Effect

Source: Julie S. Matthews and James B. Adams, "Ratings of the Effectiveness of 13 Therapeutic Diets for Autism Spectrum Disorder: Results of a National Survey," *Journal of Personalized Medicine* 13, no. 10 (September 29, 2023): 1448, https://doi.org/10.3390/jpm13101448; overall benefit was on a scale of 0 to 4, and adverse effect was on a scale of 0 to 3.

Which symptoms did the diets improve? Here is a list of the symptom improvements that were rated best for all therapeutic diets averaged together, with 1 indicating the largest number of people improving:

1. General benefit, no one particular symptom
2. Attention
3. Cognition (ability to think)
4. Irritability
5. Health (fewer illnesses and/or less severe illnesses)

6. Hyperactivity
7. Aggression/Agitation
8. Anxiety
9. Constipation
10. Diarrhea
11. Language/Communication
12. Eczema/Skin problem
13. Stimming/Perseveration/Desire for sameness
14. Sensory sensitivity
15. Social interaction and understanding
16. Falling asleep
17. Staying asleep
18. Reflux/Vomiting
19. Depression
20. Lethargy (easily tired)
21. OCD
22. Self-injury
23. Seizures
24. Tics/Abnormal movements

It's important to keep in mind that this list averages the effects of all the diets together. Different diets provided different symptom improvements—and the best overall benefit rating for a diet does not always correspond with greatest improvements in specific symptoms. For example, while the ketogenic diet is eighth on the list for overall benefit, it came in first place for nine different symptom improvements. This finding highlighted the importance of personalizing the approach to the individual. Considering symptoms when choosing a diet can be beneficial. (We'll get into the symptom improvements of each diet when we discuss the diet in detail at the appropriate step of the program.)

We also found that individuals who used therapeutic diets had a decrease (improvement) in autism severity over time, while those who did not use diet had an increase in autism severity. While they were slight changes, they were statistically significant.

What's more, the overall benefit of therapeutic diets was significantly higher than psychiatric and seizure medications, and adverse effects were significantly lower. When comparing therapeutic diets with supplements, the diets rated as more effective, but both the diets and nutraceuticals had similarly low rates of adverse effects. Put simply, this data shows that there is superior benefit to both diets and nutritional supplements with very little downside. (Of course, this doesn't mean medications cannot be helpful when needed.)

DIETS VS. NUTRACEUTICALS AND MEDICATIONS

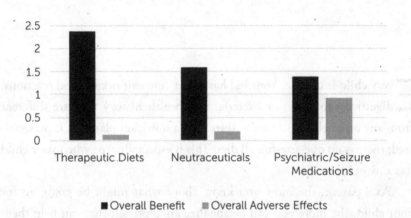

Data from: Julie S. Matthews and James B. Adams, "Ratings of the Effectiveness of 13 Therapeutic Diets for Autism Spectrum Disorder: Results of a National Survey," *Journal of Personalized Medicine* 13, no. 10 (September 29, 2023): 1448, https://doi .org/10.3390/jpm13101448.

We concluded that therapeutic diets are a generally safe, effective, and relatively inexpensive option and that therapeutic diet plans should (1) include healthy food, and (2) exclude problematic foods. This sounds simple enough—but determining *which* foods are problematic for your child can involve some trial and error.

That's where the rest of this book comes in! I'll give you the information you need to make sure your child's diet includes those healthy foods (and supplements), excludes the foods that are problematic for them, and helps them to thrive with few or no adverse effects.

PERSONALIZING NUTRITION

How to Follow the Program for Success

Every child is unique. Your kid has genes, nutrient needs, food reactions, digestive capacity, gut bacteria, and health history that are different from any other child's. As such, they need a nutrition plan that is personalized; there is no one-size-fits-all diet. This is especially true when your child has autism.[1]

As a parent, the more you know about what might be going on for your child, the more you can personalize an approach that can help them improve. Differences in your child's biochemistry, microbiome, metabolism, digestion, and genetics (which we explored in "What Causes Autism?") affect how they process food, what nutrient deficiencies they have, and what diet and nutrition approach is best. This is the essence of personalized nutrition. Each piece of the underlying puzzle is a clue that will aid you.

This program allows you to be the nutrition detective your child needs and determine what diet and nutrients are best for them. The program has two parts. The first half, "The Nourishing Hope Essentials," comprises foundational strategies that most people will find beneficial. The second half, "BioIndividual Nutrition and Therapeutic Diets," is where you will customize the diet and nutrition needs to your individual child. The diets in those chapters are arranged in the order that is typically most effective to try or consider first. For example, I find phenols are one of the biggest offenders (after gluten, casein, and soy), which is why it is the first diet presented in this part; I also recommend trying a grain-free diet (step 9) before something as restrictive as the ketogenic diet (step 11).

PROGRESSING THROUGH THE STEPS

The steps of Nourishing Hope progress in a way that's generally easiest to follow and produces results quickly. That said, you don't have to follow the steps in order. This process, just like nutrition itself, is meant to be personalized.

It's also up to you whether you want to read the whole book before you start making changes for your child, or jump right in with changes as you read step 1. I find it works well to read and implement as you go for the Nourishing Hope Essentials. With BioIndividual Nutrition, it is beneficial to read steps 7 through 12 before implementing so you have a game plan before beginning. But if your intuition tells you that a particular diet principle is key, and you want to start it right away before reading more, you can do that, too.

A section at the end of each step will help you figure out when you're ready to move on to the next. It's best to do only one new thing at a time so you can see what's working; over time, the right diet or combination of diets will become evident from the improvements your child is making.

WHICH DIET IS RIGHT FOR MY CHILD?

"Which diet is right for my child?" is one of the most common questions parents ask. There are many therapeutic diets, and it can be confusing to know where to start, what to do next, and which to choose. This book lays out the most effective therapeutic diets to help you dial in and make the right choices for your child. A personalized nutrition plan involves (1) choosing the right diet/diets, and (2) customizing it/them to your child's needs. Some people need only one therapeutic diet, while others benefit from a combination of multiple diets or dietary principles.

As you go through each chapter, you'll learn more about the different therapeutic diets: how the diets work and what underlying factors they address, the foods removed, the common symptoms relieved from the diet, how to determine if this diet is right for your child, what to eat, and how to implement the diet. There are specific symptoms and symptom clusters that are common with different food intolerances. These common reactions are important clues as to which foods are causing symptoms and which diet may help.

Your job is to be a food detective and determine the likely suspects. Look at which symptoms your child has, which foods most often result in those symptoms, and which foods they eat frequently. If your child has symptoms and the foods they eat align with common symptoms related to those foods, you have yourself a likely suspect. From here, you can choose the therapeutic diet that removes the problematic foods. Each dietary step of the program includes questionnaires to assess whether your child is experiencing these symptoms and whether they may improve with that intervention.

At the end of this chapter, you'll find a chart of the common symptoms associated with certain foods/food compounds and the diets that help improve them most. You'll see a three-tiered rating system with ✪ being a top diet to improve that symptom, ● being a great diet, and ○ being a good diet for improving that symptom. (Please note that I could have probably marked every diet for every symptom, so just because a diet isn't marked for that symptom doesn't mean it cannot help; if the top diet didn't work for your child's symptom, another one could. Everyone is unique.) This chart can help you look at the common symptoms and begin to explore diets more closely. Also be sure to read the chapter on the diet since there are some specific symptoms that relate to only one or two diets that I describe in the chapter and symptom checklists. For example, red cheeks is not a highly problematic symptom so it's not in the chart, but it's very often associated with salicylates.

DO WE NEED ANY TESTS?

Lab testing is one way to determine food and diet choices. Results can provide quantitative information on reactions and underlying biochemistry. Certain food reactions, such as food sensitivities and allergies, can be measured by immune system markers. Others, such as oxalate, can be measured by the level of an organic compound in the urine. This can provide measurable data, which is objective.

However, lab testing is not always the best way to determine the right diet and is not required for this program. Not all food reactions have laboratory values, and some are not always accurate. And lab tests can be invasive, requiring finger pricks, blood draws, or other methods that might not be possible or worthwhile.

In fact, many experienced integrative physicians consider dietary trials the best way to determine a diet's benefit. And from my many years of experience, I find symptoms and observation some of the best ways to determine which diet is right for a child.

And fortunately, observation of reactions to foods and symptoms are accessible to everyone, anywhere in the world! So regardless of whether there are lab tests or not, you can still determine the best diet for your child.

That said, should you desire the objectivity of a lab test, I will share tests that may be beneficial to ask your doctor about. Keep in mind, most conventional doctors may not have experience with these functional laboratory tests. You may have to find an integrative or functional medicine doctor to help.

EXTRA RESOURCES

You will find extra resources like worksheets, product recommendations, and more that will support you on your journey at www.PersonalizedAutism NutritionPlan.com/extras. These are resources that I either don't have room to include in the book or that are helpful to download and print. Throughout the book, I'll introduce these materials to you as they related to the steps.

TRACK YOUR PROGRESS

I will share handouts in this book and online that families can use to track their progress, so you know what is working and where you still need support. There will be a diet journal to help you track diet results. You will also find a Nourishing Hope Progress Tracker with each step of the program and an area for notes that you can download at PersonalizedAutism NutritionPlan.com/extras. These worksheets are tools you can look back on and share with your doctor and health care/nutrition team to support your journey.

I also highly recommend keeping a journal, along with photos and videos, to document your child's journey and their progress. We all tend to focus on what we are trying to improve and lose sight of the progress we have made. This will help you remember how far you have come and which interventions have helped the most. And if you need more support, these tools can be valuable to share with your team.

Before you start your Nourishing Hope journey, fill out the Parent Global Impressions survey created by Dr. James Adams. It's included in the appendix and is also downloadable on the book extras webpage. It includes ratings for language, behavior, mood, attention, cognition, physical symptoms, and more. This survey can be used as a tool to track progress any time along the way. I recommend parents fill it out every six months, after they tried an intervention, or before they start a new one. You might also consider the Autism Treatment Evaluation Checklist (ATEC) by the Autism Research Institute to evaluate your child's symptoms and progress.

MAKING IT WORK WITH RELATIVES, TEACHERS, AND THERAPISTS

Throughout this book, you'll find tools and tips you can share with loved ones and professionals that explain what you are doing regarding diet and why you are doing it. This will help you get buy-in and compliance from other caregivers. People don't always realize "one little bite" of something could hurt. Too often, well-meaning family members accidentally give an excluded food that results in a regression of symptoms that's frustrating for the child and their parent. Here is a short explanation that you can share with grandparents, relatives, and teachers so everyone understands how important diet is.

> [My child] is on a special, therapeutic diet to help them feel better. It's important that this diet is followed. Any small infraction (even the size of a grain of rice) can have big ramifications. These dietary infractions can cause reactions, symptoms, and suffering for my child that can last days or even weeks. Please do not give my child any food outside of what I send them to school with [or detailed in the letter]. If you have any questions, please ask.

You could include some information about how you are working with your doctor as well, if you want. You can also include a list of foods they can and can't have. This is beneficial for family and friends, particularly grandparents, since they often enjoy feeding their grandchildren.

There are multiple ways to engage with and inform teachers and therapists. Some families want to share what they are doing so there are no dietary infractions. Others prefer not to tell them, so they have an unbiased "blinded" trial. If there's no chance a particular caregiver will be giving your kid food, a blinded trial is a great strategy for you to get unbiased perspective. If a teacher or therapist doesn't know you've made a change but notices a difference in your kid (or not!), that's useful data for you.

THERAPEUTIC DIETS AND SYMPTOM IMPROVEMENTS

Key

✪ Top Diet
● Great Diet
○ Good Diet

	Low Sugar	Healthy	GFCF	Low Salicylate	Low SAG*
Mood and behavior symptoms					
Aggression/Irritability	✪	○	●	✪	✪
Anxiety	●	○	●	✪	✪
Depression	●	●	○	○	○
Hyperactivity	✪	○	✪	✪	●
Social interaction	●	○	✪	●	●
Stimming/Repetitive behaviors	○	○	✪	●	○
Learning					
Attention/Focus	●	○	✪	✪	●
Thinking/Cognition	●	●	✪	✪	●
Language/Communication	○	○	✪	●	
Digestion					
Constipation	○	●	✪	●	○
Diarrhea	○	○	✪	●	○
Gas/Bloating	○		✪		
Reflux/Nausea/Vomiting	○	○	●		●
Health/Physical Symptoms					
Congestion	●	○	✪	✪	✪
Fatigue/Lethargy	○	○	●		○
Headache	○	○	●	●	✪
Health/Less illness	✪	✪	✪	●	●
Pain/Inflammation	✪	●	✪	●	●
Seizures			○		○
Self-injury	●		●	●	
Sensory sensitivity	●	○	✪	✪	●
Skin rashes/Eczema	○	○	✪	●	●
Sleep	●	●	●	✪	✪

* Low SAG = Low Salicylate, Amine, and Glutamate

	Low Histamine	Elimination/Food Sensitivities	Corn-Free	Soy-Free	SCD/GAPS	Paleo	Low Oxalate	Low FODMAP	Ketogenic	Low Candida/Body Ecology
	○	○	●	●	●	○	●	○	●	○
	●	●	○	○	✪	●	●	○	✪	
	○	○		○		●		○	●	
		●		●	○	○		○	●	○
		○		○	●	●		○	✪	
		○	●		●	●	●		✪	
		○		○	✪	●			✪	
		○	○	○	✪	●	○		✪	●
		○		○	●	○			✪	
		●	✪	○	○	●	●	✪	✪	○
	●	●	✪	✪	✪	●	●	✪	●	○
		●	○	●	●	●	●	✪	○	●
	✪	✪	○	●	○	●	●	●	●	○
	✪	●	○	○			○			○
	●	○		○			✪		✪	●
	●	●	○	●	○	○	✪	○		○
	●	●	○	●	●	●	●	○	●	●
	✪	✪	●	●	●	●	✪	●	●	●
				○	○	●	●		✪	
					●	●			●	
		●	○	○	○	●	○	○	○	
	●	✪	○	○	○	○	●	○		○
	✪			○	○	○	○		✪	○

SECTION 2

The Nourishing Hope Essentials

STEP 1
Avoid Junk Food and Toxins

In my professional BioIndividual Nutrition training program, I teach nutrition practitioners this key concept: A main goal of special, therapeutic diets is to *relieve* the burden on the body by removing foods that are not tolerated and that deplete the system. From there, you can *restore* the body's systems and improve nutrient deficiencies.

While step 1 is not a therapeutic diet per se, it is a huge move toward achieving that first goal: relieving the burden on the body. Here we do that by tackling two types of stressors on the body: junk food and toxins.

GET RID OF JUNK FOOD

Avoiding junk food is crucial to the Nourishing Hope program. It's difficult to improve your child's symptoms without removing unhealthy, low-nutrient foods.

Which foods are the culprits? They're often referred to as processed foods, though that broad term also technically includes foods such as canned fish and roasted sunflower seeds, which can be perfectly fine for your child to eat. What we're really targeting here are *ultra-processed* foods. These are junk foods containing five or more industrial food additives, such as artificial colors, flavors, preservatives, and texturing agents. These are some examples of ultra-processed foods that children often like:

- Artificially colored candy
- Chicken nuggets
- Flavored potato chips
- Hot dogs
- Sugar-filled breakfast cereals
- Sugar-sweetened beverages

Many ultra-processed foods are full of sugar, refined carbohydrates, unhealthy fats, high levels of sodium, and artificial ingredients, while being low in vitamins, minerals, fiber, and good fats such as omega-3s. In fact, many of these ingredients rob the body of needed nutrients. They can negatively affect our health: Ultra-processed foods are associated with mental health conditions such as anxiety and depression.[1] And a diet high in desserts, fried food, and salt is associated with attention, learning, and behavioral problems.[2] (While moderate levels of salt are fine for most individuals, many snack foods contain very high levels of sodium, much more than you would put in home-cooked meals.)

Let's talk more about these additives' negative effects on individuals with autism and how to identify these additives so you can avoid them.

Artificial Colors, Flavors, and Preservatives

Artificial colors, flavors, and preservatives cause hyperactivity, sleep challenges, irritability, behavioral reactions, and even aggression in many children, especially those with autism and ADHD.

Artificial food additives can affect ASD symptoms in multiple ways. They contain neurotoxic chemicals that can negatively affect the brain and mental health. A study of 153 children aged three to nine years old found the preservative sodium benzoate or artificial colors (or both) caused hyperactivity in the children consuming a beverage containing them.[3] In a meta-analysis of food colors and autism, researchers explain how blue 1, blue 2, green 3, red 3, red 40, yellow 5, and yellow 6 contain chemicals toxic to the brain and deplete important nutrients causing mental health issues, ADHD, and behavioral symptoms in children.[4] (As discussed in the first chapter, ADHD symptoms can increase autism severity. So, reducing hyperactivity can benefit children with ASD.) Most artificial colors and artificial flavors are petroleum based, which makes them high-phenol compounds that contribute to behavioral symptoms (we discuss phenols in step 7). Artificial colors also contain formaldehyde and other chemicals like sulfuric acid from the manufacturing process, and may even contain lead, mercury, or arsenic. These toxins can directly damage the brain, as well as cause oxidative stress and inflammation and deplete nutrients such as zinc.

Unfortunately, despite these troubling findings, in the United States these additives are categorized by the US Food and Drug Administration as "generally regarded as safe," and the food industry is still allowed to use them. For this reason, many parents are not aware that these artificial additives may be harmful or cause behavioral and other symptoms in their children.

Fortunately, cutting out artificial colors, flavors, and preservatives is usually pretty easy and can often provide fairly immediate relief and improvement of symptoms.[5] That makes it a great place to start when reviewing your child's diet.

Identifying artificial colors, flavors, and preservatives: Some artificial colors, flavors, and preservatives are easier to recognize than others. In the United States there is no consistency in naming these artificial ingredients. Throughout the EU, Australia, and New Zealand, Europe numbers, or E numbers, are used to name artificial additives on ingredient labels, making them easier to identify. Artificial colors, flavors, and preservatives to avoid include, but are not limited to:

- Artificial colors: red 40, blue 1, blue 2, yellow 5, yellow 6, any color with a number, E numbers in the 100s, such as E102
- Artificial flavors: vanillin, artificial strawberry flavor, and similar
- Preservatives: BHA, BHT, TBHQ, propionic acid, benzoates such as sodium benzoate and benzoic acid, sorbates such as potassium sorbate and sorbic acid, propionates such as calcium propionate

and propionic acid, sulfites such as sodium sulfite or bisulfate and sulfur dioxide, and E numbers in the 200s such as E280.

MSG and Other High Glutamate Flavor Enhancers

Monosodium glutamate (MSG), on nutrition labels in Europe as E621, is a flavor enhancer and common additive high in a substance called glutamate. It is somewhat notorious because excess MSG consumption has long been blamed for causing a host of health problems, but it's not the only high glutamate flavor enhancer that can be problematic in ASD. There are many food additives by different names that are also high in free glutamate (I like to call them the cousins of MSG), such as autolyzed yeast and hydrolyzed vegetable protein. Because only ingredients that are 99 percent MSG require an MSG label, products with these other free glutamate analogs can read "no added MSG," so be sure to read the ingredient list.

Glutamate is both an amino acid and an excitatory neurotransmitter, which means that this naturally occurring amino acid can directly affect the brain, causing hyperactivity. We also produce this amino acid in our body and convert it to the calming neurotransmitter GABA. However, studies show that children with autism have genetic variants in glutamate metabolism and glutamate receptors and a disruption in the glutamate/ GABA balance, negatively impacting excitatory and inhibitory actions in the brain,[6] which can cause the hyperactivity, cognitive deficits, sensory processing challenges, and seizures we see in autism.[7]

These challenges make children and adults with autism even more susceptible to reactions from foods with glutamate, either from MSG, other similar flavor enhancers, or the glutamate that occurs naturally in some foods (discussed in step 7). MSG is an excitotoxin, a substance that can cross into the brain and overstimulate our glutamate receptors. In step 1, avoiding these flavor enhancers is key to addressing hyperactivity, behavior, and physical symptoms.

Identifying MSG and high glutamate flavor enhancers: These products are not considered artificial ingredients. Therefore, labeling can be confusing; a product can say that it "contains no artificial ingredients" even if it contains MSG or one of its cousins. Some of the high glutamate flavor enhancers to avoid include:

- Monosodium glutamate (MSG)
- Glutamate
- Glutamic acid
- Autolyzed yeast
- Yeast extract
- Yeast nutrient
- Hydrolyzed proteins or gluten (e.g., hydrolyzed wheat protein, hydrolyzed corn gluten)
- Monopotassium glutamate
- Textured vegetable protein
- E numbers E620 through E625

Emulsifiers and Other Industrial Food Additives

Emulsifiers are used as additives in ice cream, mayonnaise, chocolate, and other foods to ensure oil and water mix and stay stable to give a processed food a good texture and keep it from separating. Emulsifiers, such as carboxymethylcellulose, can damage the microbiome and cause leaky gut.[8] Emulsifiers, nanoparticles, and other food additives in industrial processed food have also been found to increase gut permeability and are now implicated in the rise of autoimmune diseases.[9]

Although not all my clients have noticed the need to avoid all emulsifiers (some are okay with xanthan gum or guar gum used in gluten-free baking, or lecithin, which is common in chocolate candy), it's good to be aware of these additives so you can look for any signs of negative reaction.

Additives such as potassium bromate added to flour for bread and baked goods, brominated vegetable oil in some citrus-flavored sodas and sports drinks, and azodicarbonamide used as a bleaching agent for flour to whiten breads have been found to cause health concerns and have been banned in various states or countries.

This conversation on additives wouldn't be complete without discussing nitrates and nitrites used to retain the pink color of cured meats like ham, salami, and bacon and as a preservative. Some research shows an increased risk of cancer in some groups of people consuming higher levels of nitrates and nitrites, but there are contradictory opinions among nutrition colleagues about consuming these foods. In my opinion, it's good to be aware of these concerns and minimize consumption. However, if these are not serious health concerns in your family and the diet is otherwise healthy with lots of vegetables, I don't think they need to be strictly avoided. I like to use bacon to get more tasty vegetables into kids' diets. In my family, we consume bacon once every few months, and that's usually with our Sauteed Cabbage with Apple and Bacon recipe (page 292).

Identifying problematic emulsifiers and additives: Look for the following in a processed food's ingredients list:

- Azodicarbonamide
- Brominated vegetable oil
- Carboxymethylcellulose
- Carrageenan
- Methylcellulose
- Mono- and diglycerides
- Nanoparticles such as titanium dioxide and silicon dioxide
- Polysorbate 80
- Potassium bromate
- Sodium or calcium stearoyl-2-lactylate
- Sucrose esters, polyglycerol esters, and other esters

Artificial Sweeteners

In the past, many people used artificial sweeteners as a "better, healthier" alternative to sugar, particularly for blood sugar and weight management concerns. However, in recent years, researchers and health experts have raised many concerns about their health effects (including the concern that they may be carcinogenic). Many of these sweeteners alter the microbiome, causing increased blood glucose, glucose intolerance, and/ or weight gain,[10] the very things people are trying to avoid by consuming them. Research also finds a potential link to ASD: one study suggested that males with ASD had more than three times the odds of having been exposed to diet sodas or the artificial sweetener aspartame in utero or while breastfeeding.[11]

Identifying artificial sweeteners: Look for the following on a food label:

- Acesulfame-K
- Aspartame
- Neohesperidin DC
- Saccharin
- Sucralose

There are other sweeteners, such as allulose, that occur in nature, so they are sometimes considered "natural." However, allulose that you can buy to use as an ingredient in recipes is synthesized in a lab. Allulose can cause the growth of the pathogenic bacteria *Klebsiella pneumoniae* and more study is needed on other potential concerns.[12] Given this, I think it's a good time to mention that it's best to tone down the sweet content of treats and use moderate amounts of naturally sweet foods such as fruit when possible, rather than replacing heavily sweetened dishes with yet another refined concentrated sugar substitute.

GMOs and Pesticides

I also recommend avoiding GMO foods and pesticides including crops commonly treated with glyphosate, the active ingredient in Roundup.

GMOs are genetically modified organisms. A GMO is different from a hybrid, one natural fruit that has been propagated with another. GMOs have been altered at the gene level through genetic engineering, adding genes from bacteria, viruses, insects, and fish that would never occur naturally in plants. There are significant concerns regarding health effects on livestock that eat GMOs as well.[13]

There is great concern over the environmental impact of GMOs tainting the wild gene pool, which alone is an important reason to avoid supporting GMO consumption. However, a bigger concern for most parents is the potential negative impact on health. There is a lot of controversy over GMOs and whether they have adverse effects. I believe the research shows GMOs are of concern because of their potential toxicity, allergy, and antibiotic resistance risk.[14] One of the most important issues is the use of the herbicide glyphosate (i.e., Roundup) on GMOs. Glyphosate is considered a potential carcinogen and there is compelling data indicating that it causes cancer, particularly non-Hodgkin lymphoma.[15] As such, many health professionals have serious concerns over the consumption of GMOs and other Roundup-treated crops.

There are three points the research highlights that are particularly relevant to autism. In addition to being an herbicide, glyphosate is a patented antibiotic. Unfortunately, not only does it kill the good bacteria including *Lactobacillus*, *Bifidobacterium*, and *Bacillus*, it doesn't kill pathogenic bacteria such as *Clostridia* and *Salmonella*, instead allowing them to overgrow. Glyphosate disrupts the microbiome, particularly in children before puberty.[16] Glyphosate may contribute to the development of autism because of *Clostridia* overgrowth.[17] Glyphosate also gives rise to oxidative stress, mitochondrial dysfunction, and neuroinflammation; these effects can cause death of neurons.[18]

Unfortunately, concern about toxic chemicals in our food supply doesn't stop at Roundup. Besides this weed killer, we can also be exposed to pesticides; many are used on food, in our homes (to discourage pests and protect our pets), in our yards, and at schools and public buildings. There are many types of pesticides, all of which can be harmful to humans, and particularly children. Studies show that pesticides affect brain development, attention, and ADHD, and can cause birth defects, cancer, and neurodevelopmental delays.[19] Research suggests that pesticides can negatively affect the blood-brain barrier and cause neuroinflammation,[20] and that children exposed to pesticides in utero and early childhood are more likely to be diagnosed with autism.[21]

While we don't have control over every pesticide that we come in contact with, we can reduce exposure to pesticides with the food we eat and avoid using them in and around our home. An organic diet can reduce levels of pesticides in the urine rapidly,[22] including glyphosate in only three days.[23] This shows that pesticide exposure, including glyphosate, comes primarily from food consumption, and we can dramatically reduce exposure through our dietary choices.

The Environmental Working Group issues a list of the Dirty Dozen, the most pesticide-containing foods. As of this writing, the most recent list included the following (in order, with #1 being the most pesticide-laden):

1. Strawberries
2. Spinach
3. Kale, collard, and mustard greens
4. Grapes
5. Peaches
6. Pears
7. Nectarines
8. Apples
9. Bell peppers and hot peppers
10. Cherries
11. Blueberries
12. Green beans

These are crops commonly treated with glyphosate (asterisks indicate they are also common GMOs) in countries like the United States that allows these agricultural products:

• Alfalfa*	• Beets
• Almonds	• Blueberries
• Apples	• Canola*
• Asparagus	• Cantaloupe
• Avocados	• Cherries
• Barley	• Chickpeas, AKA garbanzo beans
• Beans/Legumes	• Corn*

- Cottonseed*
- Dates
- Grapefruit
- Grapes
- Green beans
- Kiwi
- Lemons
- Lentils
- Oats
- Peanuts
- Pecans
- Quinoa
- Rice
- Raspberries
- Soy*
- Spearmint
- Sugar beets*
- Sugarcane
- Sunflower
- Teff
- Walnuts
- Wheat
- Wheat/Barley

Note that not all GMOs are treated with glyphosate. If you're choosing to avoid GMOs, know that squash, potatoes, and papaya are also often genetically modified.

As of 2022, US law requires manufacturers to label products that have genetically modified ingredients with a label indicating a food is "bioengineered" or "made with bioengineered ingredients." The label doesn't have to indicate which ingredients are bioengineered; it will simply indicate that one or more ingredients are genetically modified. Up to 5 percent can be bioengineered without requiring a label at all.

Sugar and Refined Carbohydrates

Sugar is one of the most harmful substances in many children's diets. Sugar causes inflammation and depresses the immune system. Sugar can lead to weight gain and even cause insulin resistance, high cholesterol, and elevated blood sugar, leading to type 2 diabetes and heart disease over time. Sugar can also contribute to hyperactivity, inattentiveness, anxiety, and depression. One study showed that more emotional symptoms were associated with higher intake of sugar-sweetened beverages in children with ASD.[24]

Conversely, a low sugar diet improved hyperactivity in 43 percent of individuals with ASD, attention in 25 percent, aggression in 23 percent, irritability in 23 percent, and anxiety in 18 percent.[25]

Nearly three in four US children are way above the recommended daily sugar intake.[26] The average American kid consumes seventeen to twenty teaspoons of added sugar per day, which is about sixty-four pounds of sugar per year.[27] The American Heart Association recommends limiting sugar to less than six teaspoons of added sugar per day, which is less than one-third of the average child's current sugar consumption.[28]

This consumption starts as soon as children wake up; sugary cereals and other typical sugar-filled breakfast foods give them around half their daily limit.[29] And sugar-sweetened beverages contribute a lot, too. It's not only sodas that are high in sugar: fruit juice, sports drinks, and even many nondairy milks have about as much sugar as soda.

Fortunately, dietary changes can result in health improvements quickly. Researchers found that reducing the sugar intake of children with obesity and metabolic syndrome by about two-thirds improved weight, blood pressure, LDL-cholesterol, triglycerides, insulin levels, and glucose tolerance in only nine days.[30]

Refined carbohydrates lack vitamins, minerals, and fiber and cause a rise in blood glucose similar to sugar. Refined carbohydrates are foods such as white flour, white rice, and other grains and starches found in most crackers, breads, and cereals. Diets higher in refined carbohydrates, glycemic index, and sugar are associated with anxiety.[31] So, limiting refined carbohydrates is beneficial to children's mental health and overall wellness.

A good rule of thumb is to eat to keep blood sugar stable. Certainly, seek medical help for blood glucose (sugar) control issues. Even for healthy people, day-to-day eating habits can balance or destabilize our blood sugar. Normal swings in blood sugar can cause mental and physical symptoms. Limiting high sugar foods and refined carbohydrates is important to helping our bodies maintain stable blood sugar.

Identifying sugar and refined carbohydrates: In addition to sugar, check food and beverage labels for high fructose corn syrup, fructose, and agave, as well as flour, white flour, white rice, potato starch, and cornstarch.

GET RID OF JUNK CHEMICALS—TOXINS

As discussed early in this book, because of reduced detoxification capability, children with autism and neurodevelopmental delays can react more strongly to, and are more harmed by, toxins in our body care products and home.

It is important to choose body care products wisely because they can contain chemicals that absorb through the skin—the body's largest organ. Many body care products contain toxic, cancer-causing, endocrine-disrupting chemicals. Many products we put on our bodies contain harmful chemicals that affect health and our mood, including preservatives such as parabens, chemical sunscreens, toluene in nail polish, and triclosan in anti-bacterial soap. Artificial fragrances found in perfume, shampoo, soap, and other body care products contain dozens of toxins that can damage the brain and liver. They can also cause physical, emotional, and behavioral symptoms, such as headaches, nausea, crying, mood swings, and hyperactivity.

Some body care products also contain heavy metals (for instance, lead in red lipstick and aluminum in antiperspirants). If your dentist gives you a silver (amalgam) filling, it contains mercury. Heavy metals are also common in our environment—there's mercury in batteries, light bulbs, and thermometers; aluminum in pots and pans; arsenic in mattresses and arsenic-treated wood; cadmium in cigarettes and inexpensive children's jewelry; and antimony in the flame retardant found in some infant and children's sleepwear. Heavy metals are also found in food, such as mercury in fish and arsenic in chicken and rice. Heavy metals are very damaging to the whole body, particularly the brain. The body requires zinc and glutathione to detoxify heavy metals, two nutrients low in those with autism. Higher levels of lead and aluminum[32] and mercury and arsenic[33] are found in those with autism.

Fluoride is a substance added to toothpaste and to the drinking water in many communities. While fluoride is added for the prevention of dental cavities, most people are not aware that elevated levels of fluoride exposure in babies, toddlers, and young children from fluoridated water, formula, and toothpaste can result in neurotoxicity and significant intellectual deficits.[34]

Two of the largest sources of chemical exposures are the water we drink and air we breathe. Tap water and indoor air can contain hundreds of chemicals and toxins. Our tap water can contain heavy metals, agricultural chemicals, and pharmaceutical drugs, and our indoor air can include chemicals off-gassing from furniture and mold toxins. Fortunately, there are water filters and air filters that can help. I understand that these can be expensive and not accessible to everyone, but by being aware of these potential factors, you may be able to address the crucial issues that could be affecting your child.

Toxins you should avoid include:

- Aluminum: pots and pans, antacids, antiperspirants
- Antimony: infant sleepwear, mattresses
- Arsenic: mattresses, arsenic-treated wood, conventionally farmed chicken meat, rice
- Cadmium: cigarette smoke, children's jewelry
- Chemical sunscreens: oxybenzone, octinoxate, octisalate, avobenzone
- Diethanolamine DEA and TEA, MEA, ETA: soaps and detergents
- Fluoride: in water supply, toothpaste, fluoride tablets
- Formaldehyde: in particleboard, plywood, and household products
- Fragrance: candles, body care, perfume
- Hydroquinone: lightener
- Hydroxybenzoic acid: phenolic preservative in cosmetics
- Lead: paint, pipes, pottery, children's jewelry, PVC toys, some dyes and lipsticks
- Mercury: silver fillings, fish, batteries, light bulbs, thermometers
- Nanoparticles: some blocking sunscreens

- Parabens: preservatives found in body care and food
- Per- and poly-fluoroalkyl (PFAS): nonstick cookware
- P-phenylenediamine: henna dyes
- Phthalates: plastics
- Sodium lauryl/laureth sulfate (SLS/SLES): toothpaste, shampoo, soap
- Talc-based baby powder
- Toluene: nail polish
- Triclosan: antibacterial soap

Fortunately, there are natural and alternative products for all of these. To find safer and healthier body care products, the Environmental Working Group's Skin Deep database has ratings on thousands of cosmetics and body care products, including the ingredients and why they are harmful. Using the database is a great way to empower your children to take an active role in their health. My teenager loves looking for better alternatives for skincare and makeup.

GET RID OF JUNK STUFF

Plastics are endocrine disruptors. They can be damaging to a developing fetus, cause reproductive abnormalities and kidney and liver damage, and have cancerous effects. Harmful plastics are everywhere in our world—and are very common in our homes in toys, food storage containers, and other household products—and it's impossible to get rid of them entirely. However, understanding their harmful effects, and eliminating them when you can, will make a great difference.

In addition to plastics, if you are building or renovating, be sure to check the health and safety of various products such as carpeting, particle board or chip board, paint, varnishes, and so on.

Some of the plastics to be aware of and avoid when possible:

- Baby bottles
- Carpeting

- Food storage containers
- Mason jar lids
- New cars (dashboard, upholstery)
- Plastic toys
- Plastic water bottles
- Recycled paper products
- Retail shopping receipts
- Teethers
- The lining of canned food
- Time-released pharmaceutical drugs

TEN WAYS TO REDUCE TOXINS

I know these are a lot of toxins to keep track of, but it's easier than you think. There are plenty of ways you can reduce toxin exposures for your child:

1. Stop eating artificial colors or flavors.
2. Stop eating MSG derivatives and other food additives.
3. Avoid spraying pesticides in your house and yard.
4. Eat organic and GMO-free.
5. Remove all air fresheners from home and car.
6. Remove all scented candles and replace with only pure options.
7. Avoid all perfume and fragrance in body care products.
8. Throw away fabric softener.
9. Switch deodorant to natural brand.
10. Remove antibacterial soaps.

READY FOR THE NEXT STEP?

Families usually spend about a week or two on step 1 before going to step 2. This gives you time to get rid of junk food and toxic products and bring in safer alternatives.

It also gives you time to see how your child responds to a cleaner diet and environment. Take a moment to jot down any improvements you see in a journal or calendar, or in the Nourishing Hope Progress Tracker you can download in the book extras section of my website. Results often include improvements in behavior, hyperactivity, attention, sleep, and overall wellness.

Of course, you can stay on this step as long as you want before going to the next. There is no rush. It's good to give this step the time you need to remove all the artificial ingredients and replace as many products as you can, so you can start to see results and gain confidence in dietary intervention.

You will continue with step 1's principles as you continue the program and in the long term. (I don't recommend reintroducing old junk foods and toxic products to test them.) Removing these items is good for everyone. You will likely even get more product savvy over time, improving on food choices, body care, and household items as you discover new ones.

STEP 2

Eat Healthfully

Eating healthfully is a cornerstone of the Nourishing Hope program. Diet affects the health and well-being of all children, particularly those with autism. Good food supplies important nutrients that reduce inflammation, fuel the brain, support mental health,[1] feed the microbiome,[2] and support intestinal health and digestion.

Unfortunately, only 3 to 7 percent of US children three to five years old consume the recommended daily intake of vegetables, and most are deficient in their intake of protein as well.[3] And atypical eating patterns, such as picky eating, in autism contribute to a reduced intake of healthy foods.[4] One study revealed that a diet high in sugar and low in vegetables, fruits, and other healthy foods was correlated with lower executive function, such as working memory, in children with ASD,[5] and Dr. Adams and I found that a healthy diet improved cognition, attention, irritability, constipation, anxiety, hyperactivity, and health.[6] Additionally, in children with ASD, fast-acting carbohydrates, such as sweets and bread, have been associated with a decrease in health, and intake of vegetables, meat, and eggs have been associated with improvement in language.[7]

In our study on therapeutic diets, a healthy diet for individuals with autism was rated the best diet in overall benefit of all therapeutic diets reported on by parents.[8] A healthy diet was defined as a diet containing good amounts of fruits, vegetables, and protein and a low intake of junk food.

While there are times nutrient supplementation is advantageous (we'll cover those later in the program), supplements do not replace healthy eating. As a colleague once said, "You can't out-supplement a bad diet." However, I recognize that getting the right nutrients from food alone is not always easy, especially if your child is a picky eater. We will discuss how to help a picky eater in step 4. For now, let's discuss what a healthy diet looks like for a child (or adult) with autism.

Eating healthfully means:

- Getting a healthful balance of macronutrients (protein, carbohydrates, and fats)
- Choosing foods rich in micronutrients (vitamins and minerals)
- Choosing high-quality foods: whole foods, organic fruits and vegetables, and grass-fed meat
- Using good preparation methods: soaked grains and legumes, fermented foods, a mixture of raw and cooked as appropriate
- Choosing non-GMO, additive-free, and nontoxic options (as covered in step 1)

NOURISHING HOPE FOOD PYRAMID

The Nourishing Hope Food Pyramid is the core of the nourishing portion of my program, and it is the starting point of each of the therapeutic diets you will learn about in this book.

The Nourishing Hope Food Pyramid is significantly different from the old USDA food pyramid many of us grew up with: Instead of building its foundation on grains and flour-based foods, it focuses on consuming larger amounts of vegetables and protein-rich foods that are nutrient dense, easy to digest, and least likely to cause a reaction. Skipping the bottom row, the foundations, for now, the food base starts with nonstarchy vegetables and protein, then proceeds to good fats, fruits, and nuts and seeds (for those not allergic), and finally gluten-free grains and legumes (for those who tolerate

The Nourishing Hope Food Pyramid

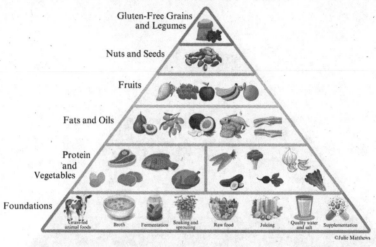

them). It works for children and adults alike and can be adapted to any special diet; we'll talk about how to do that in later chapters. Using this as your base will help you prioritize what to eat and make the best nourishing choices for yourself and your family.

I like to teach children what foods do to make us strong and healthy: I call protein our "growing foods," vegetables our "stay-healthy foods," and fats our "brain foods." When my daughter would want another helping of a starch before she finished the protein on her plate, I would say, "You need to eat your growing foods first." She understood that and was much more willing to agree to eat her protein because the reason made sense to her. For the next part of this chapter, we'll use those categories to explore these types of foods and their roles in step 2 (and throughout the program).

Protein: Our Growing Foods

The amino acids in protein are the main building blocks that help us grow. Meat, eggs, and other animal proteins are very dense in nutrients, contain all essential amino acids, and are a source of fat-soluble vitamins.

Kids' Food Pyramid

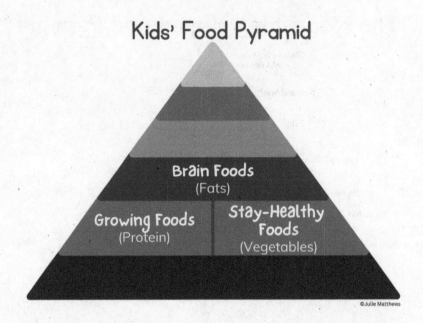

©Julie Matthews

Animal protein is low on the Nourishing Hope Sensitivity Rating Scale, a scale I use to indicate how well a food is typically tolerated. A lower value indicates a food that is generally better tolerated; higher values reflect foods that individuals with ASD commonly react to.

Because animal protein is often more easily digested and assimilated than other proteins, such as legumes and nuts, it is recommended for some (or even a majority) of protein intake. Examples of animal protein choices include grass-fed beef, grass-fed lamb, wild game like venison and elk, pastured poultry such as chicken, turkey, pheasant, and quail, wild fish, and pastured organ meats such as liver. Choose grass-fed/pastured animal products free of pesticides, hormones, and antibiotics. If you are not allergic or sensitive to eggs, they are a wonderful inclusion in the protein category; they are also a great source of good fats and brain nutrients like choline.

Although the Nourishing Hope Food Pyramid focuses on animal sources of protein, the Nourishing Hope program could be done on a vegetarian or vegan diet (though I generally don't recommend a vegan diet for children). You'll want to seek plant-based protein sources that comply with your dietary needs to ensure enough protein and proper nutritional supplementation, such as vitamin B_{12}, vitamin D, zinc, iodine, iron, and/ or calcium.

We discuss how much protein is needed later in this chapter.

Vegetables: Our Stay-Healthy Foods

Vegetables, particularly nonstarchy vegetables, share the bottom rung of the pyramid with animal proteins. For most people with digestive problems and food reactions, these foods are the easiest on the body.

Vegetables are loaded with crucial vitamins, minerals, and phytonutrients that help us to stay healthy. Vegetables contain important carbohydrates, allowing many people with inflammatory bowel conditions and other health conditions to get needed fiber and carbohydrates in a food that is easier to digest (especially when cooked) and less inflammatory than grains.

For now, prioritize nonstarchy vegetables like broccoli, carrots, and green beans. In later steps of the program, vegetable choices will be customized based on bioindividual and therapeutic diet needs.

I recommend eating at least six servings from a rainbow of vegetables every day. For children, a serving is ½ cup for vegetables and 1 cup for lettuce and leafy greens—double it for adolescents and adults. Eating by the colors of rainbow is a fun way to get your children excited about eating vegetables. And it's also delicious! Be sure to check out my Rainbow Salad (page 289) in the recipe section. It's one of my favorite recipes that my daughter and I look forward to making and eating. It's crunchy and so flavorful—not to mention beautiful and packed with nutrients.

Red	Red beet	Radish
	Red bell pepper	Red onion
	Tomato	Red potato
	Red carrot	
Orange	Carrot	Orange bell pepper
	Winter squash	Sweet potato
	Golden beet	Turmeric root

Yellow	Yellow carrot	Yellow tomato
	Yellow squash	Rutabaga
	Yellow bell pepper	Yellow beans
Green	Kale	Brussels sprout
	Collard greens	Cucumber
	Green cabbage	Zucchini
	Broccoli	
Purple	Purple carrot	Red cabbage
	Purple potato	Eggplant
	Purple kale	Radicchio

Fats and Oils: Our Brain Foods

Essential fatty acids, fat-soluble vitamins, and other nutrients found in fats are nourishing for the brain and a great source of energy. The Nourishing Hope Food Pyramid encourages a diet rich in a wide range of fats, such as fish, plant-based fats, and animal fats, including some saturated fat. Options for healthy fats include cod liver oil, fish oil, fish eggs, olive oil, nuts and seeds, avocado, coconut oil, lard, tallow, and chicken fat (assuming your child is not allergic to these). Ghee, made from dairy, is another possible option for some people on gluten-free and casein-free diets, which we discuss more in step 5.

Fruit

Fruit has wonderful phytonutrients, is tolerated by many people, and can be an important source of carbohydrates. I recommend consuming fresh (or frozen) fruit and keeping dried fruit and fruit juices to a minimum. Fruit is higher up the pyramid than vegetables because some people can't tolerate the sugars in fruit, or at least need to consume them in moderation. People often personalize their choices based on those that meet their therapeutic diet needs (e.g., low salicylate, low FODMAP, or low oxalate fruits), but more on this when we get to steps 7 and beyond. For now, focus on two to four servings (½ cup or medium size) of a variety of whole fresh fruit.

Nuts and Seeds

Nuts and seeds are higher up the pyramid because they are higher on the sensitivity rating scale; many people are allergic to nuts. Additionally, nuts and seeds are harder to digest than animal protein, especially if not soaked properly. On the other hand, nuts and seeds contain protein and good fats, and can be easier for some to tolerate than grains, so I recommend keeping them in your child's diet in moderation unless you discover a reason not to when you're personalizing their diet. Nut and seed options include almonds, walnuts, hazelnuts, pecans, cashews, macadamia nuts, Brazil nuts, sunflower seeds, and pumpkin seeds.

Legumes and Gluten-Free Grains

Because grains and legumes are difficult for many people to digest, they are at the very top of the pyramid. However, they do have good nutritional properties, so when they are tolerated, they can be a worthwhile addition to the diet (note that you may find you need to eliminate them in later steps of the program).

Legumes are high in antioxidants and fiber, making them nutrient dense and good for supporting the microbiome. However, many beans are high in oxalate and phytates, and high in FODMAPs—which create digestive issues in some people. All dried beans and legumes should be soaked in water at room temperature for eight hours before cooking. For those that tolerate them, bean and legume choices include lentils, navy beans (white), lima beans, split beans, and chickpeas, among others.

Whole grains are high in fiber, folate and other B vitamins, vitamin E, magnesium, and selenium. However, grains are the most irritating of the food categories, generally speaking. That does not mean everyone is intolerant to them or should avoid them. Grains are best as whole grains, soaked, and ideally fermented. There are a variety of flexible, nutrient-dense options, including brown rice, millet, quinoa, amaranth, buckwheat, and sorghum, if you want to try adding some of these to your diet now.

Food Pyramid Foundations: Nutrition-Boosting Principles

We'll now finally talk about the base of the pyramid. These eight principles can add more nutritional value and increase the digestibility of foods on the pyramid:

1. **Grass-fed animal foods and organic produce**: Grass-fed and pastured meat, liver, and eggs are beneficial for reaching optimal nutrition. Produce should use organic principles and not be sprayed with anything toxic.

2. **Bone broths**: Homemade bone broths from chicken, beef, or other sources are nutrient-rich and help boost digestion. Serve broth to drink or incorporate it into a meal.

3. **Fermented foods**: Consuming live-cultured foods such as raw sauerkraut or other cultured vegetables, yogurt, and kefir (dairy-free if needed) daily can be beneficial for many individuals.

4. **Soaking and sprouting**: Soaking and sprouting grains increase their digestibility and available nutrients. Another form of sprouted plants, broccoli sprouts, are a very nutrient-rich choice. More on the active ingredient in these, sulforaphane, in step 12.

5. **Juicing and blending**: Homemade vegetable and fruit juice is a wonderful way to get lots of nutrients in an easy-to-digest form that children love. Blending vegetables and fruit into smoothies is another great way to get healthy food into children, and when they're blended rather than juiced, all the fiber stays intact, too. Just be sure you're keeping high sugar veggies and fruits (like beets, carrots, and grapes) to a minimum, and instead opt for lower sugar options. Cucumbers, celery, kale, blueberries, and strawberries are great choices.

6. **Raw foods:** Raw vegetables, fruits, nuts, and seeds (ideally soaked) are rich in enzymes and nutrients, making them supportive for digestion. (That said, people with weak digestion and inflammation may need to cook their food to break it down more until a certain amount of healing takes place.) While raw foods make a wonderful addition to a healthy diet, 100 percent raw food diets (for more than a few days to weeks) can be depleting.

7. **Supplementation:** While we'd like to get all the nutrients from our food, many of us need an extra boost from supplements because our bodies or cells are not able to make or absorb sufficient amounts. Much more on this in steps 3 and 12.

8. **Quality water and salt:** Purified water is devoid of chemicals and other toxins often removed through a filtering process and is essential for good health. Drinking purified water ensures adequate hydration without additional toxins that may be present in tap water. A mineral-rich salt (such as Celtic Sea salt or Himalayan crystal salt) supplies sodium and trace minerals, while avoiding additives in standard table salt such as calcium silicate and dextrose. However, these salts do not contain added iodine. Since iodine is an essential nutrient for health, if you use a non-iodized sea salt or crystal salt, be sure your kids are getting their iodine needs met through supplementation or other sources.

Nourishing Hope Stories

"My biggest challenge prior to starting the program was not having enough options to eat on a restricted diet. I loved how Julie had the veggies list and different ideas on how we can incorporate it into our child's diet. My son's major improvement came through the diet thanks to Julie's step-by-step approach on how to nail it further down. With the use of supplements, my son's symptoms have improved, and I am glad I found this course and found Julie." —*Parent of a two-year-old with autism* ■

TIPS FOR INCREASING INTAKE OF VEGETABLES AND FRUITS

As we've talked about the nutritional importance of fruits and vegetables, here are several strategies that I find beneficial with my clients and Nourishing Hope families.

Increase Portion Size of Vegetables

In a randomized controlled trial, researchers increased the portion size of fruits and vegetables on young children's plates to see if it would lead them to eat more.[9] It turns out it does! In one scenario, they simply increased the portion size by 50 percent, which increased intake of vegetables by 24 percent and fruit by 33 percent. In the other scenario, they increased the fruits and vegetables by 50 percent while decreasing the portion sizes of other foods by a similar amount, and this resulted in a 41 percent increase in vegetable consumption and 38 percent increase in fruit consumption.

So, at your child's next meal or snack, try serving a larger portion of vegetables (and fruit if they need more).

Serve Vegetables First

In a study of preschool-aged children, eating vegetables first during a meal was associated with higher consumption of vegetables.[10] So try offering vegetables first at a meal. If your child is hungry as dinner is being prepared, serve some vegetables while they wait. Or while everyone is seated, dish out the vegetables as a first course, before the main. This works well in my family.

Make It Kid Friendly

Texture, taste, aroma, and visual presentation are all important for getting children to eat more vegetables. In step 4, I will go into detail on all these areas and provide tried-and-true strategies that work.

V123

Six servings of vegetables is a lot, particularly if we wait and try to fit it all into dinner. So, to make this more manageable, I created the V123 system, or Veggies 1, 2, 3:

- 1 vegetable at breakfast
- 2 vegetables at lunch
- 3 vegetables at dinner

I also recommend a vegetable as a snack. But V1123 is not as catchy as V123.

If it takes a bit of time to get your kid's veggie palate warmed up for the day, for breakfast, try naturally sweeter options like butternut squash hash browns, roasted root vegetables, carrot soup, or lightly steamed sugar snap peas. For lunch, find foods easy to eat on the go, like sliced raw red bell peppers, cucumbers, jicama, and/or homemade veggie chips (you may even be able to buy parsnip, carrot, sweet potato, or rutabaga chips at the store); consider adding a dip to make them more fun and tastier. For a snack, a smoothie with frozen cauliflower rice or kale is a great way to get a serving of vegetables. For dinner, salads, vegetable side dishes, and carb substitutes like cauliflower rice or tortillas, carrot fries, zucchini noodles, and rutabaga fries are great options.

MACRONUTRIENTS AND CALORIES

One of the most common questions I get from parents is how much their child should be eating, especially when it comes to protein. When it comes to children, I'm usually less concerned about calories and more concerned with quality food. With that said, calories do come in handy as a quantitative measurement when a child is under- or overweight. If your doctor is concerned that your child is underweight, the first question to answer is, "Are they eating enough calories?" The next is whether the calories are from healthy foods. If they are eating plenty, the foods are healthy, and the diet is well rounded with quality protein, fats, and carbohydrates, then you might question whether digestion is allowing for adequate breakdown and absorption of foods and nutrients. Calculating and having the calorie data can help you and your health care team determine whether your child simply needs more calories for their metabolism or whether they could use some gut healing or other support.

The following table shows the average total calories needed per day as well as protein intake for multiple age ranges. Some children (and adults) may need more than what is indicated, as vigorous activity and injury/healing require more protein.

Average Calorie and Protein Needs by Age

Age (Years)	Total Calories	Protein (Grams)
1–2	1,000	13–30
3–8	1,600	19–50
9–13	1,800–2,200	34–75
14–18	2,000–2,400 (women) 2,200–3,000 (men)	46–80 52–95
19+	1,600–2,400 (women) 2,000–3,200 (men)	44–68 58–90

The macronutrients are protein, carbohydrates, and fats. Like all of nutrition, macronutrient needs are bioindividual.

Protein

Protein needs differ based on age, since protein is required for growth. While protein charts for children commonly show protein needs based on age, a more accurate measurement can be calculated with their weight. I've included both the table based on age and more specific information based on weight for those who want to consider both options. The recommended dietary allowance (RDA) for protein for children and adults is less than what many nutritionists recommend. For example, the RDA for protein for children is 0.9 grams of protein per kilogram of body weight per day and for adults is 0.8 grams of protein per kilogram of body weight per day. However, some researchers feel that protein requirements are significantly underestimated in children and suggest that 1.3 to 1.55 grams of protein per kilogram of body weight is more accurate.[11] And several organizations recommend 1.2 to 2 grams of protein per kilogram of body weight for active adults and elderly individuals. This works out to be 30 to 35 grams of protein for a child weighing 50 pounds (22.7 kilograms). My preference for Nourishing Hope families is calculating protein based on weight, using the RDAs for minimum targets, and using higher ranges for more optimal levels in most cases.

Protein-Rich Food	Protein (Grams)
3.5 ounces chicken breast	31
3.5 ounces beef	27
3.5 ounces salmon	26
3.5 ounces shrimp	25
1 cup beans	16
2 eggs	14
2 tablespoons peanut butter	7

Carbohydrate and Fiber

Carbohydrates come in two forms: simple (sugars) and complex (starches and fiber). Carbohydrates provide us with a source of fuel, and those we can't digest (fiber) feed our good bacteria.

As we discussed in step 1, it's best to limit refined carbohydrates and sugar. When consuming carbohydrates, it's beneficial to consider their glycemic index. This is the measure of how quickly they cause a rise in blood glucose. Examples of low-glycemic foods include apples, blueberries, oranges, strawberries, legumes, almonds, sunflower seeds, broccoli, cauliflower, zucchini, and more. High-glycemic foods include packaged cereal, bread and crackers from refined and white flours, white rice, cookies, donuts, cake, potatoes, and French fries.

Fiber is found in vegetables, fruit, and whole grains such as avocados, popcorn, legumes, and sweet potatoes. Some forms are fermented in the digestive tract by beneficial bacteria, which supports the health of our digestive tract, brain, immune system, and other organs. Diets rich in high-fiber foods support a healthy microbiome.[12] Fiber also adds bulk to the stool. A scientific paper on fiber in children showed that low amounts of both types of fiber (fermentable and bulking) contributed to an imbalanced microbiome and functional gastrointestinal disorders such as constipation, diarrhea, and abdominal pain.[13] Fiber also supports weight control, aids blood sugar regulation, and lowers cholesterol.

We discuss fermentable fiber (prebiotics) more in this chapter under "Gut- and Microbiome-Healing Foods" (page 75). For now, let's talk about total fiber in general.

How much fiber should we strive for? For children, I like to use the calculation of age plus 10 grams. So, a five-year-old would need around 15 grams per day, a ten-year-old would need 20 grams per day, and a fifteen-year-old would aim for 25 grams per day. Adults need around 25 to 38 grams per day.

Fiber-Rich Food	Fiber (Grams)
Lentils, 1 cup cooked	11.6
Chickpeas, 1 cup cooked	9.7
Figs, 3½ ounces	6.9
Pear with skin	5.6
Oats, 1 cup cooked	5.4
Quinoa, 1 cup cooked	5.2
Carrots, chopped, 1 cup	4.3
Almonds, ¼ cup	4.1
Strawberries, chopped, 3½ ounces	3.8
Prunes, 5	3.4

Brussels sprouts, 1 cup	3.3
Broccoli florets, 1 cup	3.2
Brown rice, 1 cup cooked	3.2
Sunflower seeds, ¼ cup	3.1
Apple with skin	3.0

Fat

Fat often gets a bad rap, but it is a rich source of energy for our brain and cells. Understanding the different types of fats and fatty acids will help you choose the best fats. Fortunately, it's easier than it seems. I recommend getting a variety of good fats and consuming all of them in moderate amounts to keep a balance.

Olive oil and avocados contain mostly monounsaturated fats, omega-9, a healthy fatty acid. Fatty fish and fish oil offer omega-3 polyunsaturated fatty acids, EPA and DHA. EPA and DHA are important fatty acids that are essential for brain growth and development, as well as many other functions that we will discuss in detail in step 3. Flax oil contains an omega-3 fatty acid, ALA; however, it needs to be converted to EPA and DHA.

Omega-6 fatty acids are another type of polyunsaturated fat. Most of this comes in the form of linoleic acid from vegetable oils, such as corn oil, soybean oil, canola oil, safflower oil, and sunflower oil, as well as nuts and seeds. Our western diet has an overabundance of omega-6s and is lacking omega-3s. However, one omega-6 fatty acid, GLA, is often in short supply and beneficial to get in the diet or as supplementation.

Meat, dairy, and coconut contain more saturated fatty acids than other foods. Even saturated fat can be part of a healthy diet. Not all saturated fats contain cholesterol, and they affect cholesterol levels very differently. An interesting study compared coconut oil to butter and olive oil and found that the two saturated fats (coconut oil and butter) led to different responses in the body.[14] LDL cholesterol ("bad cholesterol") was raised with butter but

not coconut oil (or olive oil). And coconut oil significantly raised HDL cholesterol ("good cholesterol") more than butter (or olive oil). This means that
not all saturated fats function the same way in the body nor are all bad. Additionally, cholesterol is not all bad—it has important functions in the body,
including supporting brain development, making hormones, and producing
vitamin D.

The only fats I recommend avoiding are man-made trans fats and vegetable oils. Vegetable oils such as corn oil, canola oil, cottonseed oil, and
soybean oil contain GMOs, glyphosate, high amounts of omega-6, and/
or are highly processed. When vegetable oils are made into solids via an
industrial process, they become partially hydrogenated oils, which contain
these man-made trans fats that have been found to contribute to heart
disease. (Fortunately, they have been banned in the United States, but
vegetable oils themselves remain widely available and are ubiquitous in
processed food.)

Other than those, consuming a wide range of fats from whole foods and
healthy sources provides nutrients your child needs. Eating high-quality
sources of fat should be the goal. Choose pasture-raised meat and eggs, fish,
organic oils when possible, and plant-based oils such as extra virgin olive
oil, avocado oil, coconut oil, and flax oil.

ANTI-INFLAMMATORY PRINCIPLES

Inflammation is at the root of conditions like autism. Building your diet
with anti-inflammatory foods is a great way to design a healthy diet. Most
of the foods and principles of the Nourishing Hope food pyramid are anti-
inflammatory by nature: A diet low in inflammatory foods, including sugar,
refined carbohydrates, fried foods, trans fats, and processed foods, is a good
start. Also, whole foods, such as nonstarchy vegetables, leafy greens, fresh
berries and fruits, fish, nuts, and olive oil, are wonderful anti-inflammatory
foods. Here's a list of good options:

- Avocados
- Berries
- Broccoli sprouts
- Cacao/Cocoa
- Cherries
- Cinnamon
- Citrus/Flavanones
- Cloves
- Cruciferous vegetables
- Garlic
- Ginger
- Grapes
- Olive oil
- Onions
- Peppers
- Rosemary
- Salmon/Fatty fish
- Thyme
- Tomatoes
- Turmeric
- Anthocyanidins: purple, blue, red foods

Remember, everyone is unique and even some of these "healthy, anti-inflammatory foods" can cause inflammation for some people. For this reason, a Nourishing Hope anti-inflammatory diet is also personalized. At this stage, I suggest feeding as many healthy foods that you know are tolerated as possible. Then you can refine it once you learn more in steps 7 and beyond.

GUT- AND MICROBIOME-HEALING FOODS

As previously discussed, the gut and microbiome are key pieces of the ASD puzzle and food can be a beneficial tool for healing them.

Anti-inflammatory foods help reduce inflammation in the gut and help the healing process. And many of the therapeutic diets in this book include principles aimed at reducing inflammatory substances and healing the gut. (We will discuss this throughout the steps and summarize it in step 11.)

In addition, some foods contain high levels of nutrients that heal the gut and support the microbiome. Some of my favorite gut-healing foods include bone broths, salmon, coconut, lemon, raspberries, honey, probiotics, and prebiotics. Let's pause a moment on those last two.

Probiotics are beneficial bacteria that have many important functions and aid a healthy gut and brain. There are many probiotics found in fermented foods, including various strains of *Lactobacillus* and *Bifidobacterium*.

In a study on autism, kefir, a fermented form of dairy, increased regulatory T cells and SAM and reduced repetitive autism-like behaviors in mice.[15] Strive to include some fermented foods in your child's diet each day. While many fermented foods contain dairy, many dairy-free options are available. Probiotic foods include:

- Fermented vegetables (such as raw sauerkraut and kimchi)
- Kombucha
- Raw apple cider vinegar
- Sauerkraut juice
- Yogurt and kefir

You can make wonderful probiotic snacks and meals with these probiotic-rich foods, including my Mango Ginger Probiotic Smoothie (page 310) and Cherry Apple Cider Vinegar Drink (page 311).

Prebiotics are the food for our beneficial bacteria. They help keep our beneficial bacteria and our gut healthy and strong. Aim to include some prebiotics at each meal. Prebiotic, fermentable fiber-rich foods include:

- Apples
- Asparagus
- Avocados
- Bamboo
- Beans
- Cassava flour
- Chickpeas
- Chicory
- Cooked and cooled potatoes
- Cooked and cooled rice
- Dandelion greens
- Flaxseed
- Garlic
- Green banana flour
- Green bananas
- Honey
- Hummus
- Jicama
- Leeks
- Lentils
- Onion
- Pears
- Peas
- Plantains
- Pomegranates
- Raspberries
- Sunchokes
- Sweet potatoes
- Whole gluten-free grains

READY FOR THE NEXT STEP?

If you are very experienced with diet and already eating lots of healthy foods, you might move on quickly. So even if your family has a healthy diet, consider any ways you can improve your diet with the suggestions and principles in this chapter.

If your child eats very few vegetables and you are very new to dietary intervention, consider spending a month or two on this step and see what good nutrition alone can do to help your child. Removing sugar, junk food, and pesticides (from step 1) and adding good healthy foods like vegetables, whole fruit, and protein in this step can go a very long way toward improving your child's health and symptoms.

If your child is a picky eater and you're having difficulty making any progress with healthy eating after several weeks, it may be advantageous to move ahead to the next steps. The next several steps have principles that can help, such as nutrient supplementation and picky eating strategies. Keep these healthy foods and nutrition facts in your back pocket and come back to them later.

This step—eating healthfully—is really an ongoing process in anyone's life. So, there is no getting it perfect or being done with this step per se. Remember to track symptoms and your progress, and now you're ready to proceed to step 3.

STEP 3

Boost Nutrition with Supplements

While good food choices are an important way to improve your child's nutrient intake, a child with autism often needs additional help through nutritional supplementation. Nutritional supplements are a useful tool for picky eaters who may be hesitant about trying new healthier foods right away. And for those who have genetic variants or chemical imbalances that affect their nutrient absorption, supplementation can provide nutrients in amounts greater than they can get with food. Supplements can aid your child's body in repairing itself, as well as in growth and daily needs. They can also help reduce inflammation and minimize gastrointestinal symptoms.

Nutrient differences and deficiencies are common in autism and can affect symptoms and autism severity.[1] Kids with autism can also have *higher* levels of some nutrients, but this isn't necessarily beneficial; for instance, high copper is associated with low zinc and ADHD.[2] Additionally, even when nutrient levels fall within normal ranges, individuals with ASD can have underlying issues in which biochemical pathways that rely on certain nutrients aren't working optimally.[3] All of this affects kids' energy, growth, cognition, detoxification, oxidative stress, and overall physical and mental health. In all these instances, nutrient support is likely beneficial for improving their condition. Physicians and researchers recommend a personalized nutrient approach.[4]

In this chapter, we will cover some foundational supplements that have been found to be beneficial for many people with ASD, then talk about individual vitamins, minerals, and other nutrients we all need daily. In step 12, we will discuss other supplements that can help further personalize your supplement approach.

How to implement supplements? My motto with supplementation is "low and slow." That means start with a low dose and slowly increase it to give your child's body time to adjust and confirm there is no reaction.

In the appendix, I have included lists of natural food sources for these individual nutrients so that you can see what your child might already be getting from their diet and figure out where a supplement can help to close a gap while a child is getting acclimated to healthier food choices.

THREE FUNDAMENTAL NUTRITIONAL SUPPLEMENTS

We know that children with autism often do not meet their nutritional needs through diet and have diets that are nutritionally deficient when compared to their neurotypically developing peers. The three supplements I recommend most families start with are a multivitamin/mineral formula, essential fatty acid blend, and digestive enzymes. All three of these were part of the six interventions used in the first study I described in "The Science Behind Nourishing Hope." A multivitamin/mineral formula and essential fatty acids were the top two nutrients that parents reported to be most effective for their child. Digestive enzymes were another supplement used in our study, and I have found them to be very helpful for digestive support in my nutrition practice with clients and in our Nourishing Hope for Healing Kids program.

Let's look at all three of these.

If you find that your child cannot tolerate any of the supplements, decrease the amount and go slowly or stop the supplement and get support from your physician or nutrition professional.

Multivitamin/Mineral Formulas

Multivitamin/mineral formulas are an efficient way to get many of the nutrients your child needs, and I recommend parents start supplementing with these. One supplement provides many nutrients that are required to build our bones, muscles, brains, and neurotransmitters (to name only a few of thousands of functions). Also, some nutrients help others be absorbed, and some nutrients work together with others for needed biochemical processes.

Supplementation with a multivitamin/mineral formula has been found in multiple studies to be helpful for people with autism, improving nutrient status and reducing autism symptoms.[5] A multivitamin/mineral supplement has also been shown to help significantly improve symptoms in children with ADHD.[6] The multivitamin/mineral formula used in our randomized controlled trial[7] was reported by caregivers to improve speech and language in 32 to 39 percent of individuals with ASD, and the following symptoms in 23 percent or more: anxiety, emotion regulation, irritability, attention, play, social interaction, and cognition.[8]

Choosing a Good-Quality Brand

Not all multivitamin/mineral formulas are equal. Some multivitamins in stores are just that: a few vitamins but no minerals. Many children's vitamins are filled with lot of sugar. Some have artificial colors or flavors. Others have gluten and other allergens.

Multivitamin/mineral supplements formulated for children with autism in mind and professional supplement brands are good places to start looking. These may look different than multivitamin formulas you are used to, especially if you're most familiar with single-dose multivitamin tablets or chewables. These formulas are often powders or powder-filled capsules, often requiring several capsules per day to reach the recommended dose based on the weight of the child.

Compare an inexpensive multivitamin/mineral at the local grocery or drugstore to the following nutrient list. You'll likely find that in more commercial or cheaper products there are fewer nutrients listed. You'll also find that there are lower amounts and cheaper forms. Some companies include higher-quality forms or more expensive nutrients like CoQ_{10} so they can feature them on the label, but they are in such small quantities that they do not do much good. Look at what you get for the price, so you can make an informed choice.

Important vitamins, minerals, and other nutrients often found in high-quality multivitamin/mineral formulas include:

- Vitamin A
- Vitamin C
- Vitamin D
- Vitamin E
- Vitamin K
- Vitamin B_1
- Vitamin B_2
- Vitamin B_3
- Vitamin B_5
- Vitamin B_6
- Vitamin B_{12} (methylcobalamin)
- Biotin
- Folate (5-MTHF or folinic acid)

- Choline
- Inositol
- CoQ_{10}
- Calcium
- Chromium
- Iodine
- Lithium
- Magnesium
- Manganese
- Molybdenum
- Potassium
- Selenium
- Zinc

There are additional nutrients including bioflavonoids, boron, N-acetyl cysteine, L-carnitine, and other mitochondrial support that you might like to have in your multivitamin/mineral formula.

A Note on Copper and Iron

A couple of nutrients you may not find in a multivitamin/mineral supplement formulated for children with autism are copper and iron.

Copper has been found to be high in those with autism while zinc is frequently low (low zinc and high copper ratio has also been found to be associated with higher autism severity).[9] Because zinc and copper compete for absorption, for someone with low zinc levels, copper supplementation can cause even lower zinc levels and higher copper. High copper can cause copper toxicity and negatively affect the liver and neurological function.

High copper can cause aggression, poor concentration, and sensitivity to clothing tags and tight clothes.[10]

Iron is a pro-oxidant (causes oxidative stress) and found to be above the reference range in 42 percent of children with autism.[11] Excess iron in the brain has been found in neurological and neurodegenerative conditions, and some researchers suspect that excess dietary iron may be responsible for increases in autism and food allergies.[12]

With all of that said, copper and iron are minerals the body does require, and some people may have a need for supplementation on a personalized level. For instance, some children—such as vegetarians, those who do not eat adequate meat, and menstruating females—are deficient in iron. And iron deficiency negatively affects cognitive function. Your doctor can test your child for deficiency and help you determine if supplementation would be beneficial. From there, individuals that need them can supplement them on an individual basis. (Be aware that iron can be constipating, so if your child does need iron supplementation, find a good form and be sure to address any constipation that may result.)

Starting a Multivitamin/Mineral Supplement

Once you have chosen a multivitamin/mineral supplement, start low and slow with a fraction of the targeted dose (by taking less or pouring out some of the powder in a capsule, if applicable). I recommend starting with about 25 percent of the targeted daily total, once a day. Then, when you know that amount is tolerated, increase that dose to twice per day. After that, continue twice per day and increase the amount every few days until 100 percent of the recommended amount has been reached. Typically, it takes a couple of weeks to reach the full amount.

If your child can swallow pills, the administration of capsules or tablets is easy. If they don't swallow capsules, you'll want to break them open and mix the powder inside with something strong-tasting like fruit juice. Tablets are usually not the best option for kids who don't swallow pills; instead, it's better to look for a powder or capsule supplement.

A vitamin and mineral supplement is best taken with food. Normally, nutrients would be taken in from eating a meal, and food can help prevent the nausea that some supplements can cause. Also, the body can't always use or store every nutrient at the time it is consumed, so it's best to divide the daily dose into two or three parts taken throughout the day. Breakfast and dinner are often best because they are furthest apart and usually eaten at home. If your child isn't hungry or feels nauseous in the morning, try lunch and dinner. For others, three times a day is a possibility.

Some people are sensitive to certain forms of nutrients. If your child has increased behaviors or reactions after starting a supplement, decrease the dosage until it is tolerated, then try to increase it again. If your child cannot tolerate the multivitamin/mineral, talk with a physician or nutrition professional who might be able to identify the problem. You can try a different multivitamin/mineral brand. Clients of mine who reacted to one supplement did great on another. If a reaction persists even after going slowly or trying a different brand, take a step back, remove the multivitamin/mineral formula, and supplement with the nutrients one at a time to see which, and what forms, they might be reacting to. Later in this chapter, we discuss individual nutrients.

Food-Based Supplements

Alongside supplements, food-based powders, made from vegetables, greens, fruits, and/or organ meats, can boost nutrition while you work to increase the vegetables and variety of foods your child eats. Consider trying these:

- **Nutrient-dense food powders:** These include vegetable and fruit powders, green powders, and seaweed seasoning sprinklers. These are easy to add to (and hide in!) smoothies.
- **Protein powder:** Also great in smoothies. Choose options free of soy and casein; avoid whey and focus on other forms, such as pea protein, rice protein, beef broth protein,

and premade (CFSF) protein drinks. They often supply 20 grams of protein in a serving, but read the label to be sure.

- **Organ meats:** If you can't imagine getting organ meats like liver into your child (I have a great Super Nutrient Burgers recipe, page 277) or can't see preparing them yourself, then liver and other beef organ meat powders could come in handy.

For some of my favorite high-quality vitamins, minerals, and other supplements, download my list of favorite supplements at www.PersonalizedAutismNutritionPlan.com/extras.

Essential Fatty Acids

Essential fatty acids (EFAs), particularly omega-3 supplements such as fish oil, are another supplement I recommend for most, and I recommend adding these after you've successfully introduced a multivitamin/mineral formula. Most western diets are low in omega-3s, and this is true of children with ASD as well, since many do not eat fish. What's more, it is suspected that children with autism may have an issue with how they metabolize polyunsaturated fatty acids, which leads to omega-3 deficiency.[13] This can lead to oxidative stress and inflammation and can negatively affect the microbiome and the gut-brain connection.

Fish oil contains two essential omega-3 fatty acids: EPA and DHA. A third omega-3 fatty acid, ALA, is found in plants such as flaxseed and can be converted by humans to EPA and DHA. However, this process is not very efficient; it is difficult to produce adequate EPA and DHA from ALA.[14]

EPA and DHA are part of the cell membrane and help it maintain its flexibility to allow nutrients and substances in and out of the cell. They support gene expression and have anti-inflammatory effects, including lowering intestinal inflammation.[15] They can lower triglycerides and have a positive effect on heart health. The brain and retina contain a high amount of DHA, and DHA is very important for brain development.[16]

There's a lot of promising research supporting omega-3 supplementation. Meta-analysis studies looking at ASD along with other neurological conditions found that omega-3 supplementation was helpful in autism especially for hyperactivity, lethargy, stereotypical autism behaviors (rigid and repetitive), as well as irritability and social awareness and communication.[17] This study also found improvements in ADHD, depression, and schizophrenia. In a study of medical students, omega-3s reduced inflammation and anxiety.[18] Another study found that omega-3s with vitamin E supplementation improved speech in adolescents with ASD.[19] In one study of nutraceuticals in ASD, parents rated omega-3 supplementation highly; it was associated with an improvement in autism severity.[20] The top symptom improvements related to brain function, specifically cognition, attention, and language.[21]

GLA (an omega-6) may assist the brain in using omega-3s better. The EFA supplement used in our *Nutrients* study included fish oil (omega-3) and GLA. For ADHD, several studies have found that EPA and DHA combined with GLA is more effective than omega-3s alone for reducing inattentiveness and hyperactivity, as well as for improving impulsivity, reading, cognition, and working memory.[22] Omega-3s with GLA also improve autism symptoms and behaviors.[23]

Because of these studies, my essential fatty acid recommendation for most children and adults with ASD is fish oil with GLA (when tolerated—of course, do not give fish oil to someone who is allergic to fish! In the case of fish allergy, flax oil is an acceptable substitute). For children three years and under, I typically suggest cod liver oil. It has a higher ratio of DHA to EPA, and DHA is so important for brain development.

Starting Essential Fatty Acids

Like all new supplements, I recommend implementing essential fatty acids low and slow. However, children don't need as much of a runway or start-up ramp as they often do with multivitamins. Fatty acids are usually well tolerated. Start with a quarter of the suggested dose and increase to the recommended daily amount over one to four weeks.

My essential fatty acid suggestions are based on what we used in our comprehensive diet and nutrition study:

Weight	Recommend Daily Target
For children 30–50 pounds (14–23 kg)	1,200 mg total omega-3s (850 mg EPA, 220 mg DHA) and 250 mg GLA
For children 51–100 pounds (23–45 kg)	1,800 mg omega-3s (1,275 EPA, 330 DHA) and 375 mg GLA
For children and adults over 100 pounds (45+ kg)	2,400 omega-3s (1,700 EPA, 440 DHA) and 500 mg GLA

Capsules are fairly easy to take, but fish oil capsules can be large, and there is not much oil in each, so you often need to take quite a few. I prefer the liquid formulas. If you use the liquid formula, remember that oil floats, so they don't mix well with juice. It's better to mix them in a spoonful of nondairy pudding or ice cream.

Fish oil supplements can cause fishy-smelling burps. It can be best to take them along with a meal (at the beginning or middle of the meal, rather than at the end or alone). Or, if your child tends to have acid reflux or fish oil causes it, dividing the essential fatty acids into multiple smaller doses per day can help.

Digestive Enzymes

Digestive enzymes are helpful for children that need support with digestion, which is many children with ASD. I recommend adding these after starting the other two supplements. Digestive enzymes help your child's digestive system break down food more effectively. This helps reduce GI symptoms, optimize the nutrients they can absorb in the foods they eat, and decrease problematic protein chains associated with food sensitivities. Digestive enzymes include lipase to break down fat, proteases to break down protein, and amylase to break down carbohydrates. I recommend digestive enzyme formulas that include DPPIV, an enzyme that helps break down the protein in wheat and dairy that can become opioids—more on this in step 5.

Digestive enzymes have been found to be beneficial in autism. In a randomized double-blind trial in children with ASD, researchers found statistically significant improvements in gastrointestinal symptoms, autism symptoms, emotional response, and behavior with digestive enzymes.[24] And in the nutraceuticals rating survey, digestive enzymes were highly rated with very few adverse effects, and 40 percent who found digestive enzymes beneficial had improvement in constipation and 18 percent in diarrhea.[25]

I recommend a digestive enzyme supplement that includes lipase, protease, amylase, DPPIV, and often more enzymes for a broad-spectrum choice.

Starting Digestive Enzymes

Digestive enzymes are taken based on the size of the meal, rather than the size of the person. They digest the food you are eating at the time, so take them with meals. As always, go low and slow. Start with a fraction of the recommended amount at one meal and then slowly increase the number of meals and amount over the course of a week or so.

INDIVIDUAL VITAMINS AND MINERALS

Let's review some of the individual nutrients to understand their uses; signs, symptoms, and causes of deficiencies; best forms; and daily nutritional needs. This can help determine which forms you want to look for in your multivitamin/mineral supplement. Furthermore, some multivitamin/mineral formulas do not contain a full daily amount of every nutrient or may not be enough for that individual, so additional supplementation of some nutrients may be beneficial.

Remember, I also include food sources for these nutrients in the appendix, since our daily intake is a combination of what we get through food and supplementation. To know what to supplement, it can be helpful to know how much your child is getting through food, especially for nutrients such as calcium where most multivitamin/minerals do not contain the daily requirements. Also, if your child is having difficulty taking the full dose of daily multivitamin, knowing how much they are getting from food can help set your mind at ease or determine how to get extra from food. (That said, don't feel you need to calculate their food intake to balance against a multivitamin; multivitamin/mineral supplements are often formulated to meet the *minimum* nutrient requirements for the day, and it is very unlikely you'll get too much of a nutrient even with an extra boost from food.)

Folate

Folate is a critical nutrient for so many aspects of life, ensuring our red blood cells function properly, aiding the growth and production of cells, supporting nervous system development, and more. Folate is also an important nutrient for methylation (discussed in "What Causes Autism?").[26] For this, folate works with vitamin B_{12}.

While serum folate levels were not lower in children with ASD compared to neurotypical children in one study, a laboratory marker, FIGLU (formiminoglutamic acid), which indicates a functional need for more folate, was higher.[27]

Signs and symptoms of folate deficiency include cleft palate, anemia, poor appetite, weakness, headaches, behavioral conditions, and depression. Folate deficiency can be caused by poor gut absorption, chronic diarrhea, and MTHFR genetic variations, and oral contraception. We know GI issues are common in autism. Additionally, the MTHFR C677T variant, which reduces the conversion of folate to the active form, is associated with the risk of ASD.[28] Another concern about folate deficiency in autism is cerebral folate deficiency (CFD), a condition where folate levels appear normal in the blood but there is not enough of the nutrient in the cerebral spinal fluid, so there's not enough getting to the brain. CFD can cause profound cognitive deficits, challenges with speech, seizures, low muscle tone, and autism symptoms. In one study, twenty-three out of twenty-five children with autism were found to have low folate in their cerebral spinal fluid but sufficient levels in their blood.[29] However, high-dose folinic acid increased their folate levels to normal. CFD affects individuals with autism more than the broader population and is suspected to play a causative role or aggravate symptoms in some people. Fortunately, integrative and functional medicine doctors can help test for and treat CFD.

Forms of Folate

There are several types of folate, but they are not all created equal.

Dietary folate from whole foods is a great form. Sources of dietary folate include leafy greens, certain vegetables, legumes, and liver. (Find more details on food sources in the appendix.) Folate is destroyed by cooking, so when possible, eat folate-rich foods raw or lightly cooked. In the gut, the body converts dietary folate into an absorbable form. From there, it can be further converted and utilized by the body.

Naturally folate-rich foods are not to be confused with folic acid–fortified foods. Folic acid is a synthetic form of folate made in a lab and added into processed grains and flours in the United States, Canada, and Australia. Folic acid needs to be converted to the active form of folate, methylfolate, with the help of several enzymes, including MTHFR.

Unmetabolized folic acid can cause a variety of problems. The body can process only 200 to 300 mg of folic acid a day, and excess folic acid can build up in the blood, which can lead to immune dysfunction and cancer tumor growth.[30] High folic acid triggers a negative feedback loop, and the body slows MTHFR and the production of methylfolate.[31] In fact, both low and high folic acid during pregnancy has been associated with autism.[32]

About 50 percent of people have a genetic variant (a single nucleotide polymorphism, SNP) in MTHFR that doesn't allow for the conversion of folate very efficiently. For these individuals, folic acid is not a good form. In a study of thirty-three couples with the MTHFR SNP who struggled with four years of infertility (most while trying high-dose folic acid), including two-thirds who had used reproductive assistance, the high-dose folic acid was substituted with an adequate amount of methylfolate.[33] The results were amazing! Thirteen couples conceived spontaneously, most others became pregnant with reproductive assistance, and only three couples did not conceive, illustrating how the form of folate is crucial in some people.

Folinic acid, one form of folate, can be converted to methylfolate more easily than folic acid. For those with MTHFR genetic variants, folinic acid conversion to methylfolate is not impaired.[34] Methylfolate (also known as 5-methyltetrahydrofolate or 5-MTHF) is the active form and does not require conversion. Look for a high-quality nutritional supplement with either methylfolate and/or folinic acid, rather than folic acid.

Folate Daily Requirements and Supplementation

The recommended dietary allowance (RDA) of folate is 150 to 400 mcg per day, and the tolerable upper intake level is 300 to 600 mcg per day. Taking a supplement with RDA levels of folate is recommended for most individuals. However, for individuals with CFD, high-dose folinic acid (above 5,000 mcg) has been prescribed by doctors with success. Work with your doctor if you suspect high-dose folinic acid may be necessary.

In a study of nutraceuticals for ASD, high-dose and "moderate-dose" folinic acid were reported by parents to be beneficial for their children with autism. Although most people do not need high-dose folinic acid, for those that did in this study, 33 percent had improvements in cognition and 29 percent had improvements in attention. Language/communication improved in 20 and 24 percent of those taking moderate- and high-dose folinic acid, respectively.[35]

Vitamin B$_{12}$

Vitamin B$_{12}$ is an important nutrient for methylation. Vitamin B$_{12}$ is also essential for the nervous system because it is involved with the myelin sheath, the insulation around the nerves. It is needed for red blood cell production and involved with energy metabolism.

Meta-analysis research shows that methyl B$_{12}$ (methylcobalamin) for ASD increases methylation, transsulfuration, and glutathione, which improve language, hyperactivity, sleep, GI symptoms, tantrums, stereotypical autism behaviors, and more.[36]

Vitamin B_{12} deficiency can cause pernicious anemia, fatigue, depression, and poor growth in children. Severe B_{12} deficiency causes neuropathy, including numbness, tingling, poor balance and gait, and dementia. And because this neuropathy can be permanent, it is crucial to get enough B_{12}. Without sufficient recycling of homocysteine with B_{12}, homocysteine levels can build up, causing inflammation. A swollen, painful, red, fissured, and/or raw tongue is a common sign of vitamin B_{12} deficiency.

Vitamin B_{12} deficiency can be caused by a vegan or vegetarian diet. Vitamin B_{12} is produced by animals, so animal foods are the main source of it in our diets. Plant-based sources are few, and most (such as fermented foods, seaweed, and yeast) have limited bioavailability. (See the appendix for more on food-based sources.) For individuals who don't consume enough vitamin B_{12} or need more because of bioindividual factors, supplementation is required. Children with autism have been found to consume less B_{12} than neurotypically developing children.[37]

Additionally, vitamin B_{12} requires hydrochloric acid to be released during digestion. Therefore, proton pump inhibitors, low hydrochloric acid, and inflammatory bowel conditions or intestinal inflammation (both common in ASD) can cause vitamin B_{12} deficiency.

Vitamin B_{12} Daily Requirements and Supplementation

The RDA of vitamin B_{12} is 0.9 to 2.4 mcg per day. A tolerable upper limit has not been determined, as toxicity has not been found at higher doses. With oral supplementation, only a small amount is absorbed. B_{12} can be administered orally, sublingually, through injection, and through nasal spray.

Methyl B_{12} (methylcobalamin) is preferred over cyanocobalamin, since it contains a methyl group and is the active form.

In the parental survey of nutraceuticals for autism, vitamin B_{12} was reported to be beneficial. The survey study found that injections did perform better than oral supplements; however, whether it is worthwhile or the best for your child is something you should ask your physician. For vitamin B_{12} injections, 30 percent found improvement with language/communication, 28 percent with cognition, and 20 percent had improvements in attention. Among those taking vitamin B_{12} orally, 25 percent had improvements in cognition and 18 percent in language/communication.[38]

Vitamin B_6

Vitamin B_6 is another important nutrient in autism and for our overall health. Vitamin B_6 is important in the production of neurotransmitters, such as serotonin, dopamine, and GABA. It is a cofactor in over one hundred enzymes, including those for amino acid, fat, and glucose metabolism, which makes it very important for our health. To work, it requires magnesium intake as well.

Frank deficiency is not very common, but inadequate B_6 levels can lead to anxiety, depression, and other symptoms. Pyroluria is a condition where B_6 and zinc get bound up, rendering them ineffective (more on this in step 12). It is common in those with autism, as well as those with anxiety and depression. Deficiency of B_6 results in inflammation, redness, and pain of the tongue, as well as inflammation on the corners of the mouth.

Deficiency may be due to insufficient dietary intake; nuts, seeds, grains, animal protein, fish, and certain vegetables can supply B_6. But it can also be caused by poor digestion and absorption, as well as chronic stress and oxidative stress, which can deplete B_6. Hopefully these aren't factors for most children, but alcohol, cigarette smoke, and caffeine can deplete vitamin B_6, and oral contraceptives can, too.

Vitamin B_6 Daily Requirements and Supplementation

The RDA of B_6 is only 0.5 to 1.9 mg per day, which can be fairly easily obtained through food (see the appendix). However, many individuals with ASD need much higher levels that require supplementation. The tolerable upper intake is 12.5 mg for adults and lower for children, although higher levels are often used in practice. A study of a multivitamin/mineral formula in ASD included 40 mg of B_6, and it helped raise B_6 levels significantly.[39] Very high levels (500 mg daily) have been shown to cause neurological problems in adults, so it's important not to go over the doctor-recommended limit.

Pyridoxine, a common form of B_6, is converted to the active form pyridoxal-5'-phosphate (P5P or PLP). Because P5P is the active form, it is more common in high-quality supplements, recommended more often, and appears to be more beneficial, although reports from caregivers reported overall benefit to be similar. Regardless of the form, Vitamin B_6 was found to be beneficial for people with autism, and 20 to 25 percent found it improved their child's anxiety.[40]

Calcium

Calcium is an essential mineral for strong bones and healthy teeth. Calcium is an electrolyte and is important for our heart, muscle contraction, and nerve conduction. Calcium is also involved with blood clotting, enzyme activation, and cell membrane permeability. Adolescence, when children are growing significantly, is an important time to ensure enough calcium for growth and strong bones for adulthood.

Calcium is an important nutrient needed for individuals with autism, as they can often be deficient with or without a dairy-free diet (as I recommend for all in step 5).[41] In children, calcium deficiency can cause stunted growth, muscle cramps or spasms, and a pins-and-needles sensation in their hands and feet or mouth. In some cases, calcium deficiency can even be involved with seizures. Calcium deficiency can also cause osteoporosis.

Calcium deficiency can be caused by gut inflammation. Calcium also requires proper vitamin D levels for absorption. So, vitamin D deficiency can contribute to a deficit in calcium. The body will then take calcium from the bones to meet daily essential needs. Magnesium and calcium compete for absorption, so excess magnesium can lead to calcium deficiency. Magnesium and calcium are both important but need to be in balance.

Calcium Daily Requirements and Supplementation

The adequate daily intake of calcium is as follows: 500 mg for children three and under; 800 mg for children four to eight years old; and 1,300 mg for children nine to eighteen years of age. This can be attained from food and/or supplementation; a multivitamin/mineral supplement with only moderate levels of calcium (not full daily requirement) has been shown to improve calcium levels.[42]

There are various forms of calcium. My preference is calcium citrate. My least favorite choice is calcium carbonate, as the acid buffering effect in the stomach reduces calcium absorption.

The ratio of calcium to magnesium is typically 2:1. For example, 800 mg of calcium to 400 mg of magnesium.

Magnesium

Magnesium is a crucial mineral and cofactor in over three hundred enzyme reactions, including metabolism of carbohydrates and fats and energy production in all cells. Magnesium is an electrolyte involved with nerve impulses, muscle contractions, and heart function. Along with calcium, magnesium is an important building block of strong bones and teeth. It is needed in the pathway that creates glutathione and leads to sulfation. Magnesium can be helpful for muscle relaxation, stress and anxiety, and asthma.

Because magnesium can loosen stool, it is helpful for constipation. Caregivers reported 71 percent of individuals using magnesium citrate found that it helped with constipation.[43]

Signs and symptoms of magnesium deficiency include fatigue, poor appetite, muscle cramps, anxiety, rapid heart rate, speech impairment, hyperactivity, and failure to thrive. Magnesium deficiency is associated with insulin resistance and obesity in children.[44] It's also linked to certain types of seizures, and magnesium supplementation may be beneficial in children with autism who have seizures.[45]

Magnesium deficiency can be caused by inflammation in the intestinal tract, poor digestion, malabsorption, and vomiting. Deficiency can also be caused by kidney problems, diuretics, and antacids, as well as low intake of magnesium and B_6. Vitamin B_6 is important for the absorption of magnesium and uptake by the cells.

Magnesium Daily Requirements and Supplementation

The RDA of magnesium is 80 to 130 mg per day for children one to eight years old and 240 to 410 mg for children nine to eighteen years old. Too much magnesium will cause diarrhea; however, on the beneficial side, the right amount can help with constipation. As with all nutrients, kids can get magnesium from food and/or supplements. Nuts, seeds, legumes, and grains are good sources.

Zinc

Zinc is a mineral and antioxidant found in shellfish, meat, nuts, and seeds. It is essential for the immune system, healing, cell growth and repair, gene expression, vision, language, heavy metal detoxification, and energy metabolism. It is also important for our sense of smell and taste. Zinc has been found to help with childhood diarrhea.

Zinc deficiency has been found in children with autism,[46] and zinc levels have been associated with the severity of autism.[47] Zinc supplementation can improve ASD symptoms.[48] In a cross-sectional study of 203 children, picky eaters had significantly lower levels of zinc and higher prevalence of zinc deficiency (along with slightly higher copper and lower iron) than children who weren't picky eaters. Those with zinc deficiency also had lower developmental and physical activity levels.[49]

Pica is a condition of eating nonfood items like dirt or batteries and is common in ASD.[50] In a study of children with pica, zinc levels were significantly lower, nearly half that of those with pica as those without.[51]

Zinc deficiency can cause poor appetite, loss of smell and altered taste perception, hair loss, impaired wound healing, poor immune function, and poor growth in children. In addition, white spots on nails (not related to injury) are also signs of zinc deficiency. Poor cognitive function, inattentiveness, and developmental delays are found with zinc deficiency.

Zinc absorption competes with copper, iron, and calcium, so excess amounts of these minerals and heavy metals can contribute to zinc deficiency. Poor intestinal function and inflammation, as well as kidney and liver disease, can contribute to zinc deficiency.

Zinc Daily Requirements and Supplementation

The RDA for zinc is 3 to 5 mg per day for children one to eight years old and 8 to 11 mg for individuals nine years and older. The tolerable upper intake level is 23 to 34 mg for individuals nine to eighteen years old and 40 mg for adults. However, some individuals may benefit from more than the upper limit, and this is where your child's physician and testing can help.

As we discussed in the section on vitamin B_6, pyroluria can lower zinc (and B_6) levels, increasing oxidative stress and neurological conditions such as autism and ADHD. In fact, research shows that nearly half of people with autism, ADHD, and learning disabilities have pyroluria and may benefit from higher amounts of zinc than other individuals.[52] Your child's physician can do zinc plasma testing to determine whether levels are adequate and what level of supplementation is appropriate.

Because zinc competes with absorption of certain minerals, it's best to take zinc supplementation at a different time than iron and calcium and to possibly avoid copper supplementation when zinc is low. Zinc is best taken with food to prevent nausea.

Additional Important Vitamins and Minerals

Let's discuss some other important nutrients.

Antioxidants: Vitamins A, C, and E, Selenium, and Zinc

The acronym ACESZ, which stands for vitamin A, vitamin C, vitamin E, selenium, and zinc, is a useful way to remember your antioxidants. As the name implies, they inhibit oxidation or oxidative stress (an underlying factor in ASD).

We've talked about zinc, but the other antioxidants are helpful to know, too.

Vitamin A is important for immune function. One study found children with ASD had significantly lower levels of vitamins A and D, and a combination of these deficiencies contributes to autism symptoms.[53] Vitamin A is made in humans and animals by converting carotenoids, mainly beta-carotene, to vitamin A. So, we can either consume vitamin A from animal foods or beta-carotene from orange plant foods. Vitamin A is fat soluble, so it can build up in the body and become toxic. Beta-carotene is water soluble and needs to be converted; while it does not have the same toxicity concerns, some individuals are not able to convert beta-carotene to vitamin A well.[54]

Vitamin C is important for our immune system and the formation of collagen for growth, repair, and healthy gums. It helps with the production of some neurotransmitters. Severe vitamin C deficiency causes a condition known as scurvy. A case report of seven children with autism and other developmental delays found that these children ate a diet without fruits, vegetables, or vitamin supplementation and developed scurvy. Vitamin C supplementation reversed the health implications.[55] (If your kid doesn't eat fruits and vegetables, this is good reason to supplement.)

Vitamin E protects our body fat and cell membranes. Because it is fat soluble, it's absorbed like fat, requiring good GI function. Vitamin E deficiency and toxicity are fairly rare, though vitamin E levels have been found to be significantly lower for children with ASD than neurotypical children.[56]

Selenium is a trace mineral and important for our immune function. It has anti-inflammatory properties and neuroprotective benefits. In ASD, lower selenium has been associated with higher mercury and lead levels, and selenium deficiency may increase the risk of higher heavy metal levels and neurotoxicity.[57] And in a mouse model of ASD, selenium supplementation improved autism-like symptoms and cognitive function.[58] Fortunately, one or two Brazil nuts a day or supplementation can help fulfill the need.

Vitamin D

Vitamin D is a hormone created by our bodies from exposure to sunlight, so it is technically not a true vitamin. It's vital for the immune system and healthy bones. It helps ensure calcium gets absorbed and deposited into our bones and teeth. It helps reduce inflammation and produce insulin. Children with autism have lower vitamin D levels than their siblings without ASD, and vitamin D supplementation has been found to improve autism symptoms.[59]

Animals also make vitamin D, so some animal foods contain it. Other foods are fortified with it. It's challenging to get enough vitamin D from food and sunlight in most regions, so supplementation is often beneficial. Like vitamin A, vitamin D is fat soluble and can build up in the body and become toxic, so it's important to work with your physician to monitor levels.

Choline and Betaine

Choline and betaine are important as part of DNA methylation for gene expression.[60] Betaine is formed from choline. Choline is an important source of methyl groups, and as we discussed earlier, part of a secondary pathway involved with the methionine cycle (see graphic on page 19) that can be used when methylfolate is low. Choline is found in egg yolks, and betaine is high in beets. Please note that TMG is a form of betaine, but the supplement betaine HCl is something very different than we are talking about here.

Iodine

Iodine is very important for thyroid function. Iodine deficiency can cause symptoms of lethargy, reduced growth, and intellectual disability. It's important to get iodine from the diet, iodized salt, or supplementation.

Lithium

Lithium is a mineral that has important uses for the body. Lithium supports mood, cognitive function, metabolic needs, anti-inflammatory functions, cardiovascular health, and musculoskeletal needs.[61] Normally, it is found in our food and water. Lithium levels in children with autism were significantly less than neurotypical children.[62] Anxiety, aggression, and irritability were the three symptoms that improved most with low-dose lithium nutritional supplementation in individuals with ASD.[63]

When people think of lithium, they usually think of the psychiatric medication, but that is very high dose—not what we'd get on a day-to-day basis naturally or in a basic multivitamin. Low-dose lithium found in most multivitamin/mineral formulas helps meet our basic nutritional needs.

READY FOR THE NEXT STEP?

I recommend implementing one new supplement at a time before moving to the next, and going low and slow while introducing them. So it usually takes about a month to implement the main three: a multivitamin/mineral, essential fatty acid, and digestive enzymes. It can take a while to see the benefits from some nutrients, so you may not see a lot before you proceed; some see improvements in attention, cognition, irritability, anxiety, social interaction, and/or digestion. As ever, write down any improvements you've seen, symptoms/experiences you've had, and which nutrients they're from. If you are not seeing negative symptoms, it's likely a good time to progress to the next step.

If you are seeing negative symptoms, consider reducing the amount and going more slowly, stopping the supplement, and/or speaking with your physician. You *can* move forward to the next steps even if you can't implement the supplements right now.

If there are other individual nutrients you want to add from this step, you might stay here longer or do them while you are working on step 4 or step 12.

STEP 4

Address Picky Eating

After reading step 2, you may have been thinking, "How am I going to get my picky eater to eat *that*?" I have two responses. First, *you are not alone*. Picky eating is very common in children with autism.

How common? One study found 70 percent of children with autism had atypical eating patterns, compared to 13 percent of children with other disorders and only 4.8 percent of neurotypical children. In that study, 92 percent of children with autism preferred food like grain products and/or chicken (usually chicken nuggets). Does this sound familiar? I bet it might. What's more, a quarter of the children with autism had three or more atypical eating behaviors, whereas no other groups of children had that many restrictive habits. And two behaviors, pica (eating nonfood items) and pocketing food (putting food in their cheek and not swallowing it), were found only in the autism group. In fact, the researchers believed they could use these specific eating patterns as an early sign of ASD.[1]

However, and this brings me to my second point, *picky eating can be improved*. In my program, 82 percent of picky eaters improved with the strategies I recommend. And all the parents said they gained confidence to feed their child nutritiously. So there's hope! And with the right knowledge and some creativity, you can help your picky eater appreciate a broader range of foods.

WHY ADDRESSING PICKY EATING IS IMPORTANT

When it feels like some days there are so many battles to fight, you might be asking, "Why not just let them eat what they like?"

First and foremost, picky eating means limited food choices and decreased nutritional intake. This can be serious—and here are some research notes to underscore just how much. One review analyzed case reports of seventy-six children with autism who developed serious nutrient deficiencies from "self-imposed dietary restrictions." The most common deficiencies were vitamin C (almost 70 percent of the reports were about this), vitamin A, thiamine (vitamin B_1), vitamin B_{12}, and vitamin D.[2] One report detailed the case of a boy with autism who had only eaten French fries and potato chips from the ages of four through eight years old and developed severe vitamin A deficiency. This caused vision loss and night blindness. Sadly, even with vitamin A supplementation, the vision loss was irreversible.[3] Another paper described a fourteen-year-old boy who showed up at the emergency room with a swollen left leg and a fast heart rate. He had anxiety and refused to walk. Doctors discovered his diet was limited to chicken nuggets, macaroni and cheese, chocolate milk, junk food, soda, and water—no veggies or fruits (other than the occasional banana). He was diagnosed with anemia and scurvy. This severe deficiency in vitamin C required intense interventions and caused him emotional distress. Fortunately, he was able to reverse it.[4]

Most of the children referenced in the review had a body weight within normal range.[5] So we can't rely on a child being underweight as a sign of nutritional deficiency.

Another reason to address picky eating is its relation to autism behaviors and cognitive function. Of 67 percent of children with ASD found to have picky eating behaviors, these eating habits were associated with higher stereotyped autism behaviors, meaning repetitive or self-stimulatory behaviors.[6] And as mentioned before, children with autism whose diet was high in sugar and low in healthy foods had more challenges with memory.[7]

Finally, eating nonfood items (as in the condition pica, which we've discussed previously) can be very dangerous. One family I knew had to watch their child very closely because they would swallow small button batteries.

REASONS FOR PICKY EATING

Eating is a complex process. Feeding, chewing, and swallowing are a surprisingly complex set of actions that require physical and developmental abilities, attention to one's environment, posture, and many other factors. Challenges in any of these areas, as well as nutritional/biochemical reasons and sensory issues, can lead to picky eating.

People often think of picky eating as a dislike for foods. However, picky eating can also appear as an interest in only certain foods, in which all other foods are ignored or eliminated by default. Both can be challenging.

It's important to determine the causes behind your child's picky eating. This will allow to you seek out the best support and strategies.

Nutritional and Biochemical Reasons for Picky Eating

Nutritional deficiencies and biochemical factors can cause children to crave or avoid certain foods. The following are some of the main nutritional and biochemical reasons for picky eating:

- Gluten, casein, and soy form opiates that are addictive (more in step 5).
- Food sensitivities and intolerance, specific food compounds, and GI distress can cause cravings or aversions (more in steps 7 through 11).
- Sugar and carbohydrates cause cravings (addressed in step 1).
- Food additives like MSG and artificial additives can cause preference for processed foods (addressed in step 1).
- Microbiome influences eating behaviors (addressed in step 12).
- Nutrient deficiencies impact eating habits (addressed in step 3, again in step 12).

- Compounds that naturally occur in foods can cause cravings (more in steps 7 through 11).

Gluten, dairy, and soy can cause the formation of opioid compounds. These compounds are very addictive and can cause interest in consuming only those foods. Many picky eaters eat primarily pizza, milk, bread, chicken nuggets, crackers, cheese, and other wheat and dairy foods. I've found that once these proteins are removed (as we will do in step 5), many individuals with autism lose some or much of their picky eating. In our randomized controlled trial, a gluten-free, casein-free, soy-free (GFCFSF) diet even eliminated pica in an individual.

Sometimes, like gluten and dairy, food sensitivities can cause cravings (although through different brain-altering chemicals than opioids). Food sensitivities can cause inflammation, so people can become very picky and eat very few foods because they are afraid that everything they eat is going to cause reactions. Similarly, gastrointestinal pain and upset can cause children to significantly restrict most foods or cut out the foods that hurt. Identifying and eliminating food sensitivities or triggering foods can help create more balanced eating habits.

Sugar and carbohydrates can also be addictive. Sugar alters dopamine signaling[8] and carbohydrates increase serotonin;[9] these brain chemicals cause cravings that lead some kids to choose virtually only carbohydrates and sugar in their diet. Reducing sugar and refined carbohydrates in the diet can change eating habits in the long run by balancing neurotransmitters and hormones, which reduces the struggle of sugar cravings.

Food additives such as artificial flavors can stimulate taste in a way that other food products do not. (For instance, MSG is used specifically to make food taste better by stimulating the excitatory pathways in your brain.) Food companies spend millions of dollars getting the taste, look, and texture of food just right so ultra-processed food is more appealing to children than whole foods. Unfortunately, this can lead to children consuming only certain processed food products or brands. Eliminating these food additives, as addressed in step 1, can expand whole-food choices over time.

The microbes in our gut can influence our eating behaviors and cravings to influence their survival and growth.[10] I've seen this most in my nutrition practice with yeast overgrowth. *Candida* or yeast overgrowth is more common in children with autism.[11] Although we all have a small amount of *Candida*, when this yeast overgrows, it can cause gut inflammation and digestive problems and can negatively affect the brain and behavior. In fact, *Candida* overgrowth in the gut can cause auto-brewery syndrome, which creates a type of intoxication that can negatively affect the brain,[12] such as inappropriate laughter and balance problems. *Candida* feeds off sugar and causes extreme cravings for more sugar, so eating habits consist of high amounts of sugar and little else. Clients in my practice have very limited food variety until the yeast overgrowth was addressed by their physician. One of my clients only drank fruit juice and ate sausage before his *Candida* overgrowth was addressed. Afterward, his diet expanded.

Nutrient deficiencies can contribute to picky eating behaviors (including pica). Most notable is zinc deficiency, which can cause poor sense of smell, taste, and appetite. It can also cause food to taste unpleasant, loss of the perception of salty taste leading to the oversalting of food, and even aversion to meat.[13] Iron deficiency can also lead to picky eating. Fortunately, zinc and multivitamin/mineral supplementation can improve picky eating—so you may have already noticed a difference after step 3.

Natural food compounds (glutamate, salicylates) can also contribute to cravings and food selectivity. It's hard to eat a well-balanced diet when a child eats so much of just a few foods. Therapeutic diets that avoid foods that cause cravings and reactions can be beneficial for picky eaters. These patterns will become clearer for you in part 2 of this program.

Sensory Reasons for Picky Eating

In addition to biochemical reasons, there are sensory contributors to picky eating. It is known that children with autism have sensory issues, especially when it comes to food. In fact, it is a common cause of food aversions. Smell and taste are important aspects of mealtime for picky eaters.[14] Visual and sound experiences are also sensory aspects that can help.

I find that texture is the primary sensory issue, and research backs this up: among children with ASD who had atypical eating behaviors, 46 percent were hypersensitive to the texture of their food.[15] Mushy vegetables, lumpy mashed potatoes, wet and slimy cut fruit, and tough and chewy meat are some of the biggest offenders. Fortunately, texture is fairly easy to address. There are many ways to make vegetables crispy and crunchy and to alter food texture based on what a child likes. The goal is to figure out what they like and get creative with your options; more on this later in this step. The important thing is to think like your child when you're finding solutions for food texture. Regular yogurt is not the same texture as Greek yogurt, and fruit at the bottom is not the same as when it's premixed. Pudding is not the same texture as applesauce or mashed potatoes. While these are all soft foods, their texture is different. So try to make detailed observations and look for innovative solutions.

Other Factors and Additional Professional Support

If you need additional support for your child's food aversions and selectivity, you have options. Feeding therapy can be very beneficial. Parent and child have a different dynamic than therapist and child, and feeding therapists have additional knowledge and skills to help.

Additionally, parents can aid their children directly with some specific knowledge and training. In one approach where parents were trained on how to help their children with feeding issues, almost half of the children responded well and improved their picky eating. Kids whose parents did not participate in the training had no improvement.[16] After thirty-five years in the field, Kay A. Toomey, PhD, has created a successful approach called the SOS Approach to Feeding that combines developmental, physical, oral motor, posture, sensory, medical, and other factors. You may find her programs and trained practitioners to be very helpful.

Be aware that picky eating can be due to anxiety, trauma, or other psychological issues. Or a medical issue could be to blame. Some children have blockages or inflammation in their throat (or other medical issues) that can affect swallowing (or eating) certain foods. Seek help from a feeding therapist, occupational therapist, psychologist, or your child's doctor when necessary.

Once you've determined the biochemical, sensory, and/or other factors underlying your child's picky eating, you can address any addictive factors with a therapeutic diet (as you already began and will continue in other steps) and find creative ways to prepare healthy food your child will love. We'll talk about those ideas for the rest of this step.

KID-FRIENDLY VEGETABLES AND SOLVING FOR TEXTURE

It's easy to become discouraged after a child rejects food time and time again. But there are hundreds of vegetables in the world and many more ways to cook them. We need to think outside the box and go beyond the same two or three vegetables many of us serve every day. Here is a list of forty common vegetables, which can be helpful to check out when you get stuck in a rut:

- Artichokes
- Arugula
- Asparagus
- Beets
- Bell peppers
- Bok choy
- Broccoli
- Broccoli sprouts
- Brussels sprouts
- Butternut squash
- Cabbage
- Carrots
- Cauliflower
- Collard greens
- Cucumbers
- Fennel
- Green beans
- Japanese sweet potatoes
- Jicama
- Kabocha squash
- Kale
- Leeks
- Lettuce, head
- Lettuce, iceberg

- Okra
- Onions
- Parsnips
- Peas
- Potatoes
- Radishes
- Rutabagas
- Shishito peppers
- Snap peas
- Snow peas
- Spaghetti squash
- Sweet potatoes
- Turnips
- Yellow summer squash
- Yucca root
- Zucchini

Next, begin thinking of texture and how you can prepare these vegetables in a way your child will love. Maybe your child likes crunchy vegetables, such as raw carrot sticks. Maybe they like crispy vegetables, such as chips and fries. Maybe they like their vegetables pureed in smoothies. (One of my clients liked pancakes with a sauce on top, so his mom pureed meat and vegetables to make into a pancake and sauce, and he was happy as can be with it—though it might not be a favorite menu item for the rest of the family.)

Here are some examples of ways to prepare vegetables and create a texture they like:

- Salads (raw)
- Smoothies
- Juices
- Fries
- Chips, baked
- Chips, dehydrated
- Chips, fried
- Roasted
- Added to meatballs, sauce, etc.
- Fun—visually or with dip
- Fermented
- Pickled
- Sprouted
- Boiled or simmered
- Steamed
- Sauteed
- Pureed
- Air fried
- Spiralized into noodles
- Riced
- With bacon

If you get stuck, mix and match a veggie from the first list with a prep method from the second. Of course, not all combos will work, but search online for recipes and you might just be surprised!

Ten Favorite Kid-Friendly Vegetable Ideas

The following are my and my clients' ten favorites vegetable ideas, all of which appear in the recipe section of this book.

1. Air-Fried Popcorn Cauliflower
2. Blueberry Cauliflower Smoothie
3. Brussels Sprout Chips
4. Butternut Squash Hash Browns
5. Carrot Chips
6. Cauliflower Tortillas
7. Green Smoothie
8. Ground Beef Stuffed Zucchini (Zucchin-izza)
9. Kale Chips
10. Rutabaga Fries

INTRODUCING NEW FOODS

To keep this easy at first, come up with a list of just three new foods to try. Choose foods you can introduce one at a time. In other words, don't make a casserole or mixed vegetable dish. Start with a side dish or something where the vegetable is on its own.

Think of multiple ways to prepare. For example, root vegetables are good raw and crunchy. They also make great chips and fries.

Take baby steps. If you know your child likes raw carrots, consider a small change like carrot chips. Then maybe try carrot fries. Or if you are afraid to "ruin" a food they love, try a similar food, such as rutabaga chips or fries, instead.

GROW A FAMILY GARDEN

Gardening is another way to get children to eat more fruits and vegetables. Many schools today include gardening programs, and research shows they help improve fruit and vegetable consumption and health outcomes, including improved body mass index, increased fiber intake, and increased vitamin A and C consumption.[17]

Growing food helps children become more familiar with vegetables and excited to try them. It's fun for children to watch the plants grow and water them. It makes kids more comfortable with vegetables and interested to try them. Some of our Nourishing Hope families have said that their children eat vegetables like green beans and snap peas straight out of the garden. Others like to harvest produce like tomatoes, strawberries, and peppers.

My daughter ate zucchini for the first time after growing it in our garden—and I think that experience is why she still likes zucchini today. After harvesting it, she helped me create a recipe that she called Zucchinizza. It's a pizza-like recipe that uses a hollowed-out zucchini "boat" as the pizza bottom.

If you have the space, consider growing a garden or starting a few veggies in pots on a porch or patio. There are also indoor growing setups you can buy. Or see if there's a community garden nearby that you can use.

READY FOR THE NEXT STEP?

You can spend as much or as little time on this step as you'd like and move forward at your own pace. If you feel you want more time building up your repertoire of foods, hang out here as long as you want. But remember that picky eating can also be due, at least in part, to gluten, casein, and soy or other intolerances and food compounds, which we will address in later steps. As you proceed, write down any experiences you've had or tips you want to try out as you move forward.

STEP 5

Eliminate Gluten, Casein, and Soy

If you've heard of any special diet for autism, it's likely the gluten-free and casein-free (GFCF) diet. It's the most common therapeutic diet in autism, and there are thousands of parents sharing their experiences and stories online.

Gluten is a protein found in wheat, rye, barley, spelt, kamut, triticale, and conventional oats. Technically, the *actual* component of gluten that causes reactions in celiac disease and many other conditions is called gliadin. Casein is a protein found in animal milk and dairy products made from it. Another food that can be problematic is soy. Gluten, casein, and soy can cause some similar reactions, so in this program, we will remove them together: the gluten-free, casein-free, soy-free (GFCFSF) diet.

Many parents are told erroneously that if you don't do this diet when they are young, then it's too late. I have always disagreed with this because of what I have seen in my practice and heard from families. There is no magic window of time during which you must intervene. Also, don't believe the false narrative that the diet has no science behind it. In this chapter, we'll cover the research that supports a GFCFSF diet and how to implement it.

Nourishing Hope Stories

"Our son, Adam, is thirty-six years old. It wasn't until he was twenty-nine that I helped him with diet. I did a 'test' when he was eleven. For five days I made sure no gluten was eaten. However, the last day I ran out of gluten-free foods and handed him a waffle [containing gluten], and within ten minutes, he was screaming. I realized that all week there had been no yelling, until after he consumed the waffle. I knew gluten-free was the way to go. But it took me a while to understand the diet was not a once-a-week occurrence but 100 percent adoption.

"It was the constant stomach pain after eating that I wanted to address. And feeling better physically did seem to improve his behavior. He has learned that certain foods do not agree with him and make him feel bad, and he tries to stay on the diet.

"I found Julie's work, and when he was twenty-nine, we implemented a GFCFSF, sugar-free, non-GMO, mostly organic, and no processed foods diet. He also has no soda, alcohol, or energy drinks. He has found through trial and error that even the occasional soda and/or gluten ingestion can cause some behavioral event, usually irritability or anger.

"I think it's important to know that he, himself, believes following the diet has made a big improvement in how he feels and in his behavior, through his own experience! I believe it gives our son confidence to know that diet is something he can control and use to help himself feel better. Following the diet as a family helped us all feel better, and we all continue on the diet." —*Mom of a thirty-six-year-old with autism* ▪

COMMON SYMPTOMS OF GLUTEN
AND CASEIN INTOLERANCE

A common misconception is that if a child doesn't have digestive symptoms, then they don't have any food sensitivities or need for a special diet.

While people with food sensitivities (and autism) often do have gastro-intestinal symptoms, this is not always the case. Digestive symptoms can also be caused by other food intolerances. Two telltale symptoms of gluten and casein intolerance are high pain tolerance and gluten and dairy cravings. Congestion is also very common, particularly with dairy intolerance. The following is a long list of symptoms to be alert for. Note: I still suggest a gluten-free and casein-free diet even when a client does not have GI symptoms. Many people improve on a special diet for different reasons. While I remove soy if I suspect gluten and casein intolerance, the following list has been honed for gluten and casein, in particular:

- ❏ Abdominal pain
- ❏ Bloating/Gas
- ❏ Cognitive difficulties
- ❏ Fatigue
- ❏ Cravings for gluten and dairy
- ❏ Diarrhea
- ❏ Ear infections (especially with dairy/casein)
- ❏ Constipation (especially with dairy/casein)
- ❏ Headache
- ❏ High pain tolerance
- ❏ Stuffy or running nose/mucous (especially with dairy/casein)

- ❏ Inattentiveness
- ❏ Irritability
- ❏ Language challenges
- ❏ Nausea
- ❏ Sensory sensitivity
- ❏ Hyperactivity
- ❏ Skin rash, redness, eczema, hives
- ❏ Stimming (self-stimulatory behavior)/Repetitive behaviors
- ❏ Stomachache
- ❏ Social interaction challenges

THE SCIENCE OF GLUTEN, CASEIN, AND SOY IN AUTISM

Gluten, casein, and soy can negatively affect children with autism. Let's dive into the science!

Opioids from Gluten, Casein, and Soy

Opioids are substances, like morphine, that fit in the opioid receptors in the brain, nervous system, and all over the body, making us insensitive to pain and triggering constipation, irritability, inattentiveness, foggy thinking, and opioid addiction. While most of us are familiar with pharmaceutical-made opioids, such as medications and illicit drugs, opioids can also be formed in the body from food proteins, and they fit in the same receptors. These morphine-like compounds from outside the body are called exorphins. When gluten (or gliadin) is not broken down, it forms gluteomorphin (also known as gliadorphin). Casein can form casomorphin. Soy can also form opioids, though there is no fancy name for them.[1]

This opiate effect from these exorphins can directly affect the brain and cause symptoms similar to morphine. Their addictive effect often causes intense food cravings for wheat and dairy foods that show up like strong preferences for milk, cheese, bread, pizza, and ice cream. It's true almost all children like these foods, but this strong craving and the symptoms are very different.

I have heard countless stories of how wheat or dairy created opioid effects in my clients with autism. A mother once told me how her daughter would wake up some nights and go to the refrigerator, eat a block of cheese, and go back to bed. Because she heard her daughter in the kitchen, she got up to tend to her and found her in a bit of a trance-like state, staring off, and eating frantically—as if satisfying an addiction. The frenzied quality she had while eating, then the relaxed nature she had afterward, made us strongly suspect this was an opiate reaction: She was likely addicted to the casomorphin from dairy, and once the exorphins from dinner wore off, she had to get up and eat cheese before she could fall back asleep. Tellingly, she didn't have any of those night eating episodes after going GFCF.

To understand this, let's look at how opioids form from food. In a properly functioning body, when a gluten-, casein-, and/or soy-containing food is consumed, it is broken down into amino acids, absorbed through the intestinal tract, and used for growth, repair, and daily function. These proteins are broken down by enzymes, most notably the DPP-IV enzyme (research has found lower DPP-IV activity in kids with ASD).[2]

When these foods are not properly digested, they are not broken down into amino acids. Instead, they remain partial protein chains called peptides. And the condition known as leaky gut (more on that soon) allows these peptides to leak into the bloodstream and eventually reach our opioid receptors, causing opioid activity, inflammation, and immune reaction.

These exorphins are found in people with autism. In a study of 335 children, researchers found significantly higher levels of opioids from gluten and casein in the urine of the children with autism compared to controls. Those with late onset regressive autism had higher levels than those with early onset autism.[3] One paper suggested that the gluten and casein exorphins are possible causative factors in autism and the GFCF diet could be a treatment option.[4]

While there is a bit of controversy on whether opioids are found in those with autism since there are some inconsistent results, the way the urine specimen is frozen and processed during testing affects whether the opioids remain intact or deteriorate.[5] I suspect this is the reason for the discrepancy.

Parents will often say, "Wheat and dairy are *all* that my child eats. There's no way we can do a GFCF diet." This is usually a big clue for me that wheat and dairy are likely a problem. After all, opiates are very addictive. This is true for all types, even those caused by food. When I hear of this eating behavior in children, my first thought is that gluten and casein opioids probably play a big role in their limited diet, and they likely have an intolerance. So, while it may seem challenging, or even impossible, removing gluten and dairy may be just what they need.

Zonulin and Leaky Gut

Zonulin is a protein that regulates the permeability of the gut, and too much zonulin contributes to increased intestinal permeability (i.e., leaky gut). Zonulin has also been implicated in intestinal diseases, autoimmune disorders, neuroinflammation, cancer, and metabolic issues.[6]

How is this related to gluten and dairy? Gluten and casein increase zonulin levels and intestinal permeability in autism.[7] This leaky gut can also have negative effects on the microbiome. To add more fuel to the fire, microbial dysbiosis can trigger the release of zonulin, intensifying leaky gut.[8]

Zonulin levels are high in those with autism and leaky gut contributes to the development of autism. In a study of thirty-two children with autism, zonulin levels were significantly higher than those of the control group of healthy children without ASD. This study found that the higher the zonulin level, the more severe the autism. Researchers suspect that the severity of autism (and GI symptoms) are connected to leaky gut.[9]

Gluten, Casein, Soy, and Inflammation

Food sensitivities typically make our bodies release antibodies that cause inflammation within the gut or systemically, affecting the body and brain. Gluten and casein, and even soy, are some of these foods that can cause inflammation in autism.

In a study, gluten antibodies were significantly higher in children with autism on a regular diet compared to children without autism. Casein antibodies were also higher in the ASD group, although not statistically significantly. This study also confirmed leaky gut in ASD.[10]

In another study, researchers from New Jersey Medical School Department of Pediatrics took 143 children, ranging from one to ten years old, and divided the participants into four groups: autism with GI symptoms, autism without GI symptoms, children without autism but with nonallergy food hypersensitivity, and controls, to study the association of inflammatory reactions to foods and GI symptoms in autism. Children with ASD (with and without GI symptoms) had higher levels of two inflammatory cytokines in response to whole cow milk protein and some of its components. Soy was also studied, and while there was not a statistically significant increase, some children (seven of seventy-five kids with ASD and GI symptoms) had levels of inflammatory cytokines seemingly linked to soy.[11]

In another study, the same team found elevated inflammatory markers (IFN-gamma and TNF-alpha) for all three proteins—gluten, casein, and soy—in the children with autism.[12]

Meanwhile, in a study out of the University of Florida, 87 percent of individuals with autism had high IgG antibodies (an immune system response that can cause inflammation) to gliadin (i.e., gluten), and 90 percent had high levels of IgG antibodies to casein.[13]

And food allergies and sensitivities can trigger mast cells to release histamine, which causes inflammation, and researchers believe may even be a causative factor in autism.[14]

Lactase Deficiency, Cerebral Folate Deficiency, and Dairy

There are other issues with dairy. For one, kids with autism often lack lactase, the digestive enzyme needed to break down lactose.[15] In fact, 58 percent of children with autism five years old and younger, and 65 percent of those above five, are deficient in lactase.[16] This causes lactose intolerance and symptoms of diarrhea, flatulence, gastrointestinal pain, and nausea. And as we've discussed many times, digestive disturbances can negatively impact the brain in ASD.

For another, cerebral folate deficiency (CFD, introduced in step 3) may make some individuals with autism unable to tolerate dairy. The most common cause of this condition is autoantibodies binding to or blocking folate receptors. The folate receptor is needed to transport folate from the bloodstream into the brain. When this is not working, low levels of folate are found in the brain. Research shows that 75 percent of children with ASD had folate receptor autoantibodies.[17]

How is dairy involved? Folate-binding proteins in milk cross-react with folate receptors. This cross-reaction increases folate receptor autoantibodies and decreases folate in the brain. Fortunately, eliminating dairy consumption decreases folate receptor autoantibodies in those with CFD.[18]

Other Concerns with Soy

There are other possible neurological symptoms associated with soy, and some are quite serious. Infants that developed autism who were fed soy formula had significantly higher rates of seizures—two to four times higher.[19] Some research suggests that high consumption of soy during an infant's development can negatively affect the brain, causing excitability and neuron damage,[20] which may cause seizures, among other problems.

THE SCIENCE ON GFCFSF

Given the many issues associated with gluten, casein, and soy for kids with autism, a GFCFSF diet seems like a natural solution. Happily, research supports this logical conclusion.

In a randomized controlled trial, children implemented either a gluten-free and casein-free (GFCF) diet or regular diet (as a control) and were followed for twenty-four months. At twelve months, there was a statistically significant improvement in communication, social interaction, inattentiveness, and hyperactivity in the group of children with autism on a GFCF diet.[21]

One study found high IgG antibody levels to gluten and casein in individuals with autism (and those with schizophrenia), and showed that 81 percent of the children with autism improved with a GFCF diet. In only one to three months on the diet, they had significant improvement in behaviors including hyperactivity, stereotypical behaviors, speech, eye contact, self-injury, panic attacks, and social interaction.[22]

In a randomized controlled trial, children with autism who adopted a gluten-free diet had significantly improved gastrointestinal and behavioral symptoms compared to before starting the diet; the control group did not have any significant differences.[23]

In our randomized, controlled trial, a GFCFSF diet (with other interventions) led to significant improvement in nonverbal IQ, development, and many other autism and physical symptoms. Parents said the healthy GFCFSF diet was one of the three most helpful interventions for their children.[24] In our survey study of therapeutic diets, the GFCF diet was beneficial with very low adverse effects: 31 percent had improvement in attention, 29 percent in cognition, 25 percent in language, and 22 percent in hyperactivity. There are even more improvements including diarrhea, constipation, aggression, irritability, health, stimming, sensory sensitivity, anxiety, and more.[25]

These findings are consistent with the improvements I see in my practice from this diet. One of the biggest areas of improvement is in language. One three-year-old boy went from zero words to two hundred words in three months after the GFCF diet. Some begin to have back-and-forth conversations for the first time. It's very exciting!

Nourishing Hope Stories

"We had already started organic/non-GMO diet and supplements before the series. We immediately started a gluten-free diet the first week and [progressed to] a GFCFSF, no refined sugar, no artificial ingredients or dyes diet. We stuck to that diet throughout. She is more cognizant, more affectionate, and more focused, has few digestive issues, and is happy, social, and curious. The biggest breakthrough was introducing chicken to her diet for the first time, but the next step is not to be hiding it. We have tried for more than twenty years to figure out how to counteract sensory issues and limited food intake as well as other ASD behaviors. We felt we progressed notably during this wonderful, educational series and many of our persistent questions were answered for the first time." —Mom of a twenty-two-year-old with autism ■

DOES THE GFCF DIET CAUSE NUTRIENT DEFICIENCIES?

Many parents are concerned that the GFCF will lead to nutrient deficiencies, particularly in calcium. I don't believe the science supports this.

As we discussed in step 3, children with autism on a GFCF diet *have* been found to be deficient in calcium, having a lower intake of calcium than those not on a GFCF diet.[26] However, those on the GFCF diet had higher levels of many other important foods and nutrients including vegetables, fiber, legumes, magnesium, iron, and polyunsaturated fatty acids. Additionally, children with autism are also deficient in calcium on a regular diet that includes dairy.[27] In other words, children with autism are more likely to be deficient in calcium, but this is true with or without dairy.

Furthermore, when the gut is inflamed by dairy (or for any reason), calcium absorption is inhibited.[28] So, when someone is sensitive to dairy, consuming dairy won't do much to help them meet their calcium needs.

While dairy does contain calcium, this does not mean that dairy is the best answer to meet calcium needs. There are better options—remember, the appendix has a list of calcium-rich (dairy-free!) foods. And supplementation with only 100 to 200 mg of calcium (a fraction of the recommended daily intake, available in some multivitamin/mineral formulas) can increase calcium levels;[29] revisit step 3 for more guidance.

As far as gluten is concerned, there are no nutrients found in gluten-containing grains that someone could not easily find in other grains or foods. In fact, similar to dairy, the more inflamed the gut is by gluten, the fewer nutrients will be absorbed.

Given the wonderful results families see with this diet, and the many better ways to meet kids' nutrient needs, I believe the recommendation should be to encourage a *healthy* GFCFSF diet with added calcium and nutrition supplementation as needed.

LAB TESTING FOR GLUTEN, CASEIN, AND SOY INTOLERANCE

There are several ways to test for gluten, casein, and soy intolerance. While testing can give you quantitative data, it's not always certain to yield accurate results. Since there are so many ways someone can react, if you don't test *all* the different ways, you might miss a positive result. Test methods include:

- IgG food sensitivity testing
- Cellular mediated response testing
- IgA antibody testing
- Urinary opioid testing (for gluten and casein only)

For antibody and opioid testing, a child needs to be consuming the foods to get a positive result when there is a true reaction. So, if you want to do testing, it's important to do it before your child starts the diet.

There are tests for celiac gluten reactions as well (transglutaminase IgA antibody testing; HLA-DQ2 and HLA-DQ8 genetic tests). Not everyone who is gluten intolerant has celiac disease, so these tests alone won't be the best way to determine a gluten reaction. However, they are very good if you want to know if your child's gluten intolerance is celiac related.

While it's not quantitative, a dietary trial is a good way to assess tolerance because it provides feedback on how the individual is responding when the foods are removed.

HOW TO DETERMINE WHETHER THE GFCFSF DIET IS RIGHT FOR YOUR CHILD

I include the GFCFSF diet among the Nourishing Hope Essentials (rather than with other therapeutic diets in BioIndividual Nutrition) because it has a wealth of research to support it, virtually all my clients benefit from it, and I encourage all families to try it. The GFCFSF diet is also a foundation of many other diets. However, since it does restrict some foods, you always want to determine whether it's right for your child and family.

Check the symptoms list on page 112 and consider whether any of these sound like what your child experiences. You might also consider laboratory testing to confirm a reaction.

Everything Here Is Gluten-Free, Casein-Free, and Soy-Free

Some of the diets in the BioIndividual Nutrition part of the program would technically allow gluten, dairy, and/or soy in their original formulations outside of Nourishing Hope. However, since I recommend GFCFSF for virtually everyone, I leave these foods off those diets' food lists.

IMPLEMENTING A GFCFSF DIET

The learning curve for the GFCFSF diet may be a bit steep, but it gets much easier once you and your child get familiar with the food choices available and what they like. Additionally, as your child feels better, you'll have more quality time and free time to do some cooking if you want. As one of my clients says, "I'd rather be cooking while he's happy than watching him struggle." And once you see the beneficial results for your child, you'll never look back. So, if you feel hesitant to try the diet or a bit overwhelmed, know that it's a common experience, but you can do it. Remember other Nourishing Hope families can help, too, so reach out and join our community. And here's a seven-part process to simplify implementation. It's flexible and customizable so that you can take your time to set your strategy, get confident and familiar with the diet, and *then* begin. You can find a link to our community and printable handouts for this process in the extra book resources at PersonalizedAutismNutritionPlan.com/extras.

1. Discover what to eat and not.
2. Identify what's already GFCFSF.
3. Begin creating a meal plan.
4. Choose foods to try next.
5. Refine the meal plan and prepare.
6. Begin the GFCFSF diet!
7. Write it down.

1. Discover What to Eat and Not

First, let's talk about what not to eat. Some of the foods eliminated on this diet are straightforward and obvious, such as breads, crackers, pancakes, cereal, and pasta made with wheat or gluten grains; milk, cheese, butter, and things made with them; and soy products like tofu. However, many processed foods use these components in ways you aren't expecting and cause the most accidental infractions (think potato chips, malt sweetener, and spice blends).

AVOID   Foods That Contain or May Contain Gluten

x	Wheat	x	Cookies
x	Rye	x	Pasta
x	Barley	x	Stuffing
x	Spelt	x	Couscous
x	Triticale	x	Breakfast cereals
x	Durum	x	Crackers
x	Einkorn	x	Candy
x	Farina	x	Snack bars
x	Farro	x	Malt sweetener
x	Graham	x	Malt vinegar
x	Bulgur	x	Brewer's yeast
x	Semolina	x	Soups
x	Oats (conventional)	x	Hot dogs and bologna
x	Bread	x	Sausage
x	Breadcrumbs	x	Salad dressing
x	Biscuits	x	Sauces
x	Pancakes	x	Soy sauce
x	Dumplings	x	"Flavorings"
x	Kamut	x	"Spices"
x	Sweet potato fries (flour coating)	x	Potato chips (in the manufacturing process)
x	French fries (cross-contamination from shared fryer)	x	Spice blends (e.g., chili powder, apple pie spice)

AVOID   Foods That Contain or May Contain Casein or Lactose

x	Butter	x	Canned fish
x	Buttermilk	x	Casein
x	Cheese	x	Caseinate
x	Cottage cheese	x	Chocolate
x	Cow milk	x	Sherbet
x	Cream	x	Lactose
x	Cream cheese	x	Meal replacement drinks
x	Frozen yogurt	x	Milk chocolate
x	Goat milk	x	Protein bars
x	Ice cream	x	"Natural flavor"
x	Milk, acidophilus	x	Whey
x	Milk glaze on bakery products	x	Condensed, powdered, or evaporated milk
x	Hot Cocoa (baking cocoa okay)	x	Produce wax (fresh fruits and vegetables)
x	Sheep milk	x	Milk, lactose-treated
x	Sour Cream	x	Seasoned potato chips
x	Whipped cream	x	"Seasoning"
x	Nondairy products such as whipped topping (may be lactose-free, not casein-free)	x	Yogurt

AVOID   Foods That Contain or May Contain Soy

x	Black soybeans	x	Soya
x	Edamame	x	Tamari
x	Liquid aminos	x	Tempeh
x	Miso	x	Teriyaki sauce
x	Shoyu	x	Tofu
x	Soy cheese	x	Broths
x	Soy flour	x	Energy bars
x	Soy yogurt	x	Gravies

AVOID   Foods That Contain or May Contain Soy

x	Soy ice cream	x	Imitation meat products
x	Soy isolate	x	Infant soy formula
x	Soy lecithin	x	Meal replacement drinks
x	Soy milk	x	Soups
x	Soy oil	x	Veggie burgers
x	Soy protein powder	x	Vitamin E supplements
x	Soy sauce	x	Breads and baked goods with soy flour

Foods to Choose on GFCFSF

CHOOSE   Grains and Grain-Free Flours

✓	Amaranth	✓	Potato flour
✓	Bean flours	✓	Potato starch
✓	Buckwheat	✓	Quinoa
✓	Coconut flour	✓	Rice
✓	Corn	✓	Seed flours
✓	Green banana flour	✓	Sorghum
✓	Millet	✓	Tapioca starch
✓	Nut flours	✓	Teff
✓	Oats (certified gluten-free)	✓	Wild rice

CHOOSE   Thickeners

✓	Agar	✓	Kudzu powder
✓	Arrowroot	✓	Sweet rice flour
✓	Cornstarch	✓	Tapioca
✓	Guar gum	✓	Xanthan gum
✓	Gelatin		

CHOOSE   Nondairy Milks, Yogurt, Pudding, and Ice Cream

✓	Coconut milk	✓	Rice milk
✓	Oat milk	✓	Potato milk

CHOOSE   Nondairy Milks, Yogurt, Pudding, and Ice Cream

✓ Ice cream made from nondairy milk

✓ Nut milk (almond, cashew, hazelnut, macadamia, and more)

✓ Pudding made from nondairy milk

✓ Seed milk (hemp, pumpkin seed)

✓ Yogurt made from nondairy milk

CHOOSE   Butters, Spreads, and Cheeses

✓ Casein-free and soy-free cheeses and cream cheese

✓ Coconut oil

✓ Nondairy butter spread (soy-free version)

CHOOSE   Naturally Gluten-Free and Dairy-Free Foods

✓ Eggs

✓ Fruits

✓ Meat

✓ Oils (Olive, avocado, and more)

✓ Nuts

✓ Seeds

✓ Vegetables

Note on Ghee

Ghee is clarified butter that has been cooked down to remove the milk solids. Theoretically, it shouldn't contain casein. In fact, some brands even test and certify that theirs is casein-free, so it can be an option for some. However, it is made from dairy, so for those with allergies or severe reactions to dairy, ghee is not an option. I find it best to avoid ghee when you are starting out just to be sure there are not any potential infractions that can interfere with results. These days, there are so many good dairy-free, soy-free butters that I use ghee less frequently now. The main time I consider it is when a therapeutic diet is severely limited in other fats, and ghee is one of the few choices that an individual can tolerate.

2. Identify What's Already GFCFSF

Next is to determine what your child already eats that's GFCFSF: any fruits and vegetables; natural, unprocessed meats; and any gluten-free grains and starches mentioned in the previous section. Your child may already eat some gluten-free and nondairy products that you can include here, too. Brainstorm and make a list. Here are some ideas to get you started:

Naturally GFCFSF Foods

- ❏ Apples
- ❏ Bananas
- ❏ Berries
- ❏ Grapes
- ❏ Oranges
- ❏ Broccoli
- ❏ Carrots
- ❏ Cucumbers
- ❏ Lettuce
- ❏ Potatoes

- ❏ Red bell peppers
- ❏ Sweet potatoes
- ❏ Rice
- ❏ Popcorn
- ❏ Beans
- ❏ Hummus
- ❏ Ground beef
- ❏ Roasted chicken
- ❏ Steak
- ❏ Eggs

Prepacked Products That Need GFCFSF Confirmation

- ❏ French fries
- ❏ Kale chips
- ❏ Lunch meat
- ❏ Oatmeal

- ❏ Potato chips
- ❏ Rice cakes
- ❏ Sausages
- ❏ Tortilla chips

3. Begin Creating a Meal Plan

Now you can now begin to start filling in a meal plan with GFCFSF foods your child already eats and likes. Create a chart (like the one here) with breakfast, lunch, dinner, snacks, and (optionally) desserts. If you need to avoid sugar, then don't add desserts that contain it. But if these treats are taking the place of other foods in their current diet, then it can help transition them.

Meal Planning Example

Breakfast	Scrambled eggs Oatmeal Apple slices Carrot sticks
Lunch	Lunch meat Lettuce Cucumber slices Strawberries
Snacks	Red bell pepper slices Hummus Blueberries Cashews
Dinner	Roasted chicken Burger Beef tacos with corn tortillas Potatoes Broccoli
Desserts	Nondairy ice cream Gluten-free cookies Applesauce

4. Choose Foods to Try Next

Make a list of the foods you think could be possibilities that you've never tried or would like to try again. Maybe this list includes some new products such as:

- Dairy-free milk
- Dairy-free treats
- Gluten-free bread and hamburger buns
- Gluten-free chicken nuggets
- Gluten-free pasta
- Gluten-free snack bars

Or, you might jot down a few new GFCFSF recipes. (This book has fifty, and of course, there are many more in cookbooks and online!) Try preparing and serving some of these foods before officially starting the diet. I like to add new foods before removing old foods. The more options you have and the more familiar your child is with these new foods, the easier it will be. However, if you don't have a lot of new foods, don't be discouraged. Every child is different. Some need to not have their old food as a crutch before they will try a new one.

5. Refine the Meal Plan and Prepare

Next, refine your meal plan. Some people like their meal plan to be a list of options for each meal. For example, under dinner you'd have a list of options you could try any day. Others prefer a true meal plan where they list out days and detail out every meal of every day. It could be either a full week (Monday through Sunday) or simply a three-day plan that you rotate. Do what you think is best for you and your family.

Personally, I do a little of both. I start with the list, then I'll do a more detailed plan for a few days. This way, I can adapt on the fly once I know what my daughter likes.

6. Begin the GFCFSF Diet!

You'll notice it took us until step 6 of seven steps before we start the diet. My experience is that the more preparation you do, the more confident you'll be. The more confident you are, the more your child will feel that and the more successful you will both be. That doesn't mean that it will take a long time to get here. Some people do the first five steps in a weekend, while others take several weeks. Go at the pace that works best for you. There are several options when starting the GFCFSF diet:

Cold turkey: This method involves taking out everything overnight and implementing the GFCFSF diet all at once. The benefit is that there is no crutch to fall back on. Some children will reject the new foods when any old ones are available; that's not an issue with this method. That said, this is not my preferred method. It can be difficult for the child, either emotionally or because of opiate withdrawal (if there is one).

Percentage change: This method involves adding as many new foods as you can while reducing gluten-, casein-, and soy-containing foods. This works best when you can implement 25 percent new GFCFSF foods per week or so. In other words, week 1 would be 25 percent, week 2 would be 50 percent, week 3 would be 75 percent, and week 4 would be 100 percent. This works best when a child does better with a slow transition but will still try new things.

Remove one protein, then the next: This method is the most common one I use in my nutrition practice. It involves removing gluten or dairy 100 percent in week 1, then removing the other food the next week. Usually, soy is not a big food in the diet, so I either suggest removing it with dairy or in week 3.

The downside here is that crutch concept again. But doing things one at a time gives you a mini trial for gluten and casein. If you remove casein and see big changes, then remove gluten and don't see much, it might give you a clue as to which is a bigger issue for your child. I'm not suggesting you then keep one of the foods in. But it can help in the future to better understand your child's biggest dietary triggers.

If you do one at a time, which food should you remove first? Some people remove the food that is the easiest first. Other people remove the one they suspect is the biggest offender. If a client isn't sure and asks me to make a recommendation and plan for them, I usually start with removing casein in week 1 and gluten in week 2.

Once you have fully removed gluten, casein, and soy, give this diet about six weeks to see what changes or improvements you notice. Remember, digestive enzymes can be beneficial before you start the GFCFSF diet (one of the reasons they are added in step 3), as they can help break down the proteins that cause opioid production, potentially lessening the opioid withdrawal effect.

7. Write It Down

This is the final part of the process. Keep a diet journal. Record what your child eats and their improvements and symptoms as you go. This way, you can assess how the diet is working and fine-tune it. Sometimes, we don't notice what has improved if we can't look back. And it can help us assess if there are any new symptoms that could be due to a newly added food that has been substituted in and could be a problem. For instance, corn is a common culprit, as cornstarch and other corn-derived ingredients are very common and prevalent in gluten-free food. A diet journal is a great tool for any practitioners you are working with, too. They can help you ensure that there are no infractions and help you with the diet. This is a good time to mention that strict adherence to the diet is important. Both research and my clinical experience shows a correlation between how strictly GFCF diet is followed and the overall benefit received.[30]

List the time of the meal, what the meal consisted of, and any symptoms the child has throughout the day (recording the time of the symptoms, too). The following table is an example of what I like to track. A free digital copy is available at www.PersonalizedAutismNutritionPlan.com/extras.

Diet Journal		
Breakfast Time	Foods	Symptoms/Notes
Lunch Time	Foods	Symptoms/Notes

Snack Time	Foods	Symptoms/Notes

Dinner Time	Foods	Symptoms/Notes

Dessert Time	Foods	Symptoms/Notes

One Day of GFCFSF Meals

Breakfast	Rice Porridge (page 275) Blueberry Cauliflower Smoothie (page 309)
Lunch	Squash Meatballs (page 283) Dairy-Free Mac and Cheese (page 286) Kale Chips (page 295) Sliced apple
Snack	Carrot and jicama sticks with Peanut Dipping Sauce (page 304) Sugar-Free Hot Cocoa (page 312)

Dinner	Creamy Crushed Garlic Chicken (page 281)
	Carrot Fries (substitute carrots in Rutabaga Fries, page 290)
	Air-Fried Popcorn Cauliflower (page 299)
	Chocolate Avocado Pudding (page 306)

READY FOR THE NEXT STEP?

This step typically takes six to eight weeks because it takes some time to prepare and remove each food protein and then see what happens. You can spend longer here if you want. You are looking for symptom improvements and/or some symptom stability within the diet, so that when you move on to another step, you'll be able to properly attribute any response to that new intervention. Remember to track symptoms that have improved and those that remain.

If you haven't seen the improvements that you are looking for, or if symptoms have gotten worse (which I rarely see after eight weeks!), don't give up on diet altogether. I suggest reading ahead, and possibly proceeding with another step, while sticking with the GFCFSF diet and figuring out exactly what is causing a reaction. Foods beyond gluten, casein, and soy can cause reactions (and we'll focus on those in steps 7 through 11). Often, if a child is reactive to more than one food or food compound, you have to remove all the offenders before you'll see improvements.

It's possible that something that was newly added could be causing a reaction, such as corn from gluten-free products or salicylates from certain fruits or vegetables. Additionally, seeking support from a nutrition-savvy practitioner can be helpful—this is where your food journal is important.

STEP 6
Take Care of Yourself

I know you are here reading this book to help your child, not yourself. And you are probably already stretched for time, energy, and capacity. You have a lot on your plate. So why is it important to add strategies for self-care while you and your child are on your Nourishing Hope journey?

Parenthood requires the long game, and this is particularly true for parents of children with ASD. It's a marathon, not a sprint. You need energy and emotional well-being to care for your children.

Self-care improves our health, energy levels, and emotional well-being, and reduces stress. And self-care helps us create a calmer environment for our children. Children with autism are often very sensitive to their environment. Even if they don't seem to be paying attention to their surroundings and those around them, they often are.

We all have to look after ourselves so we can have the most to give our children. Self-care is not selfish or decadent; it is an investment in you and your child. And if you need more motivation (parents are often more willing to do things for their children), know that you can use these strategies to help your child, too.

There are entire books written on self-care, so I'm going to focus on only a few key factors: reducing stress, eating well, getting sleep, finding community, and having fun. And I'll wrap this up with my favorite technique for releasing negative emotions: EFT, or tapping.

> ### Nourishing Hope Stories
>
> "When my son was first diagnosed with autism spectrum disorder, he had limited eye contact, interactive communication skills, and language. His food repertoire was not good and [he] ate limited foods. [When he was] five, we eliminated gluten and casein from his diet. He started showing improvements after two months. It was difficult for me to help [him] eat new and nutritious foods along with raising a fourteen-month-old toddler, right at the beginning of a pandemic. There was a lot of work to be done. I found out about Julie's program and began the training sessions . . . I learned that in order to help him, I should also take care of myself. I felt refreshed with the self-care strategies, and this fueled our dietary journey.
>
> "Today, my son is nine years old . . . He has improved in language, cognition, and social interaction. Diet is the basis of all the treatments that we do to help him learn and progress in his autism journey." —*Mom of a nine-year-old boy with ASD* ■

FIND STRESS-REDUCING TECHNIQUES

It's well established that stress is a silent killer. I could cite the science (a simple PubMed search will bring up thousands of studies), but I'm guessing you already know this to be true. But we all have stress in our lives and often can't avoid it. I hate it when people tell me "Don't stress!" and I would never say that to another parent. Although we can't necessarily eliminate stress, we can reduce our response to stressful events. Paying attention to what is stressful in your life and finding ways to be proactive to care for yourself can really help.

Taking a mental break is a great way to reduce your stress response. Find five minutes, or even one minute, to breathe slowly and deeply. Consider it a mini meditation or take a moment to pray. Focus on your breathing and clear your mind.

There are many mindfulness strategies you can use, such as intentional meditative walking—closing your eyes, feeling the breeze, or listening to the birds. It doesn't need to be fancy or complicated.

If you can, take a digital detox. We often think we can't get away from the devices we "need," but often we can. Choose a finite period of time and turn off your devices. Maybe it's while you're on a walk in nature or at home with your family. The other strategies in this chapter can also help reduce your stress response.

EAT WELL AND IMPROVE YOUR ENERGY

From day to day, our energy is affected by the fuel we consume. And over time, our eating patterns can have effects on our energy and mood. One of the best ways to take care of ourselves and improve our energy is to eat well. Nourishing Hope would not be complete if we didn't extend these principles to ourselves as parents.

But how to do that is the question. I'm sure as a parent, you've probably eaten while standing or driving. And that meal may have consisted of little more than snack foods. If this is not you and you already have healthy eating down pat, then well done! For the rest of us, here are ten helpful strategies:

1. When you're cooking yourself breakfast, prepare enough for more than one day, such as making a skillet full of breakfast sausages that can be easily reheated the next morning.
2. When you are cooking for your child, make enough so you can eat, too.
3. Schedule time for yourself to eat. Literally build it into your calendar.
4. If you're packing a lunch for your child, pack one for yourself, too. If you have a busy schedule where you are on the go and have to get to lots of appointments for your child, it's especially helpful to have something ready to eat.

5. Find a café that serves healthy food near your child's therapy session.
6. Begin to apply the healthy diet and therapeutic diet ideas for yourself, as well as your child, as you read through this book.
7. Come up with some simple meals that you can grab and eat that don't involve extensive preparation, that include some protein, fat, and fiber. Meals or snacks might include a hard-boiled egg, nuts, vegetable sticks, and/or hummus.
8. Chop or prepare food ahead of time, such as sliced vegetables, hard-boiled eggs, or salmon salad.
9. Keep healthy nonperishable food, such as nuts and seeds, in your handbag, car, or desk.
10. Prepare enough dinner for leftovers at lunch the next day.

GETTING SLEEP

Sleep is one of the best ways to take care of yourself. I know it can be easier said than done. If your child isn't sleeping well, see if you can find ways to improve their sleep, so you can get some sleep yourself.

Try getting to sleep early. Getting sleep in the earlier hours of the night is better for our sleep pattern.

Employ good sleep hygiene. This includes avoiding screen time too close to bedtime for everyone in your family, removing all night-lights and making the room dark, and avoiding electronics plugged in by your bed.

If you don't feel rested, try using a sleep-tracking device like an Oura Ring. It gives fascinating information on how many hours you've slept, including light, deep, and REM sleep. In tandem with a sleep journal, it can help you fine-tune things that may be interfering with a good night's sleep. For example, you might find that when you have a heavy meal too close to bedtime, you don't sleep well.

FIND COMMUNITY

Finding people who understand the challenges and worries of being a parent of a child with ASD, ADHD, and other neurodevelopmental delays takes some concerted effort. But having someone you can talk to, ask questions about nutrition and therapies, vent to when you are stressed, who understands you when you are having a big day, is beneficial.

In our Nourishing Hope program group meetings, one of the most rewarding parts for me is not only guiding parents with nutrition questions but also supporting them emotionally when they are having a bad day. And parents tell me it is one of the most valuable parts of the program. Who else will understand after a relative or teacher derails your hard work with a treat that caused a major meltdown, setback, or regression that takes weeks to remedy?

Find a community that is focused on autism or autism nutrition. This group can be online, as ours is, or in person. The Nourishing Hope community connects parents from 145 countries (and counting). This means you can connect with people anywhere in the world who are in a similar situation. You could also connect with people near you for local resources. There are online groups, social media groups, program groups, and more.

FUN AND EASY SELF-CARE IDEAS

Self-care does not have to be difficult or a drag. The following are simple activities that do not require a lot of resources. They are easy to fit into a busy life. And they are all things that can bring joy and pleasure. These are also things I like to do when I'm stressed, anxious, or depressed because they do not take a lot of time, energy, or motivation.

- Listen to music
- Take a bath
- Light a candle
- Color in a coloring book
- Grow a plant
- Pick or buy some flowers
- Take up an art or craft
- Dance
- Meditate/Pray

- Make a gratitude jar
- Take a walk
- Call a friend
- Enjoy a cup of tea
- Eat something healthy
- Envision what you want
- Grab a coffee or drink with a friend

Add your own favorites to this list.

You can make index cards with these activities on them. Place one item on each card, decorate them, or even just write them in different colored pens. When I really can't get motivated but know it would "be good for me," I pick one and do it.

EMOTIONAL FREEDOM TECHNIQUE (EFT)

Emotional Freedom Technique (EFT), also known as tapping, is a therapy that involves tapping on acupressure points while focusing on an emotion or situation that has negative feelings associated with it. EFT helps us release emotions and stress. It often involves listening to or saying words to move someone through the emotion or situation either proactively or retroactively. I find that it's great when my child is anxious or experiencing any difficult emotion. While it may seem too good to be true (maybe even a bit woo-woo), it really does often provide amazing relief very quickly. And there is research on it!

Researchers wondered whether it was the tapping that was an active component, whether something else was driving the results, or whether it was a placebo effect. They found that the tapping itself indeed provided benefit, as does the whole approach; that EFT can have a large benefit to the user for mental health conditions such as anxiety, depression, and posttraumatic stress disorder; and that the acupressure component was an "active ingredient" that makes it effective.[1] Systemic reviews show that EFT is helpful for anxiety and depression.[2] In addition to mental health conditions, EFT has been found to be helpful for physical symptoms, such

as decreasing pain and cravings, increasing happiness and immune function, and improving resting heart rate, cortisol, and systolic and diastolic
blood pressure.[3]

EFT can also be done for your child, rather than by your child. If you
can't get your child to actively do tapping, you can do it for them by tapping on yourself. One case study of a six-year-old boy with eating phobia
was found to improve from an EFT session done with a surrogate.[4] Surrogate EFT is where the tapping is done on a third party with the intention
of helping the child.

EFT is one of my favorite techniques for improving my and my child's
emotional state. I've been using EFT for many years. We have used it for
anxiety, stress, depression, anger, and fears, like fear of needles before a
laboratory appointment. We have also used it with difficulty sleeping. It's
quick to do: An average session is around eight to ten minutes, and if I am
really busy, I'll do a one-minute session. Even then, it seems to help bring
down the negative feelings a notch or two, so I can function better or have
more capacity for a longer session. And I have taught my daughter. She usually asks me to guide her through a session, which I am happy to do. And
when she doesn't want to participate, I'll tap "for her" on my own body.
Sometimes she joins in at that point. Other times, it calms me down, which
in turn helps her because our emotional states are often connected to our
children's. There are apps like The Tapping Solution and practitioners who
can guide you with a customized session.

READY FOR THE NEXT STEP?

Self-care is an ongoing process that we hopefully give attention to for life, so
there is no "completing" this step. Instead, pick one idea and try it—don't
just think about it but actually do it. If you like it, add it to your calendar
on an ongoing basis (even if it takes just a few minutes) with a reminder.
Scheduling it and remembering to do it means it will be more likely to happen. If that strategy wasn't the one for you, try something else until you find
one or more that works. Remember, this isn't just for you; it's for your child,
too, and it'll help you keep up your energy while you continue your journey.

SECTION 3

BioIndividual Nutrition and Therapeutic Diets

STEP 7

Low Salicylate, Low Amine, and Low Glutamate Diets

These three diets are some of the most helpful approaches in my clinical practice, particularly the low salicylate diet. Salicylates are a type of phenol. Most individuals with autism have low sulfate and poor sulfation,[1] and sulfation affects our ability to tolerate foods rich in phenols.

Is this sounding a little familiar?

In step 1, we removed artificial food additives in processed foods: artificial coloring, artificial flavoring, and artificial preservatives such as BHA, BHT, and TBHQ. All of these are phenols that many children (particularly children with ADHD and autism) struggle to metabolize adequately and which can then act as neurotoxins. Other food additives removed in step 1, including propionic acid, sulfites, benzoates, sorbates, and MSG, as well as artificial sweeteners and synthetic fragrances, have similar effects on the brain.

All of those are artificial or added components of foods. But as I mentioned briefly in step 1, there are also naturally occurring food chemicals or compounds that are chemically similar to these artificial ones, that are processed by the body similarly, and that create analogous reactions on the nervous system and brain, gastrointestinal tract, skin, and respiratory tract. So when someone benefits from removing those artificial additives, you may find comparable advantages by removing some of these natural food chemicals.

In this step, you'll learn about these natural food chemicals—salicylates, amines, and glutamate—and determine whether your child could benefit from a diet that eliminates them. It's likely that they could. Salicylate intolerance is common among children with autism. In my experience, many kids with ASD do not tolerate salicylates and/or related compounds such as amines and glutamates (at least temporarily)—I'd estimate this applies to 75 percent of my clients.

This step gives you a few options. You can remove just one of these compounds in a low salicylate, low amine, or low glutamate trial. Or you can do a combination (low SAG). As we'll see, histamine is a type of amine, so I address it separately in this chapter. Amines/histamines and glutamates are contained in many of the same foods. The principles of salicylates, amines, and glutamates are similar, and as many parents opt for the combination path, I'll be presenting these alongside each other, rather than making each its own step in BioIndividual Nutrition. Let's first look at each of these food compounds and how they can affect the body.

WHAT ARE SALICYLATES?

Salicylates are substances that some plants produce as part of a defense mechanism against insects and microbes. Insects and microorganisms are killed when they consume the substances in these plants. These salicylates can also affect your child when they eat foods high in them. These include apples, grapes, berries, cinnamon, and more (see the list on page 157).

As mentioned at the beginning of this chapter, salicylate is a phenol, or phenolic substance. We will talk more about these, but for now, the reason this is important is that because salicylates are phenols, the body needs an enzyme called phenol sulfotransferase (PST) to break them down. PST is an enzyme (or "transferase") that metabolizes or breaks down phenols using sulfate. We know in autism that sulfate is low, and sulfation is poor, hence the reason so many children with autism do not handle salicylates. Not only does poor sulfation affect our ability to handle salicylates, but certain salicylate-rich foods can also inhibit sulfation, furthering the problem.

Sulfation is important for controlling neurotransmitters, proper brain function, and emotional well-being. Additionally, it's suspected that salicylate intolerance contributes to inflammation,[2] and we know that inflammation is implicated in the development of autism.[3] This adds further evidence that individuals with autism might not tolerate salicylates the same as other people and that salicylates appear to affect the brain negatively.

Salicylates can exacerbate or cause autism symptoms and comorbid conditions that make the lives of individuals with ASD more difficult. They have a large effect on behavior and sensory processing, two factors that influence the day-to-day lives of children with ASD. They can also affect physical symptoms, including digestive issues, which are also common in autism.

WHAT ARE AMINES?

Some amines (including tyramine and phenylethylamine) are phenols, like salicylates. The most well-known amine is histamine. Histamine is not phenolic, so it's processed somewhat differently than phenolic amines; however, many foods high in histamine are also high in phenolic amines. Being different, there are unique nutrition strategies to increase tolerance of histamine- and phenolic amine–containing foods. Since the biochemical pathways that help process salicylates are the same as those that process phenolic amines, sometimes people that need a low salicylate diet also need a low amine or low–food chemical diet.

WHAT IS HISTAMINE?

Histamines are the most well-known type of amines—almost everyone knows someone who suffers from hay fever and has taken an antihistamine to counter those symptoms. But histamine in foods can also be a problem.

If your child has a challenge with histamine, consuming histamines in their food can lead to chronic inflammation, skin irritation, diarrhea, headaches, and other symptoms.

One way to consider whether a low histamine diet might be helpful is to look at your child's symptoms. Symptoms of histamine intolerance are somewhat different than symptoms of intolerance to other amines. And underlying factors differ between histamine intolerance and other amine intolerance. One main difference is that some people have a histamine intolerance because of mast cell activation syndrome or other biochemical reasons for high histamine. In this case, they react to histamine but not other amines.

The main reason it is important to know the distinction between the two is that they are processed differently in the body. Histamine intolerance is an inability to handle the amount of histamine present relative to our capacity to process it. Histamine is broken down in the gut with the help of the enzyme DAO. Insufficient DAO can cause reactions to histamine-containing foods. Processing histamine also requires adequate methylation; therefore, those without adequate methylation are more prone to histamine intolerance. And when someone has too much histamine being released— such as occurs with mast cell activation syndrome—histamine capacity can be overwhelmed, leading to food reactions.

Because of this, some people have more difficulty with one type of amine over another, and understanding that will help you choose the right diet. Symptoms and food reactions can help you make the distinction. In addition to the symptoms of amine intolerance, also notice the more common symptoms of histamine intolerance in the table on page 150. Also, keep in mind that amines can inhibit the breakdown of histamine, so some people do best avoiding other amine-containing foods on a low histamine diet.[4]

WHAT IS GLUTAMATE?

I discussed glutamate in step 1 in the section on MSG. While glutamate is not a salicylate or amine, I include it in this section because glutamates involve similar symptoms and nervous system reactions as amines and salicylates and are found in many of the same foods as amines. In fact, these three food compounds have been studied together at the Allergy Unit at the Royal Prince Alfred Hospital in Australia. Glutamate intolerance has similar symptoms to amines, as well as some of the more common glutamate-specific symptoms shown here. (Revisit step 1 for more on glutamate.)

COMMON SYMPTOMS OF SALICYLATE, AMINE, AND GLUTAMATE INTOLERANCE

Intolerances to these food compounds cause a lot of behavioral, neurological, and physical symptoms. Symptoms tend to be similar with some key differences that may single out one over another as a likely culprit. For instance, red cheeks and ears, hyperactivity, and aggression are common symptoms of salicylate intolerance while itchy skin and dermatographia ("writing"/scratching on skin that leaves raised marks) indicate a likely issue with histamines. Therefore, in the table beginning on page 150, I've include a ✪ for those symptoms that are most common with a specific intolerance, and a ● for common symptoms. Note that different people respond differently, so just because a symptom is not marked doesn't mean it's not a potential reaction for your child.

FOOD CRAVINGS

Food cravings can be signs of intolerance, particularly for salicylate and glutamate. A diet high in strawberries, blueberries, apples, cinnamon, herbs, spices, honey, and other salicylates points to salicylate intolerance. High consumption of soy sauce, parmesan cheese, fish sauce, mushrooms, or seaweed can indicate glutamate intolerance.

In fact, this is one way I begin to determine if these compounds are a top suspect. If a child puts ketchup on everything or loves spicy food (but doesn't come from a culture of spicy cuisine), these are potential red flags of salicylate intolerance for me. This is especially true for a food that most kids typically don't love or that seems in excess. Although this alone is not enough to know whether they have an intolerance, it is one factor that weighs into my decision of whether they may be sensitive to salicylates.

Here's an example. A client of mine, a young boy with autism, had an unusual craving for apples. He would eat mostly the skin off the apple and eat many each day, often five or more. Kids usually don't love apple skin, but most of the salicylates are in and under the skin. And that many apples is a lot for most people. His mother told me that the local grocer knew she and her husband were part of the same family, not because they came in together but because no one else was buying fifteen apples every few days! Because of his apple craving and other salicylate-intolerance symptoms, I suggested a low salicylate diet. It turned out my suspicion was correct. Once he lowered the salicylate level in his diet, he felt better and had improved behavior.

Nourishing Hope Stories

"During the Nourishing Hope program, we did do a low/medium salicylate trial, and symptoms my son had been having disappeared within days—it was incredible. No more red cheeks, no wetting himself (we had thought he had just been taking a long time to toilet train!) including no more nighttime diapers, his challenging behavior stabilized. When introducing some salicylate foods back in, all the symptoms come back almost immediately including red cheeks, wetting himself, and 'outrageous' behavior almost came back more strongly. We find the digestive enzymes help a lot in his food reactions. We find food reactions much more severe/obvious now." —*Mom of a four-year-old with ASD* ∎

SALICYLATE AND ADHD

The low salicylate diet is my go-to diet for ADHD. In fact, a diet low in salicylates and artificial food additives was first brought forth by Dr. Ben Feingold in the 1970s as an intervention for reducing hyperactivity symptoms. Dr. Feingold found approximately half of children with hyper-activity and learning disabilities in his medical practice improved from the diet. The first things to improve were hyperactivity, aggression, and impulsivity. Next, he noticed improvements in fine motor skills like writing, gross motor skills like coordination, and speech, followed by improvements in cognitive function and attention.[5]

Salicylates are always my top suspect for the symptoms of hyperactivity, irritability, aggression, and to a lesser degree, inattentiveness. Because a large percentage of children with ADHD have poor sulfation, chances are good they have salicylate intolerance.

Several studies showed good results from a limited elimination diet that I would consider a low salicylate diet. This diet eliminated all food additives and included only turkey, rice, vegetables (including cabbage, beet, cauliflower, rutabaga, sprouts, and lettuce), pear, olive oil, ghee, salt, rice milk with supplemental calcium, and water. In one study, researchers found 63 percent of children with ADHD on this limited diet had a 40 percent or more reduction in ADHD symptoms.[6] With data from brain imaging technology, their findings suggested that the diet worked at least in part by a neurocognitive mechanism.

LOW SALICYLATE DIET IN AUTISM

Parents report great benefits with the low salicylate diet. Caregivers and individuals with ASD in our survey study rated the Feingold diet (a low salicylate diet) as the second-best therapeutic diet for overall benefit. Parents reported that 45 percent of individuals had improvement in hyperactivity, 38 percent in irritability, 37 percent in attention, and 34 percent in aggression, 28 percent in anxiety, 28 percent in cognition, and 22 percent in sensory sensitivity.[7]

	Salicylate intolerance	Amine intolerance	Histamine intolerance	Glutamate intolerance
Aggression	✪	●	●	●
Anxiety	●		✪	●
Asthma	●		●	
Cognitive difficulties	●			
Congestion/Sinus problems	●	●	✪	
Constipation	●	●	●	
Cravings for high amine foods		●		
Cravings for high glutamate foods				●
Cravings for high salicylate foods	●			
Cries easily	●	●	✪	●
Dark circles under eyes/Allergic shiners	✪			
Defiance	●	✪	●	●
Dermatographia	●		✪	
Diarrhea	●	●	●	✪
Difficulty staying asleep			●	
Dizziness/Fainting	●		●	●
Dyslexia	●			
Ear infections		✪		
Fluttering and quick heartbeat		✪	●	●
GERD/Acid reflux	●	●	✪	✪
Headaches/Migraines		●	✪	●
High blood pressure		●	●	●
Hives	✪	●	✪	●
Hyperactivity	✪		●	✪
Hypotonia			●	

Symptom	Salicylate intolerance	Amine intolerance	Histamine intolerance	Glutamate intolerance
Impatience	●			
Impulsivity	●	●		●
Inappropriate laughter	✪	●		
Inattentiveness	●			
Irritability	✪	●	●	●
Itchy skin			✪	
Nausea/Vomiting		●	●	●
Nightmares	●	●	●	
Poor coordination	●			
Red cheeks or ears	✪	●	●	●
Restlessness				●
Seizures (some forms)	●			●
Self-injury	●	●		●
Sensory sensitivity and processing	●		●	
Skin rashes	●	●	✪	●
Sleep (trouble falling asleep)	●	●	●	●
Speech difficulties	●			
Stomachaches/Abdominal pain	●	●	●	✪
Sweating			●	●
Tics	●		●	●
Urinary incontinence/Bedwetting	●	●	●	●
Vertigo	✪		●	
Visual or auditory processing challenges	●	●	●	●
Wheezing or shortness of breath			●	

✪ Most common symptom   ● Common symptom

Nourishing Hope Stories

"I was at a conference listening to nutritionist Julie Matthews. She was showing a slide of various behaviors, accurately describing my son. At that time, my son had started showing some aggressive behaviors, mostly directed toward me (biting, causing bruises), and I was getting phone calls from school about him lashing out. The follow-up slide was which foods to eliminate in order to stop the behaviors. It was all of my son's favorites. I immediately texted my husband and told him, when I got home, we were doing a diet overhaul. We took out all of the problem foods, and his behaviors stopped! The change was so dramatic that his doctor, who had wanted to start medication, decided it was unnecessary. Do not discount diet!" —*Mom of a teenage boy with autism*

HOW TO DETERMINE WHETHER ONE OF THESE DIETS IS RIGHT FOR YOUR CHILD

There is overlap here, and dietary trials are beneficial. As I mentioned earlier, my experience is that (some level of) a low salicylate diet is beneficial for about 75 percent of my clients whereas about only half of those people need a low amine diet. Said another way, if someone needs low amine, they likely need low salicylate. However, if they need a low salicylate diet, they may or may not need a low amine diet. And some people have a reaction to only salicylates, while others have reactions to only amines. It's bioindividual. Most of my clients will avoid high glutamate foods, such as soy sauce (and anything containing MSG, of course). And since a low glutamate diet does not remove too many whole foods that are not already removed in a low amine diet, I'll often recommend a trial of low glutamate during or after a low salicylate and/or amine trial.

To determine a food intolerance to any of these compounds, start by simply observing your child within the hour they eat the foods containing the compound, as well as before bedtime (see the food lists later in this chapter). Do they eat a lot of foods that are high in a particular compound? Do you notice multiple common symptoms of intolerance (see page 150)? Do you notice reactions shortly after eating those foods?

If you suspect intolerance, the best way to determine whether your child has one is to do a dietary trial. We'll get to how to do that in the following sections.

If your child has reactions to foods containing these compounds, but they still seem to be having symptoms even after removing those foods, you'll want to consider one of the other categories.

If you have already tried a diet that eliminates just one of these compounds and your child still has symptoms, consider that the combination low salicylate, amine, and glutamate (low SAG) diet might be right for them. Some people have problems with all three.

Lab Testing for Intolerance

There are no definitive laboratory tests with quantitative biomarkers except high histamine. While there are a few possible laboratory markers for salicylate intolerance and sulfation capacity, I'm not convinced that they identify these intolerances well, and in other cases, laboratory testing is not available outside of the research setting. Also, I feel some of the labs cause more harm than good because they test detoxification capacity and require taking a medication. So not only are there not great tests for this, but diet trials do an excellent job identifying these intolerances. I prefer to use symptom presence and a dietary trial (such as the low salicylate diet) as my "test."

Not All Bad

With all of this said about these natural food compounds, not everything about them is bad. In fact, there are many beneficial phytonutrient properties and additional nutrients in many of these foods—see the lists later in this chapter, and you'll understand what I mean. When people limit these foods and do not replace them with other nutrient-dense foods, a child could be at risk of nutritional deficiencies. An important thing to note here is to remove *only* those foods that you notice are causing negative reactions and/or try to find ways to limit reactions or improve tolerance.

If your child does react to these food compounds, do your best to determine their threshold and keep as many of these foods in their diet as possible. If they really don't tolerate them well, there are ways you can meet their nutritional needs while limiting the amount of these foods. There are also ways to improve tolerance to these foods so that your child may be able to consume more of them (see "Supplements and Additional Consideration to Help with Food Chemical Intolerance").

Interestingly, while broccoli, kale, and mango are high in salicylate, I have found that they are often tolerated by my clients who need a low salicylate diet (except those who are very sensitive); in fact, some low salicylate diets allow these foods while others do not. Maybe this is because overall the diets are low in salicylate, so a small amount is tolerated. Or maybe there is something else about these foods' chemical makeup that helps—such as the sulfur in kale or broccoli that increases glutathione levels or aids detoxification. The point here, again, is that it's important to find your child's individual threshold and make their diet as healthy as possible within their personal parameters. Do not overly restrict their diet.

A person's salicylate threshold depends on the amount of salicylate in a food and the serving size, so if the amount in a food is moderate but you have a large serving or several servings, it may cause a reaction. However, even very small servings (like the amount in spices) can add up very quickly because their salicylate content is so high.

If you need more details on how to do any of the diets in this step, you can explore my Nourishing Hope program and my book extras for more resources, as well as the Feingold diet, RPAH elimination diet, and FAIL-SAFE diet, which are other common variations.

Is Salicylate Intolerance Lifelong?

This brings us to another common question: whether salicylate intolerance is lifelong. My experience is that it is not. Once you reduce salicylates to take the biochemical burden off the system and address underlying factors causing the reactions, salicylate intolerance often improves. Although some people may still need to pay attention to salicylates and be careful not to overdo it, most of my clients and families I work with are able to loosen up their salicylate restrictions over time.

IMPLEMENTING A LOW SALICYLATE DIET

A low salicylate diet is as simple as removing naturally high salicylate foods, along with artificial colors, flavors, preservatives, and sweeteners (which you have likely already done in step 1).

The main decision to make is whether you want to start with a more restricted food list or more variety. If you restrict more, you're more likely to have "gotten" the offending food; however, the diet is more limited on your trial. If you start with a less restrictive list, you may miss some of the offenders and not see positive results from the diet, causing you to miss important clues.

Continue with your low salicylate diet for a three- to six-week trial period. Notice and record what you observe with your child's behavior and health. When you've had five to seven days of no symptoms or highly improved symptoms, you can consider the trial and observation period complete.

The next is the test back phase. This is where you start to add foods back until you learn what is tolerated and not. This has to do with learning your child's tolerance threshold. Salicylate tolerance is bioindividual. Some people respond to specific salicylates and not others. Some salicylate-rich foods impair PST, so they may be worse for some individuals. Some people respond to a large amount at one sitting, and others will react to a buildup of salicylates over time. Think of salicylates like water in a dam—once that threshold is exceeded, the water spills over and symptoms result. Too much of a food, or too many small servings of salicylates, can push it into a reaction. Additionally, everyone's reservoir (salicylate capacity) is a different size and has factors that may cause a buildup faster.

There is more than one way to test back. One option is to add a lot of salicylates in a day (six or more) for a period of seven days (or until you get symptoms). The second way is adding a smaller number of salicylates back (for example, just one small to medium serving). This will be the first piece of data for determining your child's salicylate threshold. From there, increase the number of salicylates over seven days or until your child experiences symptoms. I prefer to proceed slowly, as it is gentler, and if your child is sensitive, it will be easier on them. Then if you are unsure and not seeing anything with the testing back phase, you may add more in at once. For this challenge, choose foods high only in salicylates, not high in other phenols and food chemicals. Examples include strawberries, cinnamon, red bell pepper, honey, and peppermint. Foods such as tomato sauce and grapes, while high in salicylates, are also high in amines and glutamate and this can confound results.

The testing back phase can take a while, so be patient. It takes multiple food trials to determine what foods and what threshold are tolerated. Wait for symptoms to clear (about three days) before starting another food challenge—whether that's adding a subsequent salicylate-containing food or moving on to amines or glutamate. For a trial, choose foods high in only that one food chemical.

Foods to Avoid and Foods to Choose on a Low Salicylate Diet

One challenge you might find when trying a low salicylate diet is that lists of foods often conflict. This is in part because the research on salicylate levels in food is not consistent. Salicylate level is affected by where a food is grown, when it is picked, and which variety it is.

The following list is based on my years of working with clients, as well as the research on the levels in foods. For example, I have always excluded bananas on a low salicylate diet in my nutrition practice, as I often found them to cause a reaction (this is likely because of their high amine content), and I don't want parents to take the chance the banana is interfering with the rest of the dietary trial.

Another challenge? There are only a few low salicylate fruits. This is probably the most difficult part of this diet. The fruit lowest in salicylate is peeled pears; however, I find peeled Golden Delicious and Red Delicious apples are often well tolerated and include them in the dietary trial, along with papaya.

The list of low salicylate vegetables includes those with the lowest level of salicylates (indicated with an asterisk) and other vegetables that are moderately low in salicylates—such as asparagus, butternut squash, head lettuce, sweet potatoes, beets, carrots, parsnips, and turnips—can often fit into a low salicylate diet. Whether you include the moderately low salicylate vegetables depends how sensitive you suspect your child is. I find most kids are not that sensitive and that the low list is very restrictive, so I often suggest starting with this larger list of lows and moderately lows. If you are still unsure after the dietary trial, I suggest restricting to only the lowest foods.

Natural flavorings such as berry flavoring in supplements and processed foods and mint flavoring in candy should also be avoided on this diet.

AVOID   High Salicylate Fruits to Avoid

x	Apricots	x	Kiwi
x	Avocados	x	Grapes
x	Bananas	x	Oranges and other citrus
x	Blackberries	x	Pineapples
x	Blueberries	x	Plums
x	Cherries	x	Peaches
x	Dates	x	Pomegranates
x	Figs	x	Melons
x	Fruit juices (most)	x	Nectarines

AVOID   High Salicylate Fruits to Avoid

x	Grapefruit	x	Raisins and dried fruit
x	Strawberries	x	Raspberries
x	Apples (except Golden Delicious and Red Delicious, peeled)		

AVOID   High Salicylate Vegetables to Avoid

x	Artichokes	x	Jicama
x	Arugula	x	Kale
x	Beet greens	x	Mushrooms
x	Bell peppers	x	Okra
x	Broccoli	x	Olives
x	Cauliflower	x	Onions
x	Chili peppers	x	Radishes
x	Corn	x	Seaweed
x	Cucumbers (with peel)	x	Spinach
x	Eggplant	x	Swiss chard
x	Escarole	x	Tomatoes
x	Fennel	x	Zucchini (with peel)

AVOID   Other High Salicylate Foods to Avoid

x	Bone broths	x	Ketchup
x	Coconut	x	Nuts and seeds (most)
x	Coconut oil	x	Olive oil
x	Grapeseed oil	x	Herbs and spices
x	Salami and other processed meats	x	Tomato sauce

CHOOSE   Low Salicylate Fruits to Choose (* are lowest)

✓	Apples, Golden Delicious (peeled)	✓ Apples, Red Delicious (peeled)
✓	Papaya	✓ Pears (peeled)*

CHOOSE   Low Salicylate Vegetables to Choose (* are lowest)

✓	Asparagus	✓ Green onion*
✓	Beets	✓ Leeks*
✓	Bok choy	✓ Lettuce
✓	Brussels sprouts*	✓ Lettuce, iceberg*
✓	Butternut squash	✓ Parsnips
✓	Cabbage, green*	✓ Peas, green*
✓	Cabbage, purple*	✓ Potatoes, white, peeled*
✓	Carrots	✓ Rutabagas/Swede*
✓	Celery stalks*	✓ Sweet potatoes
✓	Green/String beans*	✓ Turnips

CHOOSE   Other Low Salicylate Foods to Choose

✓	Arrowroot starch	✓ Lard
✓	Cane sugar	✓ Maple syrup
✓	Cashews	✓ Parsley (in small amounts)
✓	Chives	✓ Rice bran oil†
✓	Chocolate	✓ Rice vinegar
✓	Eggs	✓ Sunflower oil†
✓	Garlic (in small amounts)	✓ Tapioca starch
✓	Grains (most)	✓ Vanilla
✓	Legumes (except fava)	✓ Rice (except basmati,
✓	Fish, seafood, meat, and poultry (most)‡	jasmine, and wild)

† Canola and palm are allowed but not recommended

‡ Fish, seafood, meats, and poultry are low in salicylates—in fact, I am not aware of any varieties that you should be concerned about.

One Day of Low Salicylate Meals

Breakfast	Maple Pork Sausage (page 274)
	Rutabaga hash browns (substitute rutabaga in Butternut Squash Hash Browns, page 274)
Lunch	Egg-Free Chicken Nuggets (page 276)
	Steamed green beans
	Golden Delicious apple, peeled
Snack	Pear Sauce (page 303)
	Peas
Dinner	Burger with gluten-free bun or iceberg lettuce wrap
	Rutabaga Fries (page 290)
	Confetti Brussels Sprouts (page 288)
	Brown rice
	Baked Pears or Apples (page 308; use peeled pears or Golden Delicious apple)

IMPLEMENTING A LOW AMINE DIET

The implementation of a low amine diet is similar to doing a low salicylate diet. A low amine diet reduces high amine food, such as processed meats, broths, and fermented foods, and focuses on foods low in amines.

You can typically remove high amine foods as quickly or slowly as you like. If a child is sensitive to amines, they usually start to feel better quickly after those compounds are removed. Note: This low amine diet does not include low *histamine* diet principles, such as removing histamine-liberating foods. So, if you suspect histamine is an issue, you'll want to check out the specific dietary strategies for that.

Testing back is also similar to food trials following a low salicylate diet. After three to six weeks, add high amine foods back over seven days or until symptoms appear, adding them in either small or large amounts, depending on how sensitive you feel someone is or how gently you want to go.

Foods to Avoid and Foods to Choose on a Low Amine Diet

Amines are found in foods that involve fermentation and protein breakdown and in certain processed foods (including sauerkraut, bone broths, aged meat, slow-cooked meat, cured meats and fish, and yeast extracts), as well as certain plant-based foods and fresh produce, particularly as they ripen.

Fresh meat, many fresh fruits and vegetables (except those that are high amine), and most whole grains are low amine foods.

AVOID   Fermented/High Amine Foods to Avoid

x	Beer and wine*	x	Soy sauce
x	Fish sauce	x	Tempeh
x	Kefir	x	Tofu
x	Kimchi	x	Vegemite/Marmite
x	Miso	x	Vinegar
x	Pickles	x	Yogurt
x	Sauerkraut		

AVOID   High Amine Meats, Fish, and Stock to Avoid

x	Aged beef	x	Barbecued meats
x	Bone broth	x	Smoked meat and fish
x	Slow-cooked meat	x	Stocks and gravy
x	Cured meat and fish	x	Turkey
x	Pork	x	Vegetable stock cubes
x	Canned meat, poultry, and fish	x	Yeast-containing foods

---

* Avoiding alcohol should go without saying for children!

AVOID High Amine Fruits, Vegetables, Nuts, and Plant Foods to Avoid

X	Avocados	X	Grapes
X	Bananas	X	Kiwi
X	Blackberries	X	Mangos
X	Broccoli	X	Mushrooms
X	Cauliflower	X	Nuts/Seeds
X	Cherries	X	Oranges
X	Chocolate/Cocoa/Cacao	X	Papaya
X	Citrus	X	Pineapples
X	Coconuts	X	Plums
X	Dates	X	Raspberries
X	Dried fruits	X	Spinach
X	Eggplant	X	Swiss chard
X	Fava/Broad beans	X	Tomatoes
X	Figs		

CHOOSE Low Amine Vegetables to Choose

✓	Artichokes	✓	Ginger
✓	Asparagus	✓	Green beans
✓	Beets	✓	Jicama
✓	Bok choy	✓	Kale
✓	Brussels sprouts	✓	Lettuce
✓	Cabbage	✓	Parsnips
✓	Carrots	✓	Peas
✓	Celeriac	✓	Potatoes
✓	Celery	✓	Red bell peppers
✓	Corn	✓	Sweet potatoes
✓	Cucumbers	✓	Winter squash
✓	Garlic	✓	Zucchini

CHOOSE   Low Amine Fruits to Choose

✓	Apples	✓	Peaches
✓	Apricots	✓	Pears
✓	Blueberries	✓	Persimmons
✓	Melons	✓	Pomegranates
✓	Nectarines	✓	Strawberries

CHOOSE   Other Low Amine Foods to Choose

✓	Cane sugar	✓	Fresh white fish
✓	Carob	✓	Maple syrup
✓	Eggs	✓	Molasses
✓	Fresh beef	✓	Olive oil
✓	Fresh chicken	✓	Vanilla
✓	Fresh lamb	✓	Herbs and spices
✓	Legumes (except fava beans)	✓	Starches (tapioca and arrowroot)
✓	Grains (amaranth, buckwheat, millet, oats, quinoa, sorghum, rice)	✓	Cashews, raw or lightly roasted*

IMPLEMENTING A LOW HISTAMINE DIET

Histamine is released by our cells in response to allergies, infections, and tissue injury, as well as certain foods known as histamine-liberating foods. A low histamine diet removes foods high in histamine and those that liberate histamine. You can typically remove the foods all at once, and if sensitive, people often feel improvements in symptoms quickly.

Testing back is also similar to the food challenges after a low amine diet, except in this case, you can try separate trials of high histamine foods and of histamine-liberating foods to see if any are more problematic. If your child is feeling good and you strongly suspect a histamine intolerance, you may not

* Cashews are low amine but are histamine liberators.

want to add the foods back for a while! As with the low amine diet, after three to six weeks, you can introduce foods back slowly, then if you are still unsure, you may want to try larger serving sizes to see if your child has a reaction.

Foods to Avoid and Foods to Choose on a Low Histamine Diet

As we've discussed, many high amine foods contain tyramine, phenylethyl-amine, and histamine. So the high histamine food list is similar to the high amine list regarding fermented and processed foods but somewhat different for vegetables and other plant foods.

AVOID   High Histamine Foods to Avoid

x	Aged meats	x	Fermented vegetables
x	Avocados	x	Smoked or canned fish
x	Bone broth	x	Spinach
x	Cured/Processed meats	x	Tomatoes
x	Eggplant	x	Vinegars
x	Fermented soy	x	Yeast-containing foods
x	Fermented beverages (e.g., beer, kombucha, wine)		

AVOID   Histamine-Liberating Foods to Avoid

x	Artificial additives	x	Legumes
x	Avocados	x	Mangos
x	Bananas	x	Mustard
x	Beer, wine, and spirits	x	Onions
x	Brussels sprouts	x	Papaya
x	Cashews	x	Pineapples
x	Chocolate/Cocoa	x	Plums
x	Citrus	x	Seaweed/kelp
x	Coffee/Caffeine	x	Shellfish
x	Cumin	x	Strawberries

AVOID	Histamine-Liberating Foods to Avoid		
x	Kiwi	x	Sunflower seeds
x	Garlic	x	Tomatoes
x	Hazelnuts	x	Walnuts
x	Egg whites (from chicken eggs)		

CHOOSE	Low Histamine Foods to Choose		
✓	Egg yolk	✓	White vinegar
✓	Quail eggs	✓	Macadamia nuts*
✓	Freshly caught fish†	✓	Oils (coconut oil, olive oil)
✓	Fresh meats	✓	Grains (amaranth, corn, millet, oat, rice)
✓	Fresh chicken (without skin)	✓	Potatoes and sweet potatoes
✓	Fruits (except those on the high histamine or histamine-liberating list)	✓	Vegetables (except those on the high histamine or histamine-liberating list)

IMPLEMENTING A LOW GLUTAMATE DIET

A low glutamate diet removes foods high in glutamate and food additives, including monosodium glutamate, autolyzed yeast, yeast extract, hydrolyzed vegetable protein, and more (which were removed in step 1). The process is similar to the other diets in this step. Remove the foods that are high in glutamate, and after three to six weeks, test the foods back. You can do this over the course of three days instead of seven. In this case, it's often best to avoid the high glutamate food additives in your challenge and focus

---

* Macadamia nuts are low histamine but contain other amines.

† Freshly caught fish and freshly caught fish that has been immediately frozen are low histamine; however, histamine increases rapidly when stored. Fish stored on ice in the grocery store (which is not fresh) is high histamine.

instead on those healthful whole foods you would like to be able to add back into your child's diet if possible.

Foods to Avoid and Foods to Choose on a Low Glutamate Diet

Glutamate and amines are both found in foods that are processed by aging, curing, simmering, and fermenting as these processes break down the protein and liberate the amines and glutamates. Glutamates are not as prevalent in fruits, vegetables, and plant-based foods as amines are, but there are some.

AVOID   High Glutamate Foods to Avoid

x	Aged cheese/parmesan	x	Mushrooms
x	Balsamic vinegar	x	Peas
x	Beet greens	x	Pickles
x	Bone broth	x	Plums
x	Bouillon cubes	x	Processed meat
x	Brewer's/Nutritional yeast	x	Sauerkraut
x	Broccoli	x	Seaweed
x	Corn	x	Soy sauce
x	Fermented foods	x	Spinach
x	Grapes	x	Stocks
x	Gravy	x	Stock powders
x	Marmite/Vegemite	x	Swiss chard
x	Monosodium glutamate (MSG)	x	Wine, bourbon, brandy, cognac, rum*
x	Hydrolyzed soy/vegetable protein and the high glutamate additives on page 47	x	Tomatoes

---

* Avoiding alcohol should go without saying for children!

CHOOSE   Low Glutamate Foods to Choose

✓   Eggs

✓   Fresh fish and seafood

✓   Fresh meat

✓   Fresh poultry

✓   Fruits (except grapes, plums, prunes, raisins, and tomatoes)

✓   Vegetables (except beet greens, broccoli, corn, mushrooms, peas, seaweed, spinach, and Swiss chard)

✓   Legumes

✓   Nuts/Seeds and coconut

✓   Vinegar (except balsamic)

✓   Whole grains (except corn)

✓   Oils (most, including avocado oil, coconut oil, and olive oil)

IMPLEMENTING A LOW SALICYLATE, AMINE, AND GLUTAMATE (SAG) DIET

Similar to the low salicylate diet, there is conflicting information about what foods you can and can't have and how to implement a diet low in salicylates, amines, and glutamates. I created this low salicylate, amine, and glutamate diet, which I refer to as the low SAG diet, to solve the problem of contradicting information by pulling together research, well-known diet principles, and my professional experience.

I suggest implementing this diet similarly to the other three diets in this chapter, following a low SAG diet for three to six weeks while recording any symptom improvements or symptom changes you see. Then test back each category one at a time, waiting three days in between food challenges until symptoms subside. As with the other diets, I prefer to start food reintroduction trials slowly, including single servings of one food from the category for a few days (choosing a different food each day). If you don't notice anything from single servings of foods, then you might consider a more significant dietary challenge with several servings (up to six) of high foods from that category in one day. You can refine the diet over the course of a few months to eliminate the foods that are not tolerated and really zero in on the threshold of what amount is tolerated.

Foods to Avoid and Foods to Choose on a Low SAG Diet

The following are lists of vegetables, fruits, and other foods to avoid and choose on my low SAG diet. As with the low salicylate list, those vegetables and fruits with an asterisk are the lowest, so some people may want to restrict to only those vegetables and fruits with the asterisk, and limit or avoid the others such as asparagus, bok choy, butternut squash, and carrots. Some people can handle these foods and can include them; others may want to limit to one to two servings per day.

High SAG Foods to Avoid

Refer to the "Avoid" food lists earlier in this chapter.

CHOOSE   Low SAG Vegetables to Choose (*lowest)

✓ Asparagus	✓ Green onions*
✓ Bamboo shoots*	✓ Leeks*
✓ Bean sprouts*	✓ Lettuce
✓ Bok choy	✓ Lettuce, iceberg*
✓ Brussels sprouts*	✓ Parsnips
✓ Butternut squash	✓ Potatoes, white, peeled*
✓ Cabbage*	✓ Rutabagas/Swede*
✓ Carrots	✓ Sweet potatoes
✓ Celery stalks*	✓ Turnips
✓ Green/String beans*	

CHOOSE   Low SAG Fruits to Choose (*lowest)

✓ Apples, Gold Delicious and Red Delicious	✓ Papaya
	✓ Pears, peeled*

CHOOSE   Other Low SAG Foods to Choose

✓	Arrowroot starch	✓	Grains (except corn)
✓	Beef, fresh (not aged)	✓	Lamb
✓	Carob	✓	Legumes
✓	Cashews, raw	✓	Maple syrup
✓	Chicken, fresh (no skin)	✓	Parsley (small amounts)
✓	Chives	✓	Rice
✓	Eggs	✓	Salt
✓	Fish, white, fresh	✓	Sunflower oil
✓	Garlic (small amounts)	✓	Tapioca starch
✓	Ghee (only if needed)	✓	Vanilla

One Day of Low SAG Meals

Breakfast	Poached eggs
	Roasted potatoes
	Cashew Milk (page 311)
Lunch	Chicken thighs (without skin)
	Green beans
	Rice
Snack	Celery sticks
	Homemade hummus with chickpeas, small amount of garlic, and sunflower oil
Dinner	Steak, nonaged beef
	Confetti Brussels Sprouts (page 288)
	Rutabaga Fries (page 290)
	Quinoa
	Baked Pears or Apples (page 308; choose pears and peel the fruit)

SUPPLEMENTS AND ADDITIONAL CONSIDERATION TO HELP WITH FOOD CHEMICAL INTOLERANCE

Improving sulfation and the underlying contributing factors is the best thing to do to increase salicylate, amine, and glutamate tolerance. Methylation and transsulfuration are connected to sulfation and come before it, so cofactor nutrients for these pathways should be considered, too. The following supplements and practices can help.

Sulfation nutrients: Increasing sulfate levels can improve sulfation. Epsom salt baths or other transdermal magnesium sulfate applications increase sulfate levels and often sulfation capacity. When added to a warm bath, the magnesium and sulfate in Epsom salt can absorb through the skin and be available for biochemical needs such as sulfation. My clients and Nourishing Hope families are often able to better tolerate salicylates and amines when they are taking regular Epsom salt baths.

In our 2018 study, participants added 2 cups of Epsom salt (and ½ cup of baking soda, used to increase absorption of Epsom salt) to a bathtub and soaked for twenty minutes, twice per week.[8] There was a greater increase in sulfate levels when Epsom salt was added compared to past studies on nutritional supplements (containing sulfate) without Epsom salt baths.[9] After our study concluded, 70 percent of parents intended to continue with the Epsom salt baths. Caregivers and individuals with ASD said that Epsom salts improved anxiety, hyperactivity, irritability, sleep, and aggression.[10]

MSM (methylsulfonylmethane) provides the body with sulfur and increases sulfation. While NAC (N-acetyl cysteine) can help increase sulfate through increasing cysteine, it's unknown whether individuals with autism have low cysteine, as a study showed that two individuals with ASD both had low sulfate but high cysteine.[11] Fish oil, vitamin B_2, and vitamin B_5 can also be helpful for individuals with low sulfate. For people who can't convert sulfite to sulfate, and it gets stuck at sulfite, molybdenum supplementation can be helpful.

Phenol enzyme: Enzymes such as No-Fenol by Houston Enzymes break down the carbohydrate structure of the plant food with xylanase. This enzyme can often help children who can't tolerate phenols add some moderate ones to their diet. It may not completely eliminate reactions but often increases tolerance capacity.

DAO enzyme: This helps break down histamine from foods for people who have histamine intolerance. It can help improve tolerance and reduce reactions to histamine foods for many people.

Reducing salicylate levels: Baking soda (bicarbonate) and activated charcoal have been found to be helpful for reducing salicylate levels— baking soda by increasing clearance of salicylate, and early administration of activated charcoal in reducing absorption.[12]

Methylation nutrients: In addition to some nutrients that are commonly available in multivitamin/mineral supplements (folate, B_2, B_3, B_6, B_{12}, zinc, choline—see step 3), betaine, choline, and methionine are methyl donors and cofactors in methylation, so you might want to add those.

Nutrients for glutamate: Vitamin B_6 is required for the conversion from glutamate to GABA, and therefore, supplementation may be beneficial for those with glutamate sensitivity. Additionally, magnesium is important for regulating and decreasing glutamate transmission while increasing GABA neurotransmission; as such, magnesium can provide a calming effect.

Microbiome/Dysbiosis support: Addressing pathogenic bacteria and other microorganisms in the gut can help improve sulfation. These organisms can give off phenols that require our sulfation to mop up, depleting our sulfation capacity. This is an area where integrative and functional medicine doctors are helpful and discussed further in "Beyond Diet and Nutrition."

READY FOR THE NEXT STEP?

If you have determined that a low salicylate, low amine, low histamine, low glutamate, or my combination low SAG diet is something you want to try, it usually takes one to three months to implement one of the dietary trials, fine-tune the diet according to the foods your child can tolerate (and in what quantities), and add the additional supplementation. Look for improvements in common symptoms associated with those foods, but also any other symptom improvements your child has, and write them down to track progress.

If you've tried one of the single-compound diets and some symptoms have improved but not others or not as much as you'd like, consider some of the other intolerances in this step.

Once you have reached a stable place with symptom improvements, you are likely ready for the next step. Or you might choose to stay here and not add or change anything for a while if you're satisfied with your child's progress.

If you determine that this diet is not right during the dietary trial, then stop this diet and move on to the next step you determine is right for you.

Remember that as your child improves in various underlying deficiencies and conditions, they may gain more tolerance for foods they were once sensitive to. This is especially true for salicylates. Once you feel you've arrived at the right bioindividual nutrition plan for your child (be it a low SAG plan or a combination with diets in later steps of the program), you may want to occasionally revisit the food trials in this step to see if your child has gained tolerance and you can loosen up any of the food restrictions.

STEP 8
Food Sensitivity Elimination Diets

Sometimes, people use the terms *food intolerance* and *food sensitivity* synonymously. But in this step, we'll be using more precise definitions. Food sensitivities are immune system reactions, while (in my definition) food intolerance is a wider term that covers any food reaction. So, a food sensitivity is a type of food intolerance, but a food intolerance is not always a food sensitivity. Food sensitivities are the focus of step 8.

Food sensitivities trigger the immune system, causing inflammation and chronic symptoms like congestion, constipation, and gastrointestinal pain. Food sensitivities and food allergies are both antibody reactions of the immune system. However, although both are immune system responses, the reactions are different because the body uses a different "weapon" in each instance to counter a perceived attack. These weapons are a type of antibody called immunoglobulins.

A food allergy triggers the production of immunoglobulin E (IgE) antibodies. There is often an immediate response with symptoms including hives; itching; tingling in the mouth; swelling of the tongue, lips, and throat; wheezing; congestion; vomiting; diarrhea; dizziness; fainting; difficulty breathing; and anaphylaxis. Parents often discover their child has a food allergy quickly, as the symptoms happen soon after ingestion and are usually pretty clear.

Food sensitivities, on the other hand, are mediated by immunoglobulin G (IgG). These are delayed reactions that produce more chronic inflammation like congestion and constipation (or diarrhea). Because of the delay and chronic nature, people can go many years without realizing they may have a food sensitivity.

COMMON SYMPTOMS OF FOOD SENSITIVITIES

The following are some of the most common food sensitivity symptoms:

- ❏ Congestion or runny nose
- ❏ Dark circles under eyes
- ❏ Diarrhea or constipation
- ❏ Ear infections
- ❏ Eczema/Skin rashes
- ❏ Gas/Bloating or digestive pain
- ❏ Hyperactivity
- ❏ Immune/Autoimmune reactions
- ❏ Inattentiveness
- ❏ Incontinence/Bedwetting
- ❏ Inflammation or pain (muscle or joint)
- ❏ Irritability, anxiety, depression, or behavioral challenges
- ❏ Nausea/Vomiting
- ❏ Reflux
- ❏ Remaining digestive issues on gluten-free/dairy-free diet
- ❏ Sleep apnea
- ❏ Stomachaches

FOOD ALLERGIES AND SENSITIVITIES IN AUTISM

A meta-analysis found an association between what researchers called food hypersensitivity (which included food allergy, food intolerance, elevated IgG and IgE, and parental reports of food reactions) and autism.[1]

Food allergies are common in children and even more so in children with autism. In a survey of parents, 13.1 percent of children with autism had food allergies—a rate two and a half times higher than neurotypical children.[2] The most common food allergies in the United States (for all children, not just those with autism) are peanut, milk, shellfish, tree nut, egg, fish, wheat, soy, and sesame.[3]

While food *allergies* are common in autism, food *sensitivities* are even more common. In one study, 89.89 percent of children with autism had at least one food sensitivity and a majority had multiple sensitivities. And in this study, IgG reactions to foods were associated with higher stereotyped autism behaviors.[4] High IgG levels can cause increased food hyperreactivity. One researcher found higher levels of circulating IgG antibodies in those with autism and postulated that it is a cause of the increased food reaction (allergy) in ASD.[5] This hyperreactivity results in inflammation, which typically begins locally in the gastrointestinal tract and may affect other parts of the body such as the brain.

However, assessing IgG levels can be a bit confusing. Even healthy children can have elevated IgG levels, and they don't always cause food reactivity and inflammation. It is suspected that when individuals have good oral tolerance (no immune system response) and no leaky gut, these elevated IgG levels do not seem to cause reactions.[6]

Food Sensitivities Affect the GI Tract and Brain

Food sensitivities can contribute to intestinal inflammation and irritable bowel syndrome (IBS). In a study, a group of adults with inflammatory bowel disease (IBD) had significantly higher IgG antibodies than controls, and one-third of patients in the study had chronic low-grade intestinal inflammation (which was not due to bacterial infections). The top IgG reactions were as follows: 53.3 percent to cow milk, 40 percent to egg white, 33.3 percent to wheat, 26.8 percent to hazelnut, 26.7 percent to garlic, and 20 percent to orange and tomato.[7]

Multiple studies show children with autism have high IgG levels from food and gastrointestinal symptoms.[8] In one study of children with autism, 84 percent had a sensitivity to eggs, 65 percent had a sensitivity to milk, and 38 percent had a sensitivity to wheat. In this study, children with autism had almost twice the rates of GI symptoms compared to neurotypical children. What was particularly interesting about this study is that they also looked at aberrant eating behaviors (food refusal, feeding difficulties) and found that both picky eating and IgG levels were associated with high levels of autism behaviors.[9] By now, you're probably not surprised to hear that picky eating is associated with ASD, but the fact that higher IgG levels were associated with higher levels of autism behaviors is a significant finding.

Food sensitivities may also cause neurological symptoms. Studies have showed that children with food allergies are more likely to have autism, ADHD, and psychiatric conditions.[10] And individuals with food sensitivities are found have higher rates of anxiety, headaches, and insomnia,[11] as well as depression.[12] Antibodies from food reactions can cause autoimmune reactions and negatively affect the brain.[13]

Top Food Sensitivities in Autism

The most common food sensitivities I see in children with autism are dairy, wheat, soy, eggs, and corn, as well as citrus and nuts (many of the same foods as the top food allergies). Food sensitivity is one of the reasons that gluten, casein, and soy are removed in step 5. While these are some of the most common, I have seen people with sensitivities to many other foods, including rice, turkey, beef, cantaloupe, cucumber, lettuce, quinoa, potato, and squash. Almost anything, you name it, can cause a reaction.

As an aside, it's interesting to note that food sensitivities change by geographical region, since they are based on what the immune system interacts with most often (that is, what people eat most often). I learned about a great example when my last book, *Nourishing Hope for Autism*, was translated into Japanese. In Japan, buckwheat (not related to wheat) is a common sensitivity and allergy. This is because buckwheat is common in the Japanese diet.

Let's take a moment to look at corn and egg reactions, as these are some of the most commonly problematic foods in my practice (after gluten, casein, and soy).

Corn

Around 1 percent of the population may have a corn allergy.[14] Although it may be less prevalent as an allergen than, say, dairy or egg, it is often of big concern for many of my clients and Nourishing Hope families. I hypothesize that because we are exposed to corn so frequently, we are more likely to develop a sensitivity (especially when we have leaky gut).

One of the big problems with corn is that it is hidden in many foods. Children get exposed to corn regularly, often multiple times per day. Corn is used to make cornstarch, corn syrup, citric acid, and other ingredients, so it can be found in many foods: breads, baked goods, powdered sugar, pudding, ice cream, salad dressings, bacon, and more.

In our survey study of therapeutic diets, a corn-free diet had a moderate to good benefit rating and zero adverse effects rating.[15] After general benefits, the most common improvements in children with autism were diarrhea in 26 percent and constipation in 22 percent, and 17 percent had improvements in aggression.

Corn can cause food reactions, and they can be severe. I had a client with such severe allergies to corn that it caused seizures, even when ingested in trace amounts (such as the small amount of citric acid used to age beef). Corn is highly susceptible to fungus, particularly *Fusarium*, and the mycotoxins from this fungus in corn can cause negative health effects in humans.[16] Some corn is also genetically modified, causing concerns to doctors and livestock veterinarians because of the lack of research on its safety for humans (and the environment). Additionally, excess corn consumption while lacking in other foods and nutrition can cause niacin deficiency, called pellagra.[17] So, there are several reasons why I suggest that most of my clients minimize corn and eat only organic corn products when they do.

Ingredients to look for in foods if your child is sensitive to corn include:

- Citric acid
- Corn flour
- Cornmeal
- Corn oil
- Corn syrup
- Cornstarch
- Dextrin
- Dextrose
- High fructose corn syrup
- Hydrolyzed corn protein
- Maltodextrin
- Modified starch
- Vegetable starch
- Vodka (and other alcohol with corn such as bourbon and beer)
- Xylitol (unless made from birch bark)

Eggs

Studies show eggs are one of the top sensitivities among children with autism. In individuals with a suspected food intolerance, egg sensitivity was the highest food reaction in one study, with 54.7 percent positive for an IgG reaction.[18] Eggs are also one of the most common allergens. On the other hand, eggs have important nutritional qualities. They are a good source of protein and are high in choline for methylation. So, removing egg from your child's diet is something that should be carefully considered.

Leaky gut has been associated with egg IgG sensitivities (along with wheat and dairy), and researchers propose that leaky gut may cause the sensitivity or the sensitivity may cause leaky gut.[19]

There was also a strong cross-reactivity between egg and cerebellar peptides (i.e., brain proteins) in a study of children with autism; this condition can increase the concerns of autoimmune reactions to brain tissue with egg.[20] An egg-free dietary trial or food sensitivity testing can be beneficial to determine whether eggs are causing a problem.

ABOUT THE ELIMINATION DIET

An elimination diet eliminates foods your child reacts to or foods you suspect they might react to. There is no strict definition of an elimination diet, but most often it removes the top sensitivities such as wheat, gluten, dairy, soy, eggs, corn, citrus, nuts, seafood, chocolate, and sugar. (Gluten, casein, and soy are three of the most problematic food sensitivities and therefore are usually removed in the first half of the program, as mentioned. But if you haven't removed gluten, casein, and soy yet, now is a good time to consider doing so!)

There are two purposes for an elimination diet. An elimination diet can be a way of testing if your child might be reactive to foods. Additionally, an elimination diet is a helpful tool for addressing known food sensitivities.

Low levels of digestive enzymes, poor digestion, leaky gut, antibodies to foods in the blood are common in autism. And researchers are now recommending an elimination diet to address it. Researchers discuss their theory of the "fragile gut" in autism (that involves poor digestive enzymes and digestion, leaky gut, food IgG antibodies, and microbial dysbiosis) and suggest that designing a personalized diet based on tolerated food proteins will improve the function of the gastrointestinal system in those with autism.[21]

Let's look at some research on an elimination diet. Eighty-five percent of parents in one study found an elimination diet (which included turkey, lamb, rice, vegetables, fruit, pear juice, and water) for children with ADHD decreased symptoms by over 50 percent, and teachers found similar results with decreases in hyperactivity/impulsivity and inattentiveness.[22]

In a study on children with infantile autism (ASD that was recognized during infancy), participants were put on a casein-free diet that also eliminated any other allergens they tested positive for. After eight weeks on the diet, they had significant improvement in behavior.[23]

Regardless of what other dietary choices you make for your child, an elimination diet helps refine their overall food plan.

Once you've determined which foods your child is sensitive to, depending on how and why the reaction occurs, they may need to avoid those foods for the long term. As such, the resulting diet is personalized. It's different for everyone and is based on your child's individual reactions.

From there, these food restrictions can be continued while you move on to any additional steps of the program to create the best personalized therapeutic diet for your child.

HOW TO DETERMINE WHETHER AN ELIMINATION DIET IS RIGHT FOR YOUR CHILD

Does your child have common symptoms of food intolerance or sensitivity? Has the GFCF diet and/or the low salicylate/amine diet not improved symptoms as you'd hoped? These are some of the instances where I'd consider an elimination diet. An elimination diet can often help with gastrointestinal symptoms, headaches, congestion, pain, anxiety, and other symptoms caused by inflammatory foods.

Lab Testing for Food Sensitivities

Food sensitivity testing is one way to determine if an elimination diet would be appropriate and which foods your child might benefit from avoiding. (If you have already run food sensitivity testing, consider implementing some of those findings into your child's personalized diet and nutrition plan.) There are different tests for food sensitivities. Some test IgG antibody levels to foods, others test IgM or IgA antibodies (other types of immunoglobulins), and some test a cell-mediated response. Each can be helpful to some extent; any data can be beneficial. And lab tests for food sensitivities can be helpful if you want to test a wide range of foods.

However, I often find that these tests are not consistent across the board. Colleagues have sent split patient samples to multiple labs and received different results. There is not one test that I have found to be 100 percent accurate and inclusive of all food reactions. Tests can be inaccurate or inconsistent for a number of reasons, including the type of food the lab is testing against. For example, raw uncooked rice may react differently than cooked rice, and not all labs use the same substance. It likely involves bioindividuality—the underlying reasons the person is reacting will determine which test is most accurate and helpful. Also, again, "higher" or "lower" levels in your results don't necessarily correlate to the severity of the reaction in the body.

Additionally, food sensitivity testing typically requires a blood draw or finger prick, which may limit options for some families. You'll want to weigh the pros and cons on a blood draw or finger prick with the data you will get back and why you want to know.

If you don't want to do a finger prick or a blood draw to do testing, then a food elimination diet can be used as your "test." Even if you opt for food sensitivity testing, I find it's important to later test these results with a food elimination diet to get a more accurate sense about whether they are really affecting your child and whether they improve over time. Food elimination diets are the gold standard for food sensitivities. In our therapeutic diet study, both methods, observation and IgG/IgE testing, were helpful. While IgG and IgE testing offered slightly better net benefit, a food avoidance diet based on observation was in the top five highest-ranked diets for fifteen symptom improvements.

IMPLEMENTING AN ELIMINATION DIET

The process of implementing and following an elimination diet depends on whether you are using it to test for sensitivities or as a healing diet for known sensitivities.

If you are using the diet to test for food sensitivities, here's what you'll do. After removing foods on the "avoid" list of a standard elimination diet, look for the reduction of symptoms to see if you are on the right track. The elimination stage lasts two to three weeks. *This elimination phase is*

érieurctcheck

very broad and is not a forever diet. Afterward, there is often a testing back phase lasting another three weeks, where foods are reintroduced for a few days one at a time (sometimes people refer to this as a "provocation phase"). Here, you'll check for the return or flare-up of certain symptoms associated with food intolerance. (However, it's best to not test back foods that you know, or suspect, are a big problem. If you already know that these foods are problematic from testing or prior dietary experience, you often skip this testing phase for those foods.)

If you're using it for healing, having already identified the foods you want to remove with food sensitivity testing, you'll eliminate any food sensitivities from the diet. You'll continue to keep any identified problematic foods out of the diet for typically three to six months, unless you have evidence or feel that they are no longer causing a problem. This three- to six-month period is intended to reduce the immune system response to these foods, ideally improving tolerance over time. At this point, you might retest these foods if you are interested in adding them back. If they appear to be tolerated, you might reintroduce them or do a rotation diet if warranted.

AVOID   Foods to Avoid on an Elimination Diet

x	Wheat and gluten grains (barley, conventional oats, kamut, rye, spelt, wheat)	x	Soy (edamame, miso, soy milk, soy protein, soy sauce, tofu)
x	Dairy/casein (cow, goat, sheep, and other dairy)	x	Foods sometimes avoided: beef, coconut, and seeds
x	Sesame	x	Chocolate
x	Corn	x	Refined sugar
x	Eggs	x	Coffee
x	Shellfish	x	Alcohol
x	Fish	x	Artificial additives
x	Peanuts	x	Tree nuts
x	Personal allergies or sensitivities	x	Citrus

CHOOSE   Foods to Choose on an Elimination Diet

✓ Fruits (except citrus)

✓ Beans (any except soy): Such as black, garbanzo/chickpeas, hummus, lentils, pinto, refried beans

✓ Flours/Starches: Including arrowroot, potato starch, and tapioca starch

✓ Non-dairy milk: Such as coconut milk (if tolerated), pea milk, or rice milk

✓ Oils: Including avocado oil, coconut oil (if tolerated), and olive oil

✓ Winter squash

✓ Vegetables: Any non-starchy vegetables such as broccoli, carrots, celery, green beans, kale, etc. (except corn)

✓ Meat: Any fresh meat—beef, buffalo, chicken, lamb, pork, turkey

✓ Root vegetables: Such as potatoes and sweet potatoes

✓ Grains: Including brown rice, buckwheat, millet, quinoa, and wild rice

One Day of Elimination Diet Meals

Breakfast	Chicken Apple Sausage (page 273)
	Green Smoothie (page 310)
Lunch	Super Nutrient Burgers (page 277) with lettuce wrap
	Carrot Chips (page 291)
	Rainbow Salad (page 289)
Snack	Red bell peppers
	Strawberries
	Roasted Chickpeas (page 302)
	Cherry Apple Cider Vinegar Drink (page 311)
Dinner	Lamb Stew (page 279)
	Air-Fried Popcorn Cauliflower (page 299)
	Green salad
	Blueberries

IMPLEMENTING A ROTATION DIET

A rotation diet is another option for people with food sensitivities. In a rotation diet, a person rotates foods to avoid eating the same food each day. For example, on a four-day rotation diet, if they eat chicken on the first day, they don't eat chicken again for the remaining three days. This gives the immune system a rest, which can help reduce overall stress on the immune system and improve the hypersensitive response to foods. The short-term break from the foods can allow those foods to be better tolerated and possibly prevent new sensitivities from forming (say, if a person knows they have leaky gut and are prone to reaction).

In a study of women with IBS, participants were put in one of three diets: a rotation diet, low FODMAP diet (discussed in step 11), or no special diet as controls. While the low FODMAP group had improvements in mucus in stool and bloating, the group on the rotation diet had significantly better improvements in symptoms that included abdominal pain after a meal and upon a bowel movement.[24]

I find rotation diets are great for someone who is reactive to many foods—whether those sensitivities were identified through lab testing or an elimination diet trial. They might apply a rotation diet to the foods that don't cause reactions to reduce their chance of developing more sensitivities. Or they might do a rotation diet with low-sensitivity foods if they can't or don't want to remove them all. For example, in my practice, if a child has forty-five foods show up on their food sensitivity panel, I'd likely suggest removing the big offenders and rotating the other foods. If someone came to me with cantaloupe, broccoli, quinoa, cucumber, apple, pear, celery, lettuce, rice, beans, and another thirty-five foods that were low sensitivities on their test—and it wasn't possible to remove all of them without creating a very limited and nutrient-poor diet—I'd suggest a rotation diet.

There are different ways to do a rotation diet. Some people rotate only certain foods; others rotate all foods. Additionally, some people rotate whole food families, not just individual foods (for example carrots, parsnip, celery are all in the Apiaceae family; someone might choose to rotate them all so they're eating from among those veggies only once per rotation). The table on page 186 is an example of a four-day rotation diet of individual foods.

SUPPLEMENTS AND ADDITIONAL CONSIDERATION TO HELP FOOD SENSITIVITIES

Digestive enzymes can be helpful with food sensitivities. Digestive enzymes break down the protein causing the reaction into individual amino acids. They can be particularly helpful when digestion is weak and needs help, which is often the case with leaky gut and food sensitivities.

However, taking enzymes doesn't give your child a license to eat unlimited amounts of these foods. I still recommend my clients remove the foods and use digestive enzymes mostly to protect if there is cross-contamination with foods that are highly reactive or with foods on a rotation diet.

READY FOR THE NEXT STEP?

If you suspect your child has food sensitivities and decide to implement step 8, the amount of time to do the elimination diet before proceeding depends on the person (as with any diet!). I suggest a minimum of a few weeks, but a few months might be advantageous as well. Once you feel enough time has gone by that those foods are out of the system and no longer causing reactions in your child, you're ready to go to the next step.

Four Days of Rotation Diet Meals

Meal	Day 1	Day 2	Day 3	Day 4
	Chicken **Grain-Free** **Almond** **Egg-Free**	**Beef** **Rice** **Sunflower Seeds** **Egg-Free**	**Turkey** **Potato** **Cashew** **Eggs**	**Pork** **Gluten-Free Oats** **Nut-Free** **Egg-Free**
Breakfast	Chicken sausage Carrot fries Berries	Muffin with rice flour, pureed pumpkin, and flaxseed egg substitute Apple with sunflower butter	Eggs Turkey sausage Blueberries	Bacon Gluten-free oatmeal
Lunch	Chicken drumsticks Peas Fruit	Hamburger with a lettuce wrap Pickle Fruit	Sliced turkey Hummus and carrots Fruit	Pork sausage Carrot chips Fruit
Snack	Almonds Pear	Banana Sunflower seeds	Potato/veggie latkes Cashews	Applesauce with pureed raw sauerkraut Leftover bacon from a.m.
Dinner	Roasted chicken Butternut squash fries Broccoli	Beef stir-fry with vegetables Rice	Turkey meatballs with pureed veggies Dipping sauce Potato	Pork chop Sweet potato fries Green beans

STEP 9
Grain-Free Diets

In step 5, we remove wheat and related gluten grains because they are the grains most researched and found to be problematic. However, other grains also have compounds that are an issue for many individuals, including some of those with ASD. Nongluten grains contain gliadin-like compounds called prolamins and lectins that cause inflammation and leaky gut.[1] These grains include corn, oats, rice, and sorghum. Another component in grains that people have difficulty with is the starch. (Most of the diets we'll cover in this step remove all starchy foods, not just grains.)

Grains and other starchy foods, like potatoes, require many steps for digestion and absorption. In fact, humans cannot break down all starches ourselves. We require beneficial bacteria to break down (i.e., ferment) some carbohydrates for us. From there, we need carbohydrate-digesting enzymes to further break things down and, next, monosaccharides to transport the remaining single-molecule sugars to the bloodstream. All three of these areas—the microbiome, carbohydrate-digesting enzymes,[2] and monosaccharide transport[3]—tend to be impaired in children with autism compared to neurotypical children. All of this can cause or compound irritation, inflammation, and dysbiosis in the gut. By reducing starch and grain intake, you can give your child's gut a chance to heal.

Additionally, grains contain phytates that bind to and inhibit the absorption of nutrients. Furthermore, some grains (but fortunately not all of them) are also high in oxalates and/or FODMAPs. We will talk about oxalates and FODMAPs in the next two steps.

For these reasons, grain-free diets can be beneficial therapeutic strategies for those with autism. I typically recommend a grain-free diet after my client has tried steps 5 and 8, as it is a good next step when a child is still experiencing gastrointestinal and inflammatory conditions. And because of the gut-brain connection, these diets can provide noticeable improvements in brain function. In this step, we'll explore different grain-free diets: the Specific Carbohydrate Diet (SCD), Gut and Psychology Syndrome (GAPS) Diet, and the Paleo diet.

COMMON SYMPTOMS OF GRAIN AND STARCH INTOLERANCE

Digestive symptoms like diarrhea, constipation, and smelly gas are good clues that the gut needs more help. And your doctor can help you determine whether it's microbiome related or due to some other cause. Grains and starches can directly cause some symptoms (such as diarrhea) on the following list. With other signs (such as language difficulties), grains aren't the cause per se, but cutting them out still improves them. In either case, a grain-free diet may be beneficial.

- ❑ Cognitive challenges
- ❑ Constipation
- ❑ Diarrhea
- ❑ Digestive pain
- ❑ Gas/Bloating
- ❑ Glucose/Blood sugar metabolism
- ❑ Inattentiveness
- ❑ Language difficulties
- ❑ Learning difficulties

❏   Mood and mental health challenges accompanied by digestive
    issues
❏   Remaining digestive issues after gluten-free/dairy-free diet

HOW TO DETERMINE WHETHER A GRAIN-FREE DIET IS RIGHT FOR YOUR CHILD

Look at the list of symptoms on page 188, and consider whether your child has these symptoms. You can also consider lab testing or a grain-free diet trial to see if their symptoms improve; in that case, you will need to decide which to follow.

Lab Testing for Grain-Free Diets

Testing whether someone needs a grain-free and starch-free diet is a bit challenging. Some doctors may run tests on the microbes in the gut or a small intestinal bacterial overgrowth (SIBO) breath test to get a picture of the microbiome. This provides some data that might point people to one of these diets. There is also a comprehensive digestive stool analysis that shows biomarkers of gut inflammation that also might indicate the benefit of a diet like this.

While you can't definitively determine a condition based on symptoms alone, digestive symptoms provide clues and a simple way to monitor the health of your child's gut and assess whether a grain-free diet is working. Diarrhea, constipation, abdominal pain, bloating, and flatulence are signs that digestion and the gastrointestinal tract need support and healing.

The dietary rules are different, but the benefits are similar among grain-free diets. These diets are helpful for gastrointestinal issues. And since the gut and brain are connected and digestive conditions are common in those with autism, these diets can help improve symptoms of autism, as well as overall health and well-being.

If you decide a grain-free diet might be right for your child, the next step is to choose a specific dietary approach. These grain-free diets remove more than just grains. They each limit certain carbohydrates and sugars, but the rules are different. Which diet to choose really depends on a few factors. Let's look at each, so that you can decide which might be the best fit.

THE SPECIFIC CARBOHYDRATE DIET

The Specific Carbohydrate Diet (SCD) was developed by Sidney Haas, MD, in the 1930s and 1940s for his patients with "pediatric celiac" and various inflammatory bowel conditions such as ulcerative colitis.[4] Instead of removing only gluten for celiac disease (as we do today), Haas removed all grains, as well as other starches and sugars. As many practitioners today are recognizing digestive and other problems with all grains, he may have been ahead of his time. SCD was later popularized in the 1990s by Elaine Gottschall, a patient of Dr. Haas, with her book *Breaking the Vicious Cycle*.

SCD restricts disaccharides (double sugars) and polysaccharides (starches). It removes all grains and starches, including rice, bread, pasta, potatoes, and some beans, as well as maple syrup, table sugar, and more. However, it still includes monosaccharides, such as honey, fruits, and non-starchy vegetables.

This diet works by restricting carbohydrate foods that cannot be adequately digested. The biological reasoning behind this diet is as follows: When someone can't digest disaccharides, they linger in the gut, providing extra food for bacteria and causing microbial overgrowth. This leads to inflammation and mucous that interferes with digestive enzyme availability. The lack of enzymes further decreases carbohydrate breakdown, and a vicious cycle ensues. This contributes to more damage in the gut. Avoiding these sugars and starches helps bypass this reaction and heal the gut.

This diet has been used by many people for digestive conditions with great success. In a survey of 417 individuals with inflammatory bowel disease (IBD) including Crohn's disease and ulcerative colitis, 33 percent reported remission of their condition after two months on SCD, and 42 percent reported remission after six and twelve months. Response to SCD can be very quick, with 13 percent having remission of their condition in less than two weeks. And although 80 percent had abdominal pain before the diet, only 7 percent had abdominal pain after twelve months. Not only did symptoms improve but laboratory values improved, indicating that the gut is healing.[5]

SCD FOR ASD

The SCD has been shown to be helpful in autism. In fact, one of the most compelling studies out there is by a colleague and graduate of my Bio-Individual Nutrition Institute training program for professionals, Silvija Ābele, PhD. Her study of twenty-seven children with ASD put seventeen of the participants on the SCD/GAPS Diet. (SCD is similar to another diet, the Gut and Psychology Syndrome, or GAPS, Diet, which I'll cover in the following section; they are sometimes referred to collectively as SCD/GAPS.) Participants followed SCD/GAPS for three months along with taking omega-3s, ascorbyl palmitate, vitamin D, vitamin C, and probiotics. The participants' Autism Treatment Evaluation Checklist (ATEC) scores decreased significantly, by 23 percent, in the SCD diet group compared to before the intervention. Health/behavior, socializing, irritability, and hyperactivity were the greatest areas of improvement. Parents also felt symptoms improved significantly, 43 percent in the SCD/GAPS group compared to 14 percent in the control group.[6]

There is also the case study in the scientific literature of a four-year-old boy with ASD and fragile X syndrome who was put on SCD. On this diet, his nutritional status and GI symptoms (specifically constipation) improved. He also had improvements in sensory and repetitive behaviors, reduction in fears, and improvements in expressive and receptive language, memory, and learning.[7] This case study mirrors what I've seen in my practice: As the gut improves, so do the brain and behavior.

In our therapeutic diets/survey study, caregivers reported moderate to good benefit from SCD. Of those that found benefit, 57 percent had general benefit, 24 percent had improvements in attention, 22 percent in cognition, 19 percent in diarrhea, and 19 percent in anxiety. Irritability, language, social interaction, hyperactivity, aggression, and sensory sensitivity also improved.

GUT AND PSYCHOLOGY SYNDROME DIET

The Gut and Psychology Syndrome (GAPS) Diet, named for the connection between the gut and brain, is based on the diet principles of the SCD with some additions and changes. Created by Dr. Natasha Campbell-McBride, the GAPS Diet was specifically designed for people like her son with autism and other neurological issues.

Like SCD, the GAPS Diet restricts rice, corn, and other grains, potatoes and starches, certain beans, and most sugars except monosaccharides; in fact, nearly all of the foods *removed* are the same between both diets. But they differ in which foods and practices they encourage. Let's look at the differences to help you decide between the two.

IMPLEMENTING AN SCD OR GAPS DIET

If you feel your child has dysbiosis, still is having a lot of digestive symptoms, particularly diarrhea, or is intolerant to all grains and starches, SCD or GAPS may be the way to go. To choose between SCD and GAPS, you may want to consider your own personality in addition to other factors.

GAPS has very specific stages and rules about what to eat and when. This is helpful for people who like to have a clear set of rules to follow. This regimented structure works great for some people and not so well for others. The GAPS Diet protocol emphasizes daily consumption of wonderfully nourishing foods such as bone broths and fermented foods, as well as supplements such as high potency probiotics. (It also has further supplements and principles that you'll want to check out to see if you feel it's right for your child in the *Gut and Psychology Syndrome* book or at www .gapsdiet.com.)

SCD, meanwhile, is mostly food focused, with very few supplements allowed or suggested. For example, only very specific probiotics and amounts are allowed on SCD, with no prebiotics.

There are also a few food differences between the diets, though a vast majority are the same, so in my guidelines later in this chapter, I present shared food lists for SCD/GAPS. Both SCD and GAPS have introductory phases that some people implement when getting started. They are a way to begin with easier-to-digest foods and give the gut a chance to calm inflammation and digestive symptoms. I don't find that the introductory phases are strict requirements; however, many people find them advantageous, especially if their child has very significant GI symptoms. SCD's introductory phase is more flexible than GAPS's. Let's look at both.

The SCD Introductory Diet

SCD optionally begins with a two- to five-day introductory phase. The SCD introductory diet includes homemade broth, chicken soup, broiled meat patties or fish, carrots (well cooked and pureed), eggs, gelatin, fruit juice, and homemade yogurt and SCD cheesecake with honey (although if you're trying SCD as part of my program, I of course recommend avoiding those last two because they are made from dairy).

After this two- to five-day period, there are no specific timelines to introduce other foods; however, there are some general guidelines. Vegetables should be peeled and well cooked, and fruits should be ripe and well cooked (applesauce is a great example; bananas don't need to be cooked but should be very ripe with brown spots). Slowly add harder-to-digest foods like lightly cooked or raw fruits and vegetables over time, starting with more digestible forms. Nuts and seeds are recommended only after three months symptom-free, and should be reintroduced in their most digestible forms first. For instance, nut milks will be added before nut butter, next nut flours, and then whole nuts.

While SCD doesn't have official stages past this, there are some very helpful resources that lay out stages based on the SCD principles; you can find these at www.PersonalizedAutismNutritionPlan.com/extras.

The GAPS Introductory Diet

The GAPS Diet begins with a six-stage introductory diet. Stage 1 includes homemade stocks at each meal, homemade soups with boiled meat and vegetables, well-cooked nonfibrous vegetables, probiotic foods (like sauerkraut juice or fermented dairy; again, dairy is not recommended on my plan), ginger tea and water with lemon, and honey. Rather than moving on after a set number of days, you'd wait for diarrhea, constipation, and/or GI pain to subside before moving to the next stage(s) of the introductory diet.

The GAPS introductory diet reintroduces foods slowly, allowing more easily digestible foods before moving to those that are more difficult in the following steps:

- Stage 2 adds raw organic egg yolks, stews and casseroles, and fermented fish.
- Stage 3 adds avocado, vegetable and nut butter–based pancakes, scrambled eggs, cooked fibrous vegetables, and sauerkraut.
- Stage 4 adds roasted and grilled meats, cold-pressed olive oil, vegetable-based juices, and homemade bread made from nut and seed flour.
- Stage 5 adds cooked apple and certain raw vegetables, followed by adding certain fruits to the fresh pressed juices started in stage 4.
- Stage 6 adds certain raw fruits (beginning with peeled apple), dried fruit, sweet baked goods, soaked nuts and seeds, and coconut milk.

These are just the broad strokes; there are more specific instructions in the stages of the GAPS Diet. (You can find these resources on the GAPS

Diet website and at www.PersonalizedAutismNutritionPlan.com/extras.) After most of these foods have been successfully introduced and your child has normal stools, you'd move on to the full GAPS diet.

The Full SCD/GAPS Diet

The full SCD/GAPS Diet includes all of the allowed foods, and of course excludes all those not allowed. Some people prefer to skip the introductory stages and jump straight into the full diet.

If you skip the introductory stages of SCD or GAPS and implement the full diet from the beginning but are not seeing symptoms improve at all after several weeks, you might consider restarting with the introductory stage. Additionally, one caution with the full SCD/GAPS Diet: It can be very high in oxalate when people replace grain flours with nut flours, as these foods are extremely high in oxalate. When eating an SCD/GAPS Diet, it's important to be aware of this so as to not add too much oxalate: As we'll see in step 10, oxalate should remain moderate for all.

If you still aren't seeing results, don't assume it's because you need to do it more strictly. Sometimes a diet might not be right for that person, or it's being implemented with other foods that are not tolerated. SCD/GAPS can be high in salicylates, amines, or oxalates because it often contains broths, fermented foods, and nut flours. Some people personalize the diet, such as not including any legumes on SCD/GAPS (both diets allow a few) or reducing salicylates, amines, or oxalates.

To truly do this diet, no infractions are allowed, so I do not add additional foods to SCD/GAPS, unless you have been following it with success for some time and are evolving the diet into something more customized. This is because additions can really affect the way the diet works, rendering it ineffective. Assuming the diet is offering some benefit, I typically suggest giving the diet four to six months to see its potential, and continuing the diet for six months to a year after symptoms have subsided.

AVOID   Foods to Avoid on SCD/GAPS

x	Agave	x	Maple syrup
x	Amaranth	x	Millet
x	Arrowroot powder	x	Oats
x	Buckwheat	x	Parsnips
x	Cane sugar	x	Potatoes
x	Chia seeds	x	Quinoa
x	Chocolate and cocoa	x	Rice
x	Corn	x	Seaweed
x	Cornstarch	x	Sorghum
x	Flaxseed	x	Stevia
x	Fructose, ingredient	x	Sugar
x	Grains/Grain flours	x	Sweet potatoes
x	Gums and stabilizers	x	Tapioca starch
x	Jicama	x	Wheat
x	Legumes, most		

Foods to Choose on SCD/GAPS

CHOOSE   most nonstarchy vegetables on SCD/GAPS

✓	Asparagus	✓	Cucumbers
✓	Beets	✓	Eggplant
✓	Broccoli	✓	Green beans
✓	Brussels sprouts	✓	Kale
✓	Butternut squash	✓	Lettuce
✓	Cabbage	✓	Red bell peppers
✓	Carrots	✓	Rutabagas
✓	Cauliflower	✓	Tomatoes
✓	Celeriac	✓	Turnips
✓	Celery	✓	Zucchini

CHOOSE   most fresh fruits on SCD/GAPS

✓	Apples	✓	Grapes
✓	Apricots	✓	Oranges
✓	Avocados	✓	Peaches
✓	Bananas with brown spots	✓	Pears
✓	Blackberries	✓	Raspberries
✓	Blueberries	✓	Strawberries
✓	Grapefruit		

CHOOSE   Additional SCD-compliant foods to choose

✓	Beef	✓	Lamb
✓	Chicken	✓	Nut milks, homemade
✓	Coconut	✓	Nuts
✓	Eggs	✓	Oils
✓	Fish	✓	Nut flours
✓	Green Peas	✓	Pumpkin seeds
✓	Honey	✓	Split Peas
✓	Legumes (only navy beans, lima beans, and lentils)	✓	Sunflower seeds

PALEO DIET

The Paleolithic (or Paleo) diet is designed after the diet of our hunter-gatherer ancestors, before humans began to farm and harvest grain and process our food.

The Paleo diet was first introduced by gastroenterologist Walter L. Voegtlin in 1975 for the purpose of addressing GI disorders. Additionally, the diet helps improve the diversity of the gut microbiome.[8] Paleo has also become popular because of its positive effects on blood sugar and insulin and because it can help with weight loss.[9] For autism, the major purpose of the Paleo diet is to support and heal the gut. This will help reduce inflammation and oxidative stress throughout the body, including the brain.

The Paleo diet was reported to improve irritability, cognition, attention, anxiety, and constipation, and it was the top diet for improving tics, self-injury, and OCD in our 2023 study.[10]

Nourishing Hope Stories

"The Nourishing Hope program is working for my son. With diet and lifestyle change, it has helped improve his quality of life. When I tell close friends and family that he has Tourette's, they are all shocked because they don't see him ticcing! This has been life-changing! . . . In fact, since the summer last year, he has flown five times with the Civil Air Patrol. He has even sat on the left seat! He's working on his private pilot license. He himself loves being on the Paleo diet, and he appreciates the changes I've made around the house and in our lifestyle." —*Mom of a fourteen-year-old with Tourette's syndrome*

(In a follow-up email two years later, his mother shared that he was still following the Nourishing Hope program, had flown solo, and was about to take his first solo cross-country trip.) ∎

IMPLEMENTING A PALEO DIET

The Paleo diet is a grain-free diet that does not have as many implementation rules as SCD and GAPS. It is a straightforward list of foods with no special rules or phases to follow. This makes it easier in my opinion.

Paleo allows flaxseed and chia seeds, which are gelatinous substances. SCD and GAPS do not. SCD and GAPS allow some legumes, but Paleo does not allow any.

AVOID   Foods to Avoid on the Paleo Diet

x	Grains	x	Dairy
x	Legumes	x	Refined sugar
x	Industrial seed/vegetable oils	x	Packaged foods with additives and preservatives
x	Processed meats (hot dogs, deli meats)		

CHOOSE   Foods to Choose on the Paleo Diet

✓	Avocados and avocado oil	✓	Nuts/Seeds
✓	Coconut oil	✓	Olive oil
✓	Eggs	✓	Vegetables
✓	Fruits	✓	Wild fish
✓	Grass-fed beef and other meat	✓	Pastured chicken and other poultry

Since the Paleo diet became a popular diet championed by many different nutrition professionals and even chefs, there is not a set of strict rules or a single source of information, as some other diets have. Sweet potatoes and other tubers such as white potatoes are a gray area among Paleo dieters. Technically, our ancestors did eat them (likely in small quantities), but they are digestively problematic for some people. For those who include them, professionals tend to recommend sweet potatoes more than white potatoes. Also, even more controversial, sometimes people include starchy flour products such as arrowroot powder that definitely would not have been part of hunter-gatherers' diet. I avoid all potatoes and starchy tubers on this diet for most of my Nourishing Hope families, unless they are at a good stage of healing and can handle them in small quantities.

Since all three diets are fairly similar, here's an idea of a one-day meal plan for a grain-free diet that also meets the rules of the SCD, GAPS, and Paleo diets (the full diet, not introductory stages).

One Day of Grain-Free Meals

Breakfast	Chicken Pancakes (page 270)
	Mango Ginger Probiotic Smoothie (page 310)
Lunch	Chicken soup with nonstarchy vegetables
	Green beans
	Sauerkraut
Snack	Grain-Free Banana Blueberry Muffins (page 269)
Dinner	Pot Roast (page 280)
	Zucchini Noodles (page 297) with Low Histamine No-Mato Sauce (page 300)
	Coconut Macaroons (page 307)

FURTHER CONSIDERATIONS
FOR GRAIN-FREE DIETS

While SCD and GAPS are comprehensive diets, some of the allowed carbohydrates can be a problem for some people. Those carbohydrates are fermentable carbohydrates known by the acronym FODMAPs (more in step 11). These have similar effects to the starches and sugars discussed in SCD, as they can feed bacteria and cause gut inflammation and digestive symptoms as we will discuss in step 11. In my experience, a small number of people may need a bioindividual nutrition plan that includes SCD and low FODMAP. However, I usually help my clients and families with one diet first, and if they don't see the results they are looking for, I consider adding the other diet principles if needed.

READY FOR THE NEXT STEP?

Give these diets several months to assess whether they are helping and you want to continue them. They are often used for gut healing, and this can take some time. If the diet is helping, your child might benefit from being on the diet for months or years for healing. Once the full diet has been implemented and you feel you have reached a stable place where the symptoms you are looking to address have minimized, it's a good time to proceed to the next step.

If you are not getting the results that you are looking for, begin looking for other therapeutic diets that might need to be added to this one or that might be a better choice than this one. Consider whether other dietary compounds that may have been added during one of these grain-free diets, such as salicylates, amines, oxalates, or FODMAPs, could be an issue, and consider proceeding to those steps.

STEP 10
Low Oxalate Diet

Let's talk oxalate. You might be thinking, *What?! Oxalate is associated with kidney stones. What does it have to do with autism?* Yes, oxalate is commonly known for causing kidney stones. However, oxalate can create more systemic issues that affect many systems in the body. And research shows that oxalate can be a problem in ASD—and that high oxalate in the body may even be a *cause* of autism.[1]

This diet requires a slow removal of oxalate over time, so this diet is not one of the first dietary trials I suggest. For example, removing salicylates, eggs, or grains from the diet can be done rapidly for a fairly quick dietary trial, compared to removing oxalate. However, having the low oxalate diet as step 10 does not mean it's a less important diet. A low oxalate diet can be life-changing for those that need it.

WHAT IS OXALATE?

Oxalate molecules are found mainly in plants. Plants create oxalate to store and regulate calcium and as a defense against insects. Oxalate is found in high amounts in spinach, nuts, soy, beans, beets, and potatoes, to name a few plant foods.

Oxalate binds to certain minerals, particularly calcium, as well as to magnesium, iron, sodium, and potassium—although not zinc.[2] As such, high oxalate foods are also often high in calcium. This means that many of the vegetables people choose because of their high calcium content—for instance, spinach—also come with a big dose of oxalate. Unfortunately, the calcium is bound to that oxalate, which renders the calcium unable to be absorbed and therefore useless. We've known for nearly a century that the calcium in spinach isn't bioavailable, evidenced by a rat study from 1939. Furthermore, in this study, not only was the calcium in the spinach unable to be absorbed, but the oxalate level was so high that it inhibited the utilization of the calcium *in the rest of the meal*.[3] But this nutrition fact is rarely discussed, and even today, spinach is praised for its high calcium and nutrient content. In reality, because of its high oxalate content, spinach can contribute to reduced bone quantity and quality.[4] Oxalate inhibits mineral absorption and contributes to mineral deficiency.

Eating high oxalate foods isn't the only reason oxalate levels can be elevated in the body, however. Let's take a closer look.

WHAT CAUSES ELEVATED OXALATE AND WHERE DOES IT COME FROM?

Oxalate can come from outside the body or inside the body. Whether these sources of oxalate become a problem and cause elevated oxalate levels in the body or not depend on additional factors.

Dietary/Exogenous Oxalate

Up to 50 percent of oxalate in the body comes from the diet.[5] Normally, the body can handle oxalate in average dietary amounts (see "Moderate Oxalate for All" later in this chapter for more considerations). In a healthy individual, only about 10 to 15 percent of dietary oxalate is absorbed through the gut.[6] The oxalate we eat is bound to calcium and other minerals, limiting the amount the gut absorbs, so instead it's excreted in the stool. Also, certain beneficial bacteria, such as *Oxalobacter formigenes*, normally break down oxalate, reducing harmful effects.

However, when the gut is permeable or the oxalate is not bound to minerals, such as with a low-calcium diet, then oxalate absorption increases, causing serious problems.[7] Dysbiosis is another factor because the gut lacks the bacteria that break down oxalate. And antibiotic use is known to kill off these bacteria that degrade oxalate.[8] Because modern medicine has now experienced three generations of widespread use of antibiotics since World War II, scientists are now identifying a new type of dysbiosis that is caused by the loss of bacteria and fungus that break down oxalate and other toxins. In fact, Susan Owens, a pioneer in oxalate research and leader in a community sixty-eight thousand strong (Trying Low Oxalates, or TLO), has consulted with about two thousand individuals, and after reviewing lab tests conducted before and after antimicrobial treatment, she believes the biggest source of problems is the overuse of antimicrobial medications. Consistent with that impression, microbiologists are finding that humans and other mammals rely on a complex organization of thousands of bacteria (and fungus) to work to degrade oxalate.[9]

Moreover, oxalate can be a cause of dysbiosis, killing beneficial bacteria and greatly altering bacterial communities.[10] This dysbiosis can include SIBO,[11] or *Candida* changing from its less harmful yeast state into its more harmful state.[12] Unfortunately, leaky gut, mineral deficiencies, dysbiosis, and antibiotic use (attributed to increased rates of infection)[13] are common in autism.

Furthermore, inflammatory bowel disease (IBD) can lead to high oxalate because, when our digestion is poor, fat is not able to be absorbed.[14] This fat binds to the calcium that would normally bind to oxalate, which allows the oxalate to remain free and be absorbed into the bloodstream. As we know, digestive disorders are common in ASD.

Vitamin Deficiencies and Endogenous Oxalate Production

In addition to oxalate coming from the diet, oxalate can also be generated inside the body. This is called endogenous oxalate production, and this mainly happens in the liver. The body can convert substances such as vitamin C, glycine, xylitol, and fructose into oxalate.[15] Endogenous oxalate production also results from nutrient deficiencies of such vitamins as A, B_1, and B_6,[16] as well as glutathione[17] (all common in autism). Vitamin B_1 is crucial for oxalate-degrading bacteria to break down oxalate,[18] vitamin A and B_6 deficiencies can also lead to increased absorption of oxalate into the blood,[19] and B_6 deficiency plays an important role in elevated oxalate levels in the body because it is a main cause of endogenous oxalate production and contributes to increased absorption of oxalate from the gut.

Because oxalate problems can arise from gut dysfunction, microbiome imbalance, nutrient deficiencies, and other complexities, it's important to note that addressing oxalate is never only a matter of diet; it requires consideration of oxalate that the human body itself produces and problems degrading oxalate. After we discuss the diet, we'll cover supplements and other considerations.

Oxalate Inside the Body and Cells

Once oxalate is inside the body (i.e., absorbed through the gut into the bloodstream, tissues, or cells), it can cause many problems that contribute to the pathology of autism. Oxalate can accumulate in the body; the most well-known example of this is kidney stones. Oxalate can also accumulate in the bones, joints, heart, eyes, and other tissues and organs, which can contribute to inflammation and tissue damage.

Oxalate can also get into cells and inhibit cellular function. One way this happens is, when there is inadequate sulfate (which we find in ASD), oxalate can get into the cell on the sulfate transporter. Oxalate can also cause faulty sulfation and exacerbate the condition in autism.

Oxalate can inhibit mitochondrial function,[20] as well as cause mitochondrial damage, decreased antioxidants, and increased oxidative stress.[21] These conditions are common in autism. While many of these conditions can have multiple causes in addition to oxalate, oxalate may cause, contribute to, or exacerbate these conditions for some people.

Oxalate can contribute to ongoing inflammation by triggering inflammasomes,[22] which are part of the immune system that triggers inflammation and can sustain it, creating chronic inflammation. The inflammasome is associated with autoimmune disorders,[23] cancer and metabolic diseases,[24] and neurological and neurodegenerative conditions.[25] In fact, researchers believe the inflammasome could be a major factor in the disordered gut-brain-microbiome connection in autism and other neurological conditions.[26]

Animal studies and case studies show us that extremely high levels of oxalate or oxalate poisoning can result in seizures.[27] It should be noted that seizures have not been reported from consuming oxalate in foods in typical amounts. However, we should not overlook the importance of oxalate as a potential contributor to neurotoxicity in autism since 20 to 30 percent of children with autism have seizures. I think more research should be done on oxalate and seizures to see if it's a contributor.

WHY OXALATE MATTERS IN AUTISM

Because of the many issues oxalate can cause in the body and its links to ASD, it is important to be aware of oxalate as a potential cause or contributor to autism symptoms. However, we have more evidence.

In a study specifically examining the role of oxalate in autism, researchers found that oxalate levels were two and a half times higher in the urine and three times higher in the plasma of children with autism compared to neurotypical children. In fact, every child with autism in the study had high oxalate levels. The study was well designed to control for factors that can contribute to high oxalate or could confound the results: None of the children had IBD or celiac disease. The children and their families did not have a history of kidney stones. The children were not on any special diet. And none of the children had a history of antibiotic use or seizures. Still, the researchers found unusually high levels of oxalate. The authors concluded that these elevated oxalate levels may be a cause or contribute to the development of autism spectrum disorder.[28] As an aside, at the time this study was published, the prevailing science held that you couldn't have oxalate issues without having kidney stones. However, through the study researchers found that this was not correct, as study participants had high oxalate without having kidney stones or an increased risk of them. That finding paved the way to realizing there could be other conditions where oxalate was elevated that also carried no risk of stones. The pioneering work of Susan Owens, one of the paper's authors, continues to identify those other conditions, helping the science of oxalate (and autism) advance significantly.

I know that this is a lot of science and that you probably have no desire to be an oxalate scientist. But this information is quite new, even to most doctors. If you share this information with your physician, it might inform decisions your care team makes about your child. In my practice and those of my colleagues, a low oxalate diet has been very helpful for some people with autism.

COMMON SYMPTOMS OF ELEVATED OXALATE

- ❏ Fatigue or weakness
- ❏ Low muscle tone/Decreased mitochondrial function
- ❏ Pain and inflammation
- ❏ Burning/Sandy eyes, eye poking
- ❏ Gum/Tooth pain or problems
- ❏ Burning feet
- ❏ Bone pain, low bone density
- ❏ Bedwetting/Incontinence, frequent urination, or pain with urination
- ❏ Crystals in dried urine
- ❏ Burning stool, sandy stools
- ❏ *Candida*/Yeast overgrowth (that doesn't go away with a low sugar diet)

- [ ] Skin rashes
- [ ] Chronic injury or difficulty healing
- [ ] Brain fog
- [ ] Irritability
- [ ] Anxiety
- [ ] Poor coordination
- [ ] Poor growth

Conditions Oxalate Can Cause

- [ ] Atherosclerosis
- [ ] Interstitial cystitis
- [ ] Kidney stones
- [ ] Low thyroid function
- [ ] Osteoporosis
- [ ] Seizures
- [ ] Vulvodynia/Vulvar pain

HOW TO DETERMINE WHETHER THE LOW OXALATE DIET IS RIGHT FOR YOUR CHILD

Look at the list of common symptoms from elevated oxalate, as well as conditions that oxalate can cause (affecting your child or a family member). If you think oxalate may be a factor for your child, consider laboratory testing. Quantitative results can be beneficial in determining whether oxalate is high and whether a low oxalate diet might be helpful.

In contrast to other diets, like a low salicylate diet, where a quick dietary trial works well, a low oxalate diet trial isn't as easy. As mentioned, oxalate must be removed slowly. And when oxalate is removed, someone might not feel better right away. Instead, people can feel worse, and it may take a while to feel better. Don't get me wrong; you can still do the diet to see if it helps, but it's not the same as a "dietary trial" used as a quick method of "testing." Additionally, for someone with oxalate issues, the approach is more than just a low oxalate diet; it also involves supportive nutritional supplementation (discussed later in this chapter), addressing the underlying factors, and clearing stored oxalate over time.

Lab Testing for Oxalate

One of the more valuable tests for high oxalate levels is an organic acid test with markers for oxalic acid (oxalate) and other markers that can help determine oxalate metabolism. These markers show if the body is excreting a lot of oxalate in the urine, indicating that oxalate is high.

However, these results are not always accurate, especially when oxalate measures are low. Humans dump oxalate in cycles, and urinary levels do not always reflect the oxalate burden in the body. Therefore, a low level may be a false negative. And the range or level can be off because of the age of the individual, the lab range, or when the marker it's compared against (creatinine) is off. However, when it's high, that's usually a good indicator that oxalate in the body is high.

These tests are often run by functional or biomedical doctors. Most conventional medical doctors are not familiar with these tests. However, they are likely familiar with a twenty-four-hour urinary oxalate excretion test and laboratory tests that can examine urine under a microscope for the presence of oxalate crystals, which may be helpful.

MODERATE OXALATE FOR ALL

Before we look at the low oxalate diet, I want to stress that because oxalate can cause mineral deficiencies, I recommend that everyone consume a well-rounded diet with only moderate amounts of oxalate (or low oxalate, if needed). This is a general principle of my Nourishing Hope Food Pyramid, regardless of whether you have autism. This means avoiding extremely high oxalate foods, especially on a regular basis. (See the list of high oxalate foods on page 213 for specifics.) Since therapeutic diets can be high in oxalate, it's important to be aware of oxalate values in food so as to not inadvertently add too many. You don't want to trade one problem for another.

How much is too much? That's hard to say because some people have underlying conditions that cause them to not be able to handle as much as other people. We know a diet over 180 milligrams per day causes significant oxalate to be excreted in the urine.[29] In a study out of England, researchers found the average diet has 70 to 150 milligrams of oxalate per day,[30] and in another study, healthy individuals from around the world were found to consume on average 100 to 200 milligrams of oxalate per day.[31]

Unfortunately, many health food trends point people toward high nutrient content foods, vegan foods, or grain-free foods (think spinach juice, green smoothies with spinach and Swiss chard, nut flours, chia seed pudding, and chia seed beverages) that pack a high oxalate load. A *single serving* of these foods can have five times the daily total for healthy individuals. While most nuts are high in oxalate, almonds—with 134 milligrams in 1 ounce—have five times more than some, and chia seeds have 190 milligrams in 2 tablespoons compared to flaxseed with 1 milligram in the same serving size.

It's an extreme example, but one case report described a woman with IBS who ate 6 tablespoons of chia seeds and five handfuls of almonds every day—meaning she took in over 1,000 milligrams of oxalate daily.[32] She developed kidney stones. Fortunately, when she switched to a low oxalate diet, her laboratory markers improved.

LOW OXALATE DIET

A low oxalate diet, for those who need it, consists of 40 to 60 milligrams of oxalate per day for a 2,000-calorie diet. It includes mostly low oxalate foods, with a few moderate oxalate foods allowed every day. While you'll avoid foods high in oxalate, it is possible to meet your nutrient needs with a low oxalate diet. Note that supplements are important for addressing high oxalate (and meeting nutritional needs); see "Supplement Support and Other Considerations for Addressing Oxalate" later in this chapter.

Nourishing Hope Stories

"We were already doing organic GMO-free, GFCFSF, essential fatty acids, and digestive enzymes before the program. The biggest improvements came from the low oxalate diet. It helped to significantly reduce pains, constipation, pain-related anxiety, and self-harming behavior (head banging) . . . Now she is a much happier child with less pains and problems and more able to realize her potential for growth and development." —*Parent of a fourteen-year-old with autism* ■

IMPLEMENTING A LOW OXALATE DIET

As mentioned, it's important to remove oxalate slowly from the diet. The most common mistake I see with implementing a low oxalate diet is trying to go too fast. Stored oxalate (which builds up over time in our tissues, organs, and bones when we aren't able to clear it) can be released when the body has some relief from reducing the amount we are consuming. Unfortunately, reducing oxalate too quickly can cause a release of oxalate into circulation too quickly, a condition informally known as oxalate dumping. This can cause negative symptoms such as pain, diarrhea, urinary frequency, and electrolyte imbalance, and it can even harm body tissues.

I recommend reducing oxalate by 5 to 10 percent per week. It could take months to reduce oxalate to the level of 40 to 60 milligrams per day. For example, when clients are eating hundreds or more than 1,000 milligrams per day (which is not unusual), it can take six months or more to get down to the recommended level. Your strategy to reduce oxalate in the diet will vary depending on the level you are starting at and what your diet consists of. Some people reduce one high oxalate food from their diet at a time or a portion of that food slowly; others move from high to moderate oxalate foods before going low oxalate. In addition to the high and low oxalate foods on the list below, there are moderate oxalate foods, such as oats, green beans, snow peas, macadamia nuts, bananas, pineapple, and pears. More resources, including where to find a full list of thousands of foods with oxalate values, can be found at PersonalizedAutismNutritionPlan.com/extras.

Remember, a low oxalate diet is 40 to 60 milligrams per day for a 2,000-calorie diet. This means that if your child's diet is fewer than 2,000 calories, the range may be a bit lower. For example, if your child eats 1,700 calories a day, aim for 35 to 50 milligrams of oxalate. The range is personalized to the needs of the individual; some can handle a bit more, others less.

Foods to Avoid and Foods to Choose on a Low Oxalate Diet

Oxalate is calculated by milligrams per serving size, such as ounce, grams, teaspoons, and so on. So, it's important to know the serving size along with the level of oxalate. For my clients, I recommend simply sticking to a very low/low list (with a few moderates) rather than calculating all the time, although it is good to calculate a couple days at some point to ensure you have a true sense of your child's oxalate consumption.

"Very low" means less than 1 milligram per serving. "Low" means 1 to 5 milligrams per serving. "Moderate" is 5 to 15 milligrams. "High" oxalate foods, above 15 milligrams per serving, vary widely. (For instance, half a cup of raw carrots has about 15.5 millgrams of oxalate, whereas ½ cup of steamed spinach has 365 milligrams!) For this reason, many lists also include "very high" and "extremely high" to make a distinction of *how* high it is. Serving sizes of some foods, such as many grains, seeds, and legumes, should be ½ cup or less to remain low oxalate (as indicated on the food list). Since foods very low in oxalate typically have a ½-cup or larger serving size with less than 1 milligram of oxalate, they are marked with "VL" instead of a serving size because they can be consumed liberally.

Note, most wheat- and soy-containing foods are high in oxalate. While dairy is not, since this program is intended to be GFCFSF, those foods are not included in these lists.

AVOID   High Oxalate Vegetables to Avoid

x	Artichoke hearts	x	Plantains
x	Beet greens	x	Potatoes
x	Beets	x	Rhubarb
x	Carrots	x	Snap peas
x	Celery	x	Sorrel
x	Citrus peel	x	Spinach
x	Eggplant	x	Sweet potatoes
x	Hearts of palm	x	Swiss chard
x	Okra	x	Yucca

AVOID   High Oxalate Fruits to Avoid

x	Apricots	x	Kiwi
x	Blackberries	x	Pomegranates
x	Boysenberries	x	Prunes
x	Figs	x	Raspberries
x	Guava	x	Starfruit

AVOID   Other High Oxalate Foods to Avoid

x	Almonds	x	Cloves
x	Amaranth	x	Cornmeal
x	Arrowroot flour	x	Cumin
x	Black beans	x	Hemp seeds
x	Black pepper	x	Green banana flour
x	Brazil nuts	x	Olives
x	Buckwheat	x	Peanuts
x	Carob	x	Pecans
x	Cashews	x	Pinto beans
x	Chia seeds	x	Poppy seeds
x	Chocolate	x	Potato flour
x	Cinnamon	x	Quinoa

AVOID   Other High Oxalate Foods to Avoid

x	Sesame seeds	x	Turmeric
x	Soybeans	x	Walnuts
x	Tahini	x	White beans

CHOOSE   Low Oxalate Vegetables to Choose

✓	Acorn squash, ½ cup	✓	Kale, curly, raw, ¼ cup
✓	Arugula, VL	✓	Kale, lacinato, raw, ½ cup
✓	Asparagus, ½ cup	✓	Kale, purple, raw, ½ cup
✓	Bok choy, VL	✓	Mustard greens, raw, VL
✓	Brussels sprouts, boiled, ½ cup	✓	Mustard greens, boiled, ½ cup
✓	Broccoli, boiled, ½ cup	✓	Onions, raw, ½ cup
✓	Broccoli sprouts, raw, VL	✓	Peas, green, boiled, VL
✓	Butternut squash, ½ cup	✓	Red bell peppers, ½ cup
✓	Cabbage, ½ cup	✓	Romaine lettuce, VL
✓	Collard greens, raw, ½ cup	✓	Rutabagas, boiled, ½ cup
✓	Cauliflower, VL	✓	Rutabagas, raw, 1 cup
✓	Cucumbers, ½ cup	✓	Turnips, ½ cup
✓	Iceberg lettuce, 1 cup	✓	Zucchini, ½ cup
✓	Kale, boiled, ½ cup		

CHOOSE   Low Oxalate Fruits to Choose

✓	Apples, 1 fruit	✓	Honeydew melon, ½ cup
✓	Avocado, very ripe, ½ cup	✓	Lemon juice (no peel), VL
✓	Blueberries, fresh, ½ cup	✓	Orange juice (no peel), VL
✓	Cantaloupe, ½ cup	✓	Peaches, 1 fruit
✓	Cherries, fresh, ½ cup	✓	Strawberries, ¼ to ½ cup
✓	Grapes, ½ cup	✓	Watermelon, 1 cup

CHOOSE   Other Low Oxalate Foods to Choose

✓	Chickpea flour, ½ cup	✓	Meat, VL
✓	Chickpeas, ½ cup	✓	Most oils, VL
✓	Coconut shreds, VL	✓	Potato starch, ½ cup
✓	Coconut flour, ½ cup	✓	Pumpkin seeds, ¼ cup
✓	Coconut milk, 1 cup	✓	Split peas, ½ cup
✓	Coconut oil, VL	✓	White chocolate, 1 ounce
✓	Cornstarch, ½ cup	✓	White rice flour, ½ cup
✓	Eggs, VL	✓	Wild rice, ½ cup
✓	Fish, VL	✓	Rice, white, cooked, ½ cup
✓	Flaxseed, whole or ground meal, ½ cup	✓	Lentils, brown or red boiled, ½ cup
✓	Black-eyed peas, ½ to 1 cup	✓	Sunflower seeds, 1 tablespoon
✓	Pumpkin seed flour or butter, ¼ cup	✓	Sunflower seed butter, 1 tablespoon
✓	Pumpkin seeds, sprouted, ½ cup	✓	Rice, brown, soaked, rinsed, and cooked, ½ cup
✓	Millet, soaked, drained, rinsed, and boiled, ½ cup		

Cooking and Preparing Foods

There is a common misconception that all cooking reduces the oxalate level of foods. Methods like sauteing and baking do not reduce oxalate levels. However, oxalate can be lowered by cooking with water.

Boiling removes oxalate the best, reducing it by 30 to 87 percent; boiling can take a moderately high oxalate food and reduce it to almost low. Steaming reduces oxalate but not as much, by only 5 to 53 percent. For example, 3.5 ounces of raw Brussels sprouts have 15.2 milligrams, steamed have 13.3 milligrams, and boiled have 6.1 milligrams of total oxalate. That said, boiling does not make all foods low. Boiled spinach still has 428 milligrams of oxalate and is way too high for someone on a low oxalate diet.[33]

216 THE PERSONALIZED AUTISM NUTRITION PLAN

Normally, nutritionists recommend steaming rather than boiling vegetables to preserve more nutrients. However, for a child needing a low oxalate diet, reducing oxalate is more important—so boiling is the way to go. This does mean that the dish will lose some nutrients, but it will allow you to offer your child a wider variety of foods. Just remember to dump the cooking water and not consume it.

Soaking is another food preparation method that can be helpful. Soaking grains can reduce the total oxalate and particularly the soluble oxalate. Once again, remember to drain and dump the water. Then boil the soaked grains with excess water, like you would with pasta, and dump the water at the end to reduce oxalate to an even lower level. Also, germinating or sprouting legumes and grains is even more effective than soaking.[34]

All these food preparation methods can help your child have a diet filled with more variety and nutritional value while reducing oxalate.

One Day of Low Oxalate Meals

Breakfast	Eggs, any style Butternut squash fries (substitute butternut squash in Rutabaga Fries recipe, page 290)
Lunch	Ground Beef Stuffed Zucchini (Zucchin-izza) (page 278) Butternut Squash Soup (page 294) ¼ cup Roasted Pumpkin Seeds (page 301)
Snack	Deviled Eggs (page 305) ½ cup sliced cucumbers (skinless)
Dinner	Chicken tacos with Cauliflower Tortillas (page 293) Cauliflower Rice (page 290) Sauteed Cabbage with Apple and Bacon (page 292) Sliced peaches with coconut whipped cream

Personalizing a Low Oxalate Diet

Some people may need a low oxalate diet in combination with another approach, such as a low phenol diet or a grain-free diet. In fact, a low phenol, low oxalate diet is a common combination because both diets may be needed when sulfate is low.

Just keep in mind that combining low oxalate eating with other diets can restrict a child's available food choices significantly. And sometimes, once oxalates are addressed, a child may not need other diet principles. For example, I have heard of children on a grain-free diet for microbial dysbiosis who no longer need to avoid grains once oxalates were addressed.

SUPPLEMENT SUPPORT AND OTHER CONSIDERATIONS FOR ADDRESSING OXALATES

Dietary oxalate is not the only source of high oxalate levels in the body. Oxalate problems can arise from internal biochemistry and nutrient deficiencies, as discussed earlier in this chapter. So addressing high oxalates often includes nutritional supplementation and GI/microbiome support.

Supplements such as calcium citrate and magnesium citrate can bind to oxalate in the diet, reducing absorption of oxalate significantly.[35] Additionally, the citrate in these supplements helps dissolve calcium oxalate crystals.[36] There are also nutrients that can become depleted, such as glutathione, vitamin A, and other antioxidants. Adequate B_6 and B_1 help support the proper conversion of oxalate. Probiotics can also be beneficial. Those with high oxalate should avoid over-supplementation with ascorbic acid (a form of vitamin C) since it can convert to oxalate.

There are nutrients that can also help with dumping symptoms. For additional resources on oxalate supplements and other supportive information, check out www.PersonalizedAutismNutritionPlan.com/extras.

In addition to these nutrients, healing the gut and balancing the microbiome are important factors for many people with oxalate issues to address (see more on this in steps 11 and 12 and "Beyond Diet and Nutrition").

READY FOR THE NEXT STEP?

If you decide a low oxalate diet may be right for your child, it generally takes three to six months to bring oxalate levels down to target levels and see improvements. After that period, they may need to remain on this diet for the long term. Many low oxalate advocates feel this is a lifelong diet; however, I have some colleagues and clients who were able to use the diet short term. This likely depends on the underlying factors causing the high oxalate issue. While sometimes people initially feel a bit worse before feeling better, get professional support if you have questions and need help. Track symptom changes and improvements. When you feel symptoms are more stable, this is a good time to proceed to the next step of your choosing.

STEP 11

Gut Healing and Additional Therapeutic Diets

I n this chapter, you'll learn about other therapeutic diets that can be implemented to support your child's underlying biochemical needs and improve their health: the low FODMAP diet, Body Ecology Diet, ketogenic diet, nightshade-free diet, autoimmune Paleo diet, lectin-free diet, and low sulfur diet. And because the gut is such an important aspect in autism and because diet can be so beneficial, we will start with a special section on diets for gut healing and GI support.

This step will help you further refine your child's bioindividual nutrition plan to reduce symptoms and help them thrive. Perhaps you haven't found the diet that works best, or you need to refine their diet by layering multiple approaches. For example, you may use the GFCFSF diet established in the Nourishing Hope Essentials and decide to restrict nightshades. Reading about and trying one or more of these diets may give you a crucial piece of the puzzle.

DIETS FOR GUT HEALING AND GI SUPPORT

Because food has direct contact with the GI tract and the microbiome, it's not surprising that therapeutic diets can be of particular benefit to the gut and gut healing.

The Nourishing Hope program supports the microbiome from step 1. Sugar, white flour, and processed foods can cause negative changes to the microbiome, including contributing to the perpetuation of *Candida*,[1] an imbalance in the gut microbiome, leaky gut, and/or a depressed immune system.[2] Artificial sweeteners (aspartame, sucralose, saccharin) have been found to negatively affect the microbiome, while stevia has been shown to not cause changes.[3] Glyphosate, the active ingredient in Roundup, disrupts the microbiome, especially in children before puberty,[4] and may contribute to the development or exacerbation of autism, as discussed in step 1.[5]

Conversely, healthy diets high in good fats, fiber, polyphenols, and antioxidants help shape a balanced microbiome.[6] The probiotic- and prebiotic-rich foods we covered in step 2 foster healthy gut microbiota. The microbiome is particularly influenced by diet. In fact, in only twenty-four hours, diet can have a significant impact on the microbiome; however, those changes revert quickly once the diet is altered again.[7] Long-lasting changes to the microbiome are likely multifactorial and require time. We know that vegetables, fruit, and other fiber-rich foods support a diverse and healthy microbiome, but fiber can be tricky for some (we'll talk about that more later in this chapter).[8] Omega-3 fish oils—recommended in step 3—are also beneficial for the microbiome.[9] And coconut oil has been found to be beneficial with *Candida*.[10]

Other therapeutic diets are a crucial tool in our gut-healing arsenal. Any foods that cause inflammation for an individual are important to remove on a bioindividual gut-healing diet. We've already covered many related dietary strategies (removing gluten, casein, and soy in step 5; pinpointing and addressing sensitivities in step 8; and going grain-free in step 9). Oxalate can both contribute to inflammation and disrupt the microbiome, as we covered in step 10. Furthermore, as we discussed in step 7, salicylates can cause digestive symptoms[11] and increase GI pain from FODMAPs,[12] which we'll talk about in this step.

Diarrhea and constipation are two of the most common GI symptoms that parents need solutions for. For the basics, probiotic foods can help both conditions, and fiber (and foods like prunes) are particularly helpful with constipation (refer to step 2). As I mentioned in step 5, in my experience dairy is one of the most common causes of constipation. In our study, the most beneficial diets for constipation in individuals with ASD were the ketogenic diet, corn-free diet, GFCF diet, Paleo diet, and a healthy diet. For diarrhea, the most helpful diets were the corn-free diet, GFCF diet, food avoidance based on observation, and Specific Carbohydrate Diet.[13] Additionally, we will discuss supplement strategies for diarrhea and constipation in step 12.

With all that said, your child may need additional gut-healing support. So let's dive into two more diets that are important with the microbiome and gut health: the low FODMAP diet and the Body Ecology Diet.

LOW FODMAP DIET

FODMAP is an acronym for fermentable oligosaccharides, disaccharides, monosaccharides and polyols. These short-chain carbohydrates are fermentable fiber, sugars, and alcohol sugars that some people have difficulty digesting and absorbing or that require beneficial bacteria to digest.

Let's look at fiber first. It can be a confusing topic. When you consume fiber, it travels to the gut and serves as a food source for your microbiome. The bacteria digest the fiber for us and turn it into short-chain fatty acids that fuel our intestinal cells. We need the help of our beneficial bacteria to break these down for us.

Fiber is important for improving the diversity of microbiota in the gut; it's a prebiotic, and low fiber can reduce bacterial composition. However, for those with an imbalanced microbiome, these FODMAPs may cause negative symptoms.[14] For example, when there is small intestinal bacterial overgrowth (SIBO), a low FODMAP diet may improve symptoms by not feeding the overgrowth of bacteria.

Unlike fiber, sugars are digestible and absorbable by most humans. However, some people are unable to digest or absorb them, particularly lactose and fructose, which are FODMAPs. Sugar alcohols (another category of FODMAPs) are slowly digested. When certain gut bacteria ferment any of these lingering FODMAPs, they can produce hydrogen or methane gas—causing bloating, gas, distention, and gastrointestinal discomfort in sensitive people. FODMAPs can also trigger diarrhea by bringing liquid into the gut.

The low FODMAP diet has been well researched for gastrointestinal symptoms like bloating, gas, diarrhea, constipation, and gastrointestinal pain. Research shows improvement with irritable bowel syndrome (IBS), including abdominal pain and stool frequency.[15] The diet has also been shown to reduce gastroesophageal reflux disease (GERD) in those with IBS.[16] It's been found to be helpful in reducing abdominal pain in children.[17]

The low FODMAP diet restricts fructose, cow and soy milk, wheat, legumes, certain fruits (such as apples and cherries), and certain vegetables (including the onion family). The FODMAPs in wheat may explain another reason wheat is such a problem: in individuals with nonceliac gluten intolerance, it was found that FODMAPs worsened symptoms,[18] not the gluten.[19]

The important point here is to be your own nutrition detective. If someone had issues associated with gluten that got better with a low FODMAP diet, they might conclude the issue was FODMAPs—while the solution might simply have been removing wheat (and other grains that contain gluten). However, if someone removed gluten and still had digestive problems, that's when they might want to consider removing FODMAPs.

LOW FODMAP DIET AND AUTISM

Children with autism have low lactase, the enzyme needed to break down the FODMAP disaccharide lactose.[20] They also have reduced transport or absorption of monosaccharides (the M in FODMAP).[21] Research found that these deficiencies were associated with negative changes to the gut microbiome in these children. This mechanism may be one reason the low FODMAP diet (as well as the SCD/GAPS Diet) is beneficial for children with autism.

A randomized controlled trial was conducted for the low FODMAP diet for children with autism. Researchers found improvement in GI symptoms with the diet.[22]

There is also a case study in the literature of a seventeen-year-old girl with autism and epilepsy. The girl had not only seizures but also neurodevelopmental delays, poor growth, GI pain, and diarrhea. The therapies that doctors tried were not helpful, so they tried diet. A ketogenic diet improved her microbiome and digestive symptoms modestly but was not tolerated because of hypoglycemia. Next, her caregivers transitioned her to a low FODMAP diet, and she showed great improvement. Her glycemic levels were more stable, she had GI symptom improvement, and her seizures decreased. She also had improvement in her gut microbiome.[23]

Since the low FODMAP diet can affect the gut, which then affects the brain, it has also been found to be beneficial with anxiety and/or depression.[24]

IMPLEMENTING A LOW FODMAP DIET

Some people are only reactive to certain FODMAPs. For example, maybe it's only fructose or polyols, or a specific polyol like sorbitol, that causes problems. Others react to all of them. Some foods contain multiple FODMAPs; for instance, asparagus contains both fructans and fructose. Understanding which FODMAPs are in different foods and which ones your child is reacting to helps personalize this diet and implement it most effectively.

FODMAP Categories
- Oligosaccharides
  — Fructans
  — Fructo-oligosaccharides
  — Galacto-oligosaccharides
- Disaccharides
  — Lactose

- Monosaccharides
  - Fructose
- Polyols
  - Mannitol
  - Sorbitol
  - Xylitol

The first step of this trial is simple: observe any food reactions, without cutting any foods. Does your child get gas and bloating with beans or with onions? Too much of these foods can cause gas for anyone, but if small to moderate amounts of these foods are not tolerated and cause big symptoms, or if your child's belly is fine in the morning but gets bloated as they eat certain foods throughout the day, suspect FODMAP intolerance.

Next, a dietary trial is beneficial. A low FODMAP dietary trial helps you determine whether you or your child is sensitive to FODMAPs and which categories are the problem. A low FODMAP diet avoids all high FODMAP categories and foods for two to six weeks. Next, one FODMAP category is reintroduced every three days to determine which categories (if any) are causing a problem.

I recommend starting with a small serving size of one food high in that category and increasing the portion over three days (if tolerated) until you reach a full serving. See if your child's symptoms return at any point. Once testing is complete for that category, pull that category back out of the diet, and go to the next one. Once all are tested (except lactose, since dairy is avoided on Nourishing Hope), avoid FODMAP categories your child can't tolerate, and add back to their diet only the ones they can. Also remember that levels add up, so small amounts may be tolerated, but when small amounts of several FODMAPs are included in one sitting, there may be a reaction.

After your child has had time for the gut to heal and you've addressed any dysbiosis or other issues with your pediatrician, retest tolerance to see if any categories are tolerated. Some might be tolerated after inflammation in the gut has subsided and the microbiome is rebalanced.

Foods to Avoid and Foods to Choose on a Low FODMAP Diet

Foods can be low, moderate, or high FODMAP, depending on the serving size; others are more straightforward. In the low FODMAP lists that follow, an asterisk indicates those foods can be low FODMAP when portion sizes are limited: ½ to ¾ cup in most cases.

So, if you do this diet, keep in mind that after the elimination period, there may be more foods to choose from when you determine which FODMAPs your child is reactive to and how much of a serving they can tolerate. FODMAPs are dose dependent, so even lower FODMAP foods may have a limit.

Note: Avocado is dose dependent; 3 tablespoons is considered low FODMAP, while 4½ tablespoons is considered high.

High FODMAP Foods to Avoid

	Fructans	Galacto-oligo-saccharides	Fructose	Lactose	Polyols
Agave			●		
Almonds		●			
Amaranth	●	●			
Apples			●		●
Apricots					●
Artichokes	●				
Asparagus	●		●		
Avocados (see note)					●
Bananas	●				
Beets	●	●			
Blackberries					●
Brussels sprouts	●				
Butternut squash		●			
Cashews		●			

	Fructans	Galacto-oligo-saccharides	Fructose	Lactose	Polyols
Cauliflower					●
Celery					●
Cherries			●		●
Chickpea flour	●	●			
Chicory root	●				
Chile peppers			●		
Coconut flour	●		●		●
Corn on the cob					●
Cottage cheese				●	
Cream				●	
Fennel	●				
Figs					●
Fructose			●		
Garlic	●				
Grapefruit	●				
Grapes			●		
High fructose			●		
Honey			●		
Ice cream				●	
Legumes	●	●			
Mangos			●		
Mannitol					●
Milk				●	
Mushrooms					●
Nectarines	●				●
Onions	●				
Peaches					●
Pears			●		●
Peas	●	●			

	Fructans	Galacto-oligo-saccharides	Fructose	Lactose	Polyols
Pistachios		●			
Plums					●
Pomegranates	●				
Prunes	●				●
Red bell peppers			●		
Savoy cabbage	●				
Seaweed					●
Soft cheeses				●	
Sorbitol					●
Soybeans	●				
Sugar snap peas			●		
Watermelon	●		●		●
Wheat	●	●			
Winter squash	●				
Xylitol					●

CHOOSE Low FODMAP Vegetables to Choose*

✓	Arugula	✓	Green beans*
✓	Bok choy*	✓	Hearts of palm
✓	Broccoli heads*	✓	Kale*
✓	Cabbage, common*	✓	Olives
✓	Carrots	✓	Parsnips
✓	Celeriac	✓	Potatoes, white
✓	Chives	✓	Radishes
✓	Collard greens	✓	Romaine lettuce
✓	Cucumbers*	✓	Rutabagas
✓	Eggplant	✓	Swiss chard

* Low FODMAP when portion size is limited

CHOOSE   Low FODMAP Fruits to Choose

✓	Bananas, firm, not ripe	✓	Lemons
✓	Blueberries	✓	Limes
✓	Cantaloupe*	✓	Mandarins*
✓	Coconut	✓	Oranges*
✓	Dragon fruit	✓	Papaya
✓	Guava, ripe	✓	Passionfruit
✓	Kiwi	✓	Pineapples

CHOOSE   Other Low FODMAP Foods to Choose

✓	Arrowroot	✓	Oats
✓	Buckwheat	✓	Oils
✓	Eggs	✓	Pecans
✓	Fish	✓	Potato starch
✓	Green banana flour	✓	Rice, white and brown
✓	Macadamia nuts	✓	Tapioca starch
✓	Meat	✓	Turmeric
✓	Millet	✓	Walnuts

One Day of Low FODMAP Meals

Breakfast	Omelet with kale, black olives, and chives Roasted potatoes
Lunch	Salmon Cakes (page 282) ½ cup Candied Ginger Spaghetti Squash (page 296) Blueberries
Snack	Carrot sticks Walnuts or macadamia nuts Popped Sorghum (page 303)

Dinner	Shepherd's Pie (page 284)—omit the onion and garlic
	Sauteed collard greens
	Salad with romaine lettuce, arugula, carrots, and cucumber slices with olive oil and apple cider vinegar dressing
	Dairy-Free Low Sugar Fudge (page 306)

BODY ECOLOGY DIET

The Body Ecology Diet also supports the microbiome. It is used most commonly to reduce yeast (*Candida*) overgrowth to regain health. This diet works by avoiding the foods that feed *Candida*, adding beneficial bacteria, and balancing the microbiome for gut healing.

Parents and practitioners commonly report or suspect *Candida* overgrowth in children with autism (though, of course, not all children with autism have it). In one study, 57 percent of children with ASD had *Candida* present compared to zero controls, and the yeast was often in its aggressive form where it adheres to the intestinal mucosa.[25]

It's possible that some cases are missed because of testing methods, since the way the *Candida* is tested (stool or urinary organic acids) can affect the results. It could also be that the amount of *Candida* isn't the problem, but the pathogenic presentation in the aggressive form is. More research is needed; however, for those that do have *Candida*, diet is an important piece of the puzzle, along with appropriate treatment with the support of a physician.

When *Candida* is present in the gut it can contribute to an imbalanced microbiome (dysbiosis) and lead to inflammation. This inflammation can cause decreased nutrient absorption, increasing food reactions and negatively impacting overall health. *Candida* can cause digestive symptoms such as diarrhea, constipation, gas/bloating, and an itchy anus. Other signs of yeast overgrowth include genital itching, athlete's foot, nail fungus, and thrush (yeast overgrowth in the mouth). Additionally, dysbiosis creates symptoms such as brain fog, hyperactivity, inappropriate laughter, and other neurological symptoms. In fact, yeast can cause symptoms of drunkenness, such as slurred speech and difficulty walking straight.[26] After all, alcohol is made when yeast and bacteria ferment carbohydrates. One of the large dietary issues with *Candida* is that it causes sugar cravings, which can perpetuate more yeast overgrowth.

The Body Ecology Diet avoids foods that yeast feed on, including sugars and starches. It includes live-culture fermented foods such as young coconut kefir and cultured vegetables. Many other principles in the Body Ecology Diet are included to aid gut healing, such as a focus on alkaline-forming foods like vegetables, as well as building 80 percent of the meal with vegetables. Another concept is food combining: pairing vegetables with meat or vegetables with grain-like seeds (e.g., millet and quinoa) but not meat and grain-like seeds together. This diet was created by Donna Gates, a pioneer in the field who has been dedicated to the pursuit of a healthy gut for children for many years. These are just some of the principles of the Body Ecology Diet. You can find more about her diet, her book, and helpful resources at her website, BodyEcology.com.

KETOGENIC DIET

The ketogenic diet is a very high fat, very low carbohydrate diet aimed at getting the body to use fat rather than carbohydrates as its main fuel source. Normally, our bodies break down dietary carbohydrates into glucose for energy. When carbs are restricted, the body begins breaking down fat into a type of compound called ketones for fuel—a state called ketosis. The ketogenic diet emphasizes healthy fats, with adequate protein, and a small number of nonstarchy vegetables. It restricts most fruits, grains, sugar, honey, starches, and beans.

Macronutrient ratios are important in a ketogenic diet as it works by initiating and maintaining ketosis. There are multiple versions of a ketogenic diet. There is the classic ketogenic diet, with more restrictive rules around protein amounts; the modified Atkins diet, with more liberal protein consumption; and a medium-chain triglyceride (MCT) ketogenic diet that uses MCT oil (from coconut), which produces ketones more readily than other types of fat and allows for increased carbohydrate and protein consumption. All are intended to maintain ketosis but utilize different macronutrient ratios.

The original formulation of this diet has been used for decades to reduce intractable seizures in children with epilepsy. When glucose cannot be effectively used by brain cells, the ketogenic diet can be beneficial for brain function. Therefore, it has several neurological benefits and can improve behavior in children with autism, and several studies have investigated this.

Our study of therapeutic diets found the ketogenic ranked first for improving nine symptoms: attention, cognition, anxiety, language/communication, social interaction and understanding, constipation, seizures, lethargy, and depression.[27] The ketogenic diet has been shown to improve mitochondrial function and energy metabolism in children with autism along with selenium levels and antioxidant capacity.[28] In one study of fifteen children with autism on a gluten-free ketogenic diet that contained MCT, researchers found significant improvement in symptoms of autism including fear or nervousness, imitation, and social affect.[29] Another diet compared the ketogenic diet to the gluten-free casein-free (GFCF) diet, where both diets were found to improve symptoms in children with ASD. Overall, the ketogenic diet offered better results especially in cognition and sociability. That said, one-third of participants dropped out of the ketogenic group because the diet was difficult to follow.[30]

The ketogenic diet can offer beneficial results for some individuals. However, it is a very restrictive diet, and it's rarely the first place I would start; I'd likely suggest a gluten-free diet, then a grain-free diet, then a lower carbohydrate diet before I would try a ketogenic diet. (If you start with keto, it's difficult to say whether results are from ketosis or from going gluten-free, for instance.) When an entire macronutrient is significantly decreased from the diet, it is important to work with a qualified physician and nutrition professional.

NIGHTSHADES AND THE AUTOIMMUNE PALEO DIET

The nightshade family is a group of fruits and vegetables that contain flavonoids, phenols, and alkaloids.[31] Tomatoes, white potatoes, peppers, and eggplant are popular nightshades. Although some nightshades are known to have anticancer, antioxidant, anti-inflammatory, and antimicrobial properties, there are some concerns about toxicity.[32] Nightshades are reported to be inflammatory to some people as they contain alkaloids and glycoalkaloids. These glycoalkaloids can disrupt the cell membrane, interfere with cellular metabolism, and affect the central nervous system.[33]

While there are few studies on the effects of nightshades, some people report an intolerance to them. It's possible that, depending on their genetics and biochemistry, certain individuals are more negatively affected than others. If you suspect your child has a reaction to nightshades, you might consider a short elimination diet and see if symptoms improve.

The autoimmune Paleo diet avoids nightshades. This diet is sort of a combination between aspects of several diets: the Paleo diet, the elimination diet, and the nightshade-free diet. The autoimmune Paleo diet removes all foods excluded on the Paleo diet, including grains, legumes, dairy, refined sugars, and industrial seed/vegetable oils. It also removes nuts, seeds, eggs, coffee, alcohol, and nightshades. As the name implies, this diet is often used by people with autoimmune conditions.

LECTIN-FREE DIET

Lectins are found in beans, grains, peanuts, cashews, dairy, and nightshades such as tomatoes, potatoes, and eggplant. They are proteins that bind carbohydrates, sugar molecules, and cells. Lectins are antinutrients. Lectins in wheat and other grains can bind to organs, causing damage, and can contribute to chronic inflammation and autoimmune reactions.[34] For some people, they cause problems such as gastrointestinal distress.

Fermenting, cooking, and sprouting can reduce the lectins in foods. For example, raw beans contain high levels of lectin, which can be dangerous for humans, but once cooked, the legumes contain an amount that is manageable for most people. One of the things that makes gluten problematic are the lectins. Fermenting the gluten grains reduces the lectins,[35] and this fermentation may allow gluten to be tolerated in those with nonceliac gluten sensitivity.[36]

Many years ago, autism parents had a social media group about lectins. They felt these substances were problematic for their children. They would even ferment their own bread to reduce lectins and felt it really helped.

You'll notice that these lectin-containing foods are also foods that have several other problematic substances, such as gluten, casein, FODMAPs, and starches. It's hard to know what the underlying culprits in these foods are. As with nightshades, there is little research on lectins, so I find a low lectin diet is best for those that are observing a reaction to them.

LOW SULFUR DIET

The body needs sulfur. It's critical to health and aids detoxification. However, some people are unable to tolerate large amounts in their diet because of genetic variations that are commonly found in ASD.[37] Sulfur-containing foods include meat, dairy, eggs, seafood, cruciferous vegetables, onions, legumes, peas, and some nuts. Processed foods containing emulsifiers, phosphates, and nitrates are also high in sulfur.

Additionally, individuals who have high levels of sulfur-reducing bacteria, such as *Desulfovibrio*, can have negative reactions to diets high in sulfur-containing foods. The bacteria convert the dietary sulfur into hydrogen sulfide, and when concentrations of hydrogen sulfide in the gut gets too high, it can damage the mitochondria, mucous layer, and cells of the gastrointestinal tract.[38] This bacterium is also what causes gas that smells like rotten eggs.

However, there are multiple factors that affect whether someone reacts to sulfur in the diet, including whether the food is cooked, the cooking temperature, how well the food is chewed and ground up, and the fiber content. High sulfur vegetables do not cause the same negative reaction as animal-based sulfur-containing food, as fiber reduces hydrogen sulfide production.[39] Both the sulfur and the fiber content are important factors to consider.

Since sulfur is so important to health and there are multiple factors that can influence tolerance, I don't recommend limiting sulfur across the board for more than a short period unless you are confident there is a problem with it and are working with a qualified professional. Also, you might consider how to reduce certain types of sulfur (such as those in food additives) without avoiding all forms of sulfur-containing foods and beneficial nutrients.

HOW TO DETERMINE WHETHER A THERAPEUTIC DIET IS RIGHT FOR YOUR CHILD

To determine whether a therapeutic diet is right for your child, you need to understand the mechanism(s) by which it works and whether that mechanism might be a factor in your child's individual ASD symptoms. Also, look for research or anecdotal reports you trust of symptoms that the diet is supposed to help with, and compare that to your situation. Do a dietary trial and record symptom changes and improvements. Generally speaking, a few months is a reasonable timeframe for determining whether the diet is effective and worth continuing.

COMBINING DIETS AND CREATING A PERSONALIZED DIET PLAN

Therapeutic diets should prioritize healthy diet principles while avoiding foods that your child reacts to. You might start with just one therapeutic diet, adhering to the rules very strictly. It's best to do one diet at a time. However, you may find it beneficial to combine diets, loosen the rules, and/or incorporate a few principles from another diet after you gain some experience.

As you combine more diets, you might find it complicated to find foods that fit all your child's dietary requirements. Check the tables that follow for an at-a-glance guide.

READY FOR THE NEXT STEP?

If you decide one of these approaches could help your child, do that one strategy until you get to a place where you are familiar with the diet and have reached a plateau in symptom improvements. It's always best to only try one new intervention at a time. Then you're ready to add another or move on to the next step.

FOODS ALLOWED ON THERAPEUTIC DIETS

Key
- ● Allowed
- ○ Moderate, limit

	Elimination	Low Salicylate	Low Amine	Low Glutamate	Low SAG	Low Histamine	SCD/GAPS	Paleo	Low Oxalate	Low FODMAP	Ketogenic
Vegetables											
Beets	●	○	●	●		●	●	●			
Broccoli*	●					●	●	●	●	●	●
Brussels sprouts	●	●	●	●	●		●	●	○		●
Butternut squash	●	○	●	●	○	●	●	●	●		
Cabbage*	●	●	●	●	●	●	●	●	●	●	●
Carrots	●	○	●	●	○	●	●	●	●	●	
Cauliflower	●			●							●
Corn, fresh			●			●			●	○	
Cucumber†	●	○	●	●		●	●	●	●		●
Garlic‡	●	○	●	●	○		●	●	●		●
Green peas	●	●	●			○	●	●	●		
Kale, curly	●		●	●		●	●	●		●	●
Kale, lacinato	●		●	●		●	●	●		●	●
Lettuce, head	●	○	●	●	○	●	●	●	●	●	●
Onion	●		●	●			●	●			
Potato, white	●	●	●	●	●	●			●		
Red bell pepper	●		●	●		●	●	●	●		●
Rutabaga	●	●	●	●	●	●	●	●	●	●	
Spinach	●						●	●		●	●
Sweet potato	●	○	●	●	○	●				○	
Swiss chard	●					○	●	●		●	●
Tomato	●						●	●	○	○	●
Zucchini†	●	○	●	●		●	●	●	●	○	●

Some foods depend on portion size, cooking methods, or variety for diet compliance.

*For Low FODMAPS—broccoli heads (not stalks) and common cabbage (not Napa).

†Cucumber and zucchini are moderate salicylate when peeled, otherwise high.

‡Garlic is allowed on low salicylate in small amounts.

FOODS ALLOWED ON THERAPEUTIC DIETS

Key
●   Allowed
○   Moderate, limit

	Elimination	Low Salicylate	Low Amine	Low Glutamate	Low SAG	Low Histamine	SCD/GAPS	Paleo	Low Oxalate	Low FODMAP	Ketogenic
Fruit											
Apple	●		●	●		●	●	●	●		
Apple, Golden Delicious, peeled	●	●	●	●	●	●	●	●	●		
Avocado	●			●			●	●	●		●
Banana, green*	●	○		●				●	○	●	
Banana, ripe	●	○					●	●	○		
Blackberries	●			●		●	●	●			●
Blueberries†	●		●	●		●	●	●	●	●	
Coconut, shredded‡	○			●		●	●	●	●	●	●
Grapefruit				●			●	●			
Grapes	●					●	●	●	●		
Lemon				●			●	●	○	●	●
Lime				●			●	●	○	●	●
Mango	●			●			●	●	○		
Melon	●		●	●		●	●	●	●		
Orange				●			●	●		●	
Pear**	●	●	●	●	●	●	●	●			
Raspberries	●			●			●	●		○	●
Strawberries†	●		●	●			●	●	●	○	●
Watermelon	●		●	●		○	●	●	●		

Some foods depend on portion size, cooking methods, or variety for diet compliance.

*Green banana flour is low FODMAPs.

†Blueberries and strawberries are considered low oxalate but levels vary between lists.

‡½ cup shredded coconut is low FODMAPs but coconut flour is high FODMAPs.

**Peeled pear is low salicylate, with peel is moderate.

STEP 12

Supplements for BioIndividual Nutrition

We return to supplementation once you've made changes to your child's diet and determined which foods are problematic.

Beyond the basics we covered in step 3, other supplements can address additional individual biochemical needs, such as mitochondrial support, neurotransmitter production, microbiome balance, detoxification support, and more. These are often tried on a trial basis of a few weeks to see if there is a positive response.

As a reminder, introduce supplements one at a time and slowly. And stop a supplement if your child reacts and can't tolerate it. Keep your health care professionals informed of what your child is taking. You may benefit from using lab testing and guidance from a health practitioner. Tests may include labs for gastrointestinal health, toxins and detoxification, hormones, genetic factors, and nutritional status, such as vitamin D levels.

In this section, I will lay out the supplements by systems and symptom support:

- Gastrointestinal and microbiome support
- Inflammation, immune system, detoxification, and antioxidant support

- Anxiety, mood, mental wellness, and sleep support
- Mitochondrial support
- ADHD support
- Speech, language, and communication support

GASTROINTESTINAL AND MICROBIOME SUPPORT

Some supplements support the GI tract itself and others, the microbiome.

Probiotics, Prebiotics, and Postbiotics

Probiotics are beneficial bacteria and microorganisms that can be taken as supplements. Probiotics come in many formulas. Some are sold as single strains, and many come as broad-spectrum formulas. Probiotics include:

- Lactobacillus such as *Lactobacillus acidophilus*, *Lactobacillus rhamnosus*, and *Lactobacillus reuteri*
- *Bifidobacterium*
- *Bacillus subtilis* (spore based)
- *Saccharomyces boulardii* (a beneficial yeast)

Bacteria that affect the central nervous system and brain are called psychobiotics. Psychobiotics can improve neurodevelopmental disorders including autism spectrum disorder and autism symptoms.[1] For example, *Lactobacillus reuteri* can influence the brain and behavior by raising oxytocin levels, and bacteria can create neurotransmitters in the gut.[2] The symptoms to improve most often from probiotics in ASD were constipation and diarrhea.[3]

Prebiotics are fermentable carbohydrates or fiber that beneficial bacteria use as fuel. The bacteria feed on the prebiotics and create short-chain fatty acids such as butyrate, which is important for keeping the gut healthy. In addition to the prebiotic-rich foods we discussed in step 2, there are also prebiotic supplements.

There is a substantial amount of research on probiotics and prebiotics for autism. Findings suggest they can be beneficial for reducing GI symptoms and improving autism symptoms. Probiotics improved bacterial balance, decreased pathogenic bacteria, and reduced inflammation in children with ASD. A prebiotic improved beneficial gut bacteria and butyrate levels, and the combination of a probiotic and prebiotic reduced *Clostridia*.[4] Again, go slowly. Since prebiotics feed bacteria, they can cause symptoms such as gas and bloating in someone with SIBO.

Postbiotics are substances created by probiotics when they feed on prebiotics. Short-chain fatty acids, such as butyrate (or butyric acid), is the one we've discussed most. Butyrate not only helps the gut but also has effects on the body and brain (even mitochondria).[5]

Herbal Antimicrobials

I always recommend working with a physician when dealing with gut pathogens because it is a delicate balance and reducing one may increase another. Physicians have a larger arsenal of antimicrobial agents since they can use pharmaceuticals as well as natural and herbal remedies. Find a physician well versed in both.

Herbs have many different beneficial immune properties, such as reducing inflammation, increasing antioxidant status, modulating the immune system, and promoting antimicrobial effects. Some beneficial herbs include bilberry, shiitake mushroom, golden seal, black walnut, milk thistle, and garlic. Because herbs work synergistically, I particularly like broad spectrum formulas, which have multiple herbs to address a wider range of pathogens and functions, and they can be more effective together.

One botanical product I like, Biocidin, has been found to have antimicrobial properties and reduce biofilms.[6] Biofilms are communities of pathogens that make it more difficult for antimicrobials to work. I've used it for many years with my own family. It is a pleasant-tasting liquid, so it's easy for children to take.

Serum-Derived Bovine Immunoglobin—Immune Support and GI Repair

Colostrum, transfer factor, and/or serum-derived bovine immunoglobin (SBI) can be very helpful for those with immune conditions and gastrointestinal issues. Bovine colostrum comes from cow milk from the first days of lactation. Colostrum is important for the immune system of infants and newborn animals. Transfer factors are immune messenger molecules extracted from colostrum. SBI is a more recent supplement that has been found to help with diarrhea-predominant IBS. It appears SBI binds to pathogenic bacteria and their toxins, improves gut barrier integrity, reduces antigen absorption, decreasing immune activation, and reduces inflammation.[7]

Camel Milk

Although camel milk is a food rather than a supplement, it is a wonderful healing food for some individuals. While it is dairy and does contain casein, it has a different form of casein molecule than any other animal milk and is much more tolerated by some individuals. It has unique benefits for the immune system and many other unique healing properties. Camel milk has been shown to reduce oxidative stress, increase glutathione, decrease inflammation, and improve behavior and autism severity in children with ASD.[8] If you'd like more information on camel milk, see the article about it on NourishingHope.com (the link will be in the book extras at www.PersonalizedAutismNutritionPlan.com/extras). While camel milk may be an interesting option for some individuals, as it is a dairy product (though very different), it's best to avoid it until after the casein-free diet has been established for several months and you have more thoroughly considered the pros and cons. This will allow you to more easily see if there are negative reactions or beneficial results.

Constipation and Diarrhea

Supplements that improve gut health and the microbiome, such as those mentioned in this chapter, can also be beneficial for constipation and diarrhea. Supplements specifically found to be beneficial for improving constipation for those with ASD include magnesium citrate, aloe vera, digestive enzymes, flaxseed, fruit/vegetable powder, and the probiotic *Saccharomyces boulardii*. For improving diarrhea, digestive enzymes and the probiotic *Saccharomyces boulardii* were beneficial.[9]

INFLAMMATION, IMMUNE SYSTEM, DETOXIFICATION, AND ANTIOXIDANT SUPPORT

As we have discussed throughout this book, oxidative stress, inflammation, immune function, and detoxification challenges are common in ASD. Since many of the following nutrients support several of these systems, they are grouped together.

Sulforaphane

Sulforaphane is a supplement from a compound in cruciferous vegetables, mainly broccoli sprouts. Sulforaphane raises glutathione levels in the body and brain.[10] Therefore, it has antioxidant and anti-inflammatory properties. A variety of studies on humans and animals have shown sulforaphane to be neuroprotective, decrease neuron damage, reduce cell death, reduce seizures, and improve mitochondrial function.[11]

There are many studies on sulforaphane for many conditions, including autism. In a randomized controlled trial of children with ASD, sulforaphane improved levels of glutathione, reduced inflammation, and improved mitochondrial function.[12] One randomized controlled trial of sulforaphane with young men with autism showed improvements in behavior, verbal communication, and social interaction.[13] In a follow-up study of these subjects years later, nine of the sixteen families felt the results from the supplement were so beneficial they continued to use sulforaphane for the next three years.[14]

Not all sulforaphane is equal. Look for one with a high amount of the active ingredient and with myrosinase.

Glutathione

Glutathione is the master antioxidant and plays a role in reducing free radicals, improving detoxification, and supporting the immune system. Even a moderate decrease in glutathione can lead to neuroinflammation. Glutathione is significantly lower in children with autism spectrum disorder than neurotypical children,[15] and this may be is a key factor in ASD, either as a cause or contributing factor.[16]

Fortunately, glutathione supplementation in ASD can improve reduced glutathione levels in the body.[17] In terms of what form is best, both the standard GSH form and the liposomal form of glutathione supplementation can improve glutathione levels.[18] According to caregivers and individuals with ASD, oral glutathione was reported to help more individuals than transdermal glutathione. N-acetyl cysteine, which converts to glutathione, was also considered beneficial with a rating similar to transdermal. After general benefit, glutathione was found to improve language/communication in 18 percent of those who found benefit; cognition and social interaction were both improved in 13 percent; and attention, irritability, anxiety, and health improved in 7 to 9 percent.[19]

Health and Immunity

The highest ranking supplements according to caregivers and individuals with ASD for improving health and having fewer illnesses were high-dose multivitamins, vitamin C, olive leaf, fruit and vegetable powder, vitamin B_6, vitamin D, and zinc.[20] During this step, these vitamins and minerals (discussed in step 3) can be adjusted for bioindividual needs. For example, this is often a good time to work with a physician who can do vitamin D testing to recommend the optimal amount for your child.

ANXIETY, MOOD, MENTAL WELLNESS, AND SLEEP SUPPORT

Anxiety is common in autism, as are other mood and mental health challenges. Supplementation can often be helpful in reducing symptoms of anxiety, irritability, sadness, and poor sleep by adding vitamins, minerals, and other needed nutrient support.

Anxiety Support

Some of the highest-rated nutraceuticals for improving anxiety for individuals with ASD are Epsom salt baths and lotion, GABA, vitamin B_6, tryptophan, 5-HTP, a blend of amino acids, multivitamin/mineral formulas, herbal antifungals, magnesium, low-dose lithium as a nutritional supplement, alpha lipoic acid, and inositol.[21]

Methylation Support for Mental Health

Methylation helps ensure neurotransmitters are activated; therefore, low methylation can contribute to anxiety, depression, irritability, defiance, and hyperactivity. Important nutrients for methylation include folate, vitamin B_{12}, vitamin B_6, riboflavin, magnesium, choline, and betaine. While we covered these nutrients in step 3, in this step, you might refine the dosage of these vitamins and minerals through testing with your doctor to prescribe higher amounts when needed, choose different forms, or add nutrient cofactors.

Nutrient Therapy for Brain Chemistry

Targeted nutrient therapy is an approach that was used by Abram Hoffer and Carl Pfeiffer, physicians and cofounders of orthomolecular psychiatry, for decades and has continued to be carried on by William Walsh (a PhD and expert in nutrient-based psychiatry) and others. It involves lab testing for nutrient support, including zinc and copper levels, kryptopyrrole testing (for pyroluria), and whole-blood histamine testing (for methylation status). While we have talked about many of the following nutrients in step 3, this approach is about customizing these vitamins and minerals using lab testing (and clinical assessment).

In a paper, Dr. Walsh and colleagues applied targeted nutrient therapy to 567 consecutive patients with autism, depression, anxiety, schizophrenia, bipolar disorder, ADHD, and Asperger's syndrome. For those with pyroluria, they recommended vitamin B_6 (pyridoxine), P5P (pyridoxal-5'-phosphate), zinc, and vitamin C. For those with a high ratio of copper/zinc, individuals received zinc. For those with undermethylation (insufficient methylation), they used vitamin B_6, P5P, zinc, magnesium, methionine, and vitamin C. And those with overmethylation (too much methylation) received zinc, folic acid, P5P, and vitamins B_3, B_6, B_{12}, and C. Out of 108 individuals with autism, 45 percent had major improvement, and 35 percent had partial improvement. On average (for all the conditions), 58 percent of patients had major improvement, and 24 percent had partial improvement.[22]

Additional targeted nutrients such as essential fatty acids, vitamin D, amino acids (which we discuss next), and others are needed for supporting balanced brain chemistry. For example, vitamin D is required for the conversion of tryptophan to serotonin, and vitamin D, EPA, and DHA are needed for proper serotonin production and use in the brain.[23] While vitamin D and EPA and DHA are added in step 3, understanding their synergy is important for mental health, as well as ensuring adequate levels of vitamin D are obtained through proper testing.

Amino Acids: Building Blocks for Neurotransmitters

After basic nutrients are optimized, you might consider working with your physician on amino acids and related compounds involved with building neurotransmitters. For example, serotonin is the feel-good hormone and involved with social behavior, so it plays an important part in autism, depression, and ADHD. Serotonin is created from tryptophan, which is converted to 5-HTP then serotonin, and then to melatonin for sleep.

I recommend 5-HTP over tryptophan when someone needs supplementation because it's closer to serotonin, and tryptophan can go down the wrong pathway and have negative consequences. 5-HTP can help some people with anxiety and depression, as well as their sleep. But too much of these nutrients is not beneficial so I always recommend working with your physician.

Caregivers and individuals with ASD found 5-HTP and tryptophan to both be helpful for sleep as the number one benefit (although melatonin was by far the top supplement for sleep), followed by anxiety. Generally, 5-HTP had a higher rating than tryptophan and a lower adverse effects score.[24]

Another amino acid to consider is GABA, which can help with anxiety that often has an aspect of tension. GABA also was reported to improve sleep, cognition, attention, irritability, and hyperactivity.[25] Tyrosine is another amino acid to look at when needed, but this is the precursor to dopamine, and for some people, this is too stimulating. D-phenylalanine (DPA) can help with sadness and weeping. However, phenylalanine is not to be used for people with phenylketonuria (PKU), and inborn error of metabolism.

Sleep Support

As I mentioned earlier, melatonin is considered the top supplement for falling and staying asleep.[26] Phosphorylated serine can be incredibly helpful for falling asleep when sleeplessness is due to high cortisol levels. Please note that phosphorylated serine is different than phosphatidylserine, which we discuss in the ADHD section.

Inositol

Inositol is a nutrient that some consider part of the B-vitamin family. Inositol is important for the cellular signaling of neurotransmitters, such as serotonin and hormones. Therefore, it has been used in studies for depression with some success. While more research is needed, clients and families I've worked with have shared their praises of inositol. It can help with anxiety, particularly symptoms such as ruminating thoughts. Also, it has a sweet taste and is easy to give to kids. Caregivers and individuals with ASD reported anxiety, attention, irritability, and aggression as the top symptoms that improved with inositol supplementation.[27]

MITOCHONDRIAL SUPPORT

Mitochondrial dysfunction affects some individuals with autism, and there are supplements to consider. Carnitine, coenzyme Q10, thiamine, riboflavin, and antioxidants are often recommended and have been used in studies and by clinicians for individuals with mitochondrial dysfunction.[28]

Carnitine

Carnitine, or L-carnitine, helps shuttle fat into the mitochondria for burning energy. For various reasons, including low meat intake, someone might be low in carnitine and benefit from supplementation.

Coenzyme Q10

Coenzyme Q10 (CoQ10), along with B vitamins thiamine and riboflavin, is needed in the production of energy in the mitochondria. It is important to check your multivitamin/mineral formula because the amounts of nutrients included may be too low to have a therapeutic effect; additional supplementation may be beneficial.

ADHD SUPPORT

Various nutrient deficiencies and underlying factors can contribute to ADHD. The following are some supplements that can help relieve symptoms.

Antioxidants and Pycnogenol

As discussed in step 3, supplements can help with certain nutrient deficiencies and differences found in ADHD (zinc, iron, vitamin D_3), and omega-3s have also been shown to be beneficial. But there are other supplements to consider. Oxidative stress leads to chronic inflammation, including brain inflammation and damage, which can cause or contribute to ADHD. Antioxidants can reduce these effects and symptoms. Antioxidants, including supplements like Pycnogenol, have been shown to be beneficial for reducing symptoms in individuals with ADHD.[29]

Phosphatidylserine

Phosphatidylserine is a key brain nutrient that can regulate many functions of the cell membrane, positively affect neurotransmitters, and counteract stressors. In a randomized controlled trial of children with ADHD, phosphatidylserine supplementation led to significant improvement in ADHD, hyperactivity, inattentiveness, impulsivity, and short-term auditory memory.[30]

Attention and Hyperactivity

If your child has either inattentiveness or hyperactivity, it's helpful to look at the conditions and beneficial supplements individually. In the nutraceutical study of children with autism, the top-rated supplements for attention were high-dose folinic acid, omega-6, transdermal Epsom salt, high-dose multivitamin formula, cod liver oil, omega-3, evening primrose oil, vitamin B_6 and P5P, oral B_{12}, and fish oil. And in individuals with autism, the top supplements for hyperactivity were high-dose folinic acid, high-dose multivitamin formula, and magnesium. [31]

SPEECH, LANGUAGE, AND COMMUNICATION SUPPORT

Communication is a core area affected in ASD. Important nutraceuticals for improving language and communication include methyl B_{12}, folinic acid, and trimethylglycine (TMG), which have been rated highly by integrative pediatricians and parents for many years. Additionally, alpha lipoic acid, glutathione, cod liver oil and fish oil, omega-6, Epsom salt baths, and multivitamin/minerals are helpful for improving language in individuals with ASD.[32]

Methyl B₁₂ and Folinic Acid for Language

As we've discussed, methyl B_{12} and folinic acid are important for methylation and transsulfuration, which supports many methylation functions and glutathione. In a clinical study of children with autism, methyl B_{12} and folinic supplementation led to improvements in not only glutathione levels but also receptive, expressive, and written language. There were other benefits outside of language, too, including social skills, play, and living skills.[33]

TMG and Language

TMG is a methyl donor that supports methylation. TMG can reduce inflammation and oxidative stress and inhibit the activation of inflammasomes.[34] It is rated by parents as a top supplement for language and communication, as well as positively regarded by practitioners. In a study of five-year-old children, betaine levels (remember TMG is a form of betaine) were positively associated with language scores.[35]

For more information on high-quality supplement brands I like, have used, and/or recommend, go to www.PersonalizedAutismNutritionPlan .com/extras.

READY FOR THE NEXT STEP?

There is no real way of being done with this step because choosing supplements for your child's current needs is something you may come back to throughout their childhood. Remember, diet and nutrition needs are always evolving. You may return to fine-tuning your child's diet again after trying bioindividual supplementation. Once healing has occurred or your child's picky eating has evolved, you may find that a new dietary intervention is beneficial or that you can loosen up on dietary restrictions. As nutrition improves, you may change the supplements you are using.

Continue to revisit your child's symptoms and needs. Fill out the Parent Global Impressions survey and Autism Treatment Evaluation Checklist (ATEC) every six to twelve months to see how your child has improved and which symptoms you would like to address.

So what's next? In addition to evolving your child's diet and nutrition plan over time, continue working with your integrative physician. The next chapter discusses underlying factors, medical conditions, and laboratory testing that you can ask your doctor about and that can help you improve your child's health and happiness.

BEYOND DIET AND NUTRITION

Working with Your Child's Doctor and Other Factors to Know

As we have thoroughly discussed throughout this book, autism spectrum disorder is a complex condition. While nutrition, therapeutic diets, and supplementation can play a powerful role in helping your child live better, there are often other conditions at play that require or benefit from medical interventions and therapies. By now, I hope you're well on your way to creating a supportive personalized autism nutrition plan that can help you clear out some of the "noise" in your child's symptoms so you and your doctor can begin to see additional areas that need support, sometimes benefiting from medical interventions, if they haven't already picked up on them before.

With the multiple triggers and underlying factors involved in ASD, working with a good physician is key. A skilled physician can support your nutrition journey, run and interpret laboratory testing, and diagnose and treat medical conditions. Look for a physician who has training in integrative medicine, functional medicine, or biomedical intervention and who can take a more holistic approach.

In this chapter, we discuss underlying contributing factors, common comorbid medical conditions, and other less common medical conditions to give you and your doctor some ideas of areas that can influence symptoms and the severity of autism. Here are some of the areas to ask them about:

- Gut pathogens
- PANDAS, PANS, mold, and conditions of infections
- Mast cell activation
- Diabetes and insulin resistance
- Stressors, electromagnetic fields (EMFs), and trauma
- Toxins and detoxification

And you can also ask about lab testing, such as:

- Comprehensive digestive stool analysis
- Gut microbiome testing
- Organic acid testing
- Food sensitivity testing
- Pyroluria, zinc, and copper testing
- Genetics and nutrigenetics testing
- Nutrient testing

PERSONALIZED MEDICINE

Personalized medicine, just like personalized nutrition, is the future of ASD treatment. And although we cannot discuss all that personalized medicine entails here, we can discuss some of the factors my clients and colleagues have found are important.

The future of personalized medicine includes some exciting new areas of science. There are also many aspects of personalized medicine available to us now, such as genetics and SNP testing. Your doctor can test for genetic variants that can affect biochemical pathways and nutrient levels and use supplementation and dietary strategies to support the individual. In addition to these newer strategies, diagnostic testing and functional lab testing also provide data to help your physician personalize treatment for your child.

UNDERLYING FACTORS AND MEDICAL
CONDITIONS FOR YOU AND YOUR DOCTOR

We have spoken extensively about mitochondrial dysfunction, gastrointestinal diseases and disorders, microbiome imbalance, and many other conditions in autism. These underlying factors can be contributors to the development or the severity of autism. Your child's doctor can work with you to identify and address them.

Medical comorbidities in ASD that your doctor can diagnose and treat include asthma, allergies, immunodeficiency, systemic infections, gut pathogens, seizures,[1] mast cell activation,[2] metabolic disorders and hormonal dysfunction,[3] gastrointestinal disorders, mitochondrial dysfunction, and sleep disorders.[4] Addressing these conditions can take the burden off the body and brain and help individuals with autism feel better, be healthier, and often reduce their symptoms.

Your doctor can use clinical observation and laboratory testing to understand what areas may be factors for your child and how to address them. Sometimes your doctor might address these conditions with nutrition, diet, and supplementation. At other times, they might use medications, natural remedies, medical treatments, or other approaches. Find a doctor who is knowledgeable and open to the type of treatment interventions that interest you most.

Gut Pathogens

Addressing the microbiome can be a complex issue but an important one—hence why I mention it yet again in this chapter. *Clostridia* (a genus of bacteria known to include some highly pathogenic strains) can cause elevated dopamine levels and toxins in the brain, increased repetitive behaviors, and GI disturbances—and can possibly contribute to the development of regressive (late-onset) autism and increased severity.[5] Another pathogen more common in children with autism is *Candida*, which we've discussed previously; when overgrown it can cause gut inflammation and digestive problems, and it can even negatively affect the brain and behavior.[6] In one study, children with ASD with *Candida* or *Candida albicans* had significantly worse autism symptoms.[7]

When microbes are killed, such as with antibiotics, more pathogenic strains like *Clostridia* can take hold, or another microorganism like *Candida* can overgrow. Additionally, when one microbe is eradicated, another that was being suppressed by the first pathogen can increase. For instance, when *Clostridia* is killed, *Candida* can overgrow; when *Candida* is addressed, *Clostridia* can increase. Your child's doctor can do testing and look at the big picture to provide a comprehensive treatment approach. They also have medications in their toolbox and can determine if natural antimicrobials, pharmaceuticals, or a combination approach is best.

PANDAS, PANS, mold, and conditions of infections

PANDAS stands for pediatric autoimmune neuropsychiatric disorders associated with streptococcal infections. This is a condition where a strep infection causes autoimmune reactions that affect the brain. It typically causes abrupt neurological and behavioral symptoms such as OCD, tics, aggression, anxiety, restrictive eating, and more. There are also other, similar conditions such as PANS (pediatric acute-onset neuropsychiatric syndrome) and PITANDS (pediatric infection-triggered autoimmune neuropsychiatric disorders) that can be caused by a broader host of infections and noninfectious agents such as viruses, Lyme disease, and mold that can affect the brain in children. Rapid onset of new neurological symptoms is a key to these conditions.

Let's take a closer look at mold and its toxins because they are another environmental trigger that can cause health and neurological problems in individuals with ASD. Mold exposure often comes from homes and buildings with water damage but may also come from certain foods such as peanuts, tree nuts, corn, coffee, grains, and grapes. Mold can cause mast cell activation and a condition known as chronic inflammatory response syndrome (CIRS). This can cause sensations that feel like electric shock as well as pain and other physical symptoms. These infectious conditions can cause postural orthostatic tachycardia syndrome (POTS), a condition in which heart rate elevates quickly upon standing.

Your physician can help you identify whether your child's symptoms may be due to one of these conditions, do proper testing, and give appropriate treatment.

Mast Cell Activation

Mast cell activation was discussed in the first chapter of the book. It's a condition in which histamine and other inflammatory substances are released from mast cells, causing inflammation. This condition can cause brain inflammation and significant symptoms that increase the severity of ASD and health symptoms, including gastroesophageal reflux disease (GERD). Luteolin, a natural flavonoid, was found to be helpful with mast cell activation in ASD.[8] In addition to luteolin and a low histamine diet, there are other interventions your physician can help with.

Diabetes and Insulin Resistance

While diabetes is not one of the most common conditions you hear about with autism, there is some evidence of an association with ASD and increased risk of type 2 diabetes.[9] Type 2 diabetes involves insulin resistance and can affect the brain. Brain glucose metabolism may also be impaired in those with autism, possibly impairing neuron function in the brain (contributing to brain dysfunction).[10] The brain uses glucose for energy, and if it cannot get it or utilize it, it can negatively affect the brain unless another energy source is available. (Recall that this is one of the mechanisms of action behind the ketogenic diet, which uses fat in the form of ketones for energy.) New research is looking at insulin resistance and glucose metabolism in neurological conditions.

For individuals with insulin resistance or diabetes, working with a physician and addressing it in a medically appropriate manner is essential for the individual's health. It also may influence the symptoms of autism.

Although more research is needed, anything that affects inflammation and brain function could affect symptoms of autism.

Stressors, EMFs, and Trauma

Stressors and trauma can be both physical and emotional. One of the biggest physical stressors are electromagnetic fields (EMFs) and radio frequency radiation (RFR). EMFs are a combination of electrical and magnetic fields, and RFR is a type of EMF. Our exposure to EMFs has increased exponentially compared to decades ago because of cellular phones, headsets, electronic devices, and in-home routers. These high frequency waves can travel at the speed of light and can cause physical challenges to the body. Researchers have found that EMFs may reduce learning, memory, and attention, and increase behavior problems in children, and this may be caused by DNA damage and epigenetic changes.[11] Some researchers make the case that the physiological effects and known symptoms of EMF exposure match the behaviors and symptoms of autism.[12]

Although we may not be able to eliminate all exposure to EMFs, there are things we can do to significantly reduce our children's exposure. Do not put the Wi-Fi router in your child's room or close to where they spend a lot of time. Turn the router off at night when you're sleeping. Avoid electronics, including clocks, close to where your child sleeps. Avoid wireless baby monitors. Minimize your child's exposure to handheld devices. Turn off Bluetooth. There are also EMF meters that can help you detect sources of EMFs in your home and experts that can give you more advice.

Trauma can include emotional trauma and should not be discounted. Research into emotional trauma found that adverse childhood experiences (ACEs) can disrupt our microbiome along with causing many changes to our biochemistry and brain and affecting the way we react to stress. Fortunately, diet and nutrition strategies such as omega-3s, probiotics, and prebiotics may help reduce these stress-induced changes.[13]

Physical trauma, such as traumatic brain injury, can cause neuroin-flammation and exacerbate symptoms of autism. Always seek the support of your doctor and health care team if you suspect a possible brain injury.

Toxins and Detoxification

Toxins are a key factor in the development of ASD. While we talked about how to do your best to avoid environmental toxins such as heavy metals, pesticides, industrial chemicals, and plastics, exposures are not always within your control. Also, the synergistic nature of toxins makes small amounts of several toxins considerably more harmful than one toxin.

Additionally, when someone has poor detoxification (as is common in ASD), they may not be able to clear out small amounts of toxins that typically would not be a problem. In this case, the toxins can build up and cause serious harm.

Furthermore, the gut and brain have a barrier to prevent further exposure to the body and brain, and those with autism are more likely to have poorly functioning protective barriers, which allows toxins to cause more damage.

If healthy eating and supplementation don't seem to be enough to relieve the burden on the body and support detox function, or when someone has more toxins—such as heavy metals, mold toxins, and environmental chemicals—in their system, significant detoxification strategies may be needed.

Detoxification agents can bind to toxins in the gut or neutralize them through phase 1 and phase 2 liver detoxification. Heavy metals are so harmful that they are often stored away deep in the system. Some detoxification strategies can bind to them and pull them out of their deep storage location, causing them to circulate around the body. If the detoxification substance "drops" or becomes unbound to the toxins, they are free to damage more tissues. Therefore, I recommend working with a doctor who is very experienced and skilled with detoxification, who can help you find safe strategies and supplements.

LABORATORY TESTING

I divide laboratory testing into two categories: conventional testing and functional testing. For example, conventional tests include common laboratory tests such as a complete blood count, comprehensive metabolic panel, and lipid panel. Conventional testing helps doctors understand the blood cells, metabolism, and cholesterol levels, as well as heart, liver, and kidney function. All doctors are familiar with these types of tests and run them often.

Functional laboratory tests consist of testing that gives you and your doctor a better understanding of what is happening functionally in the body. Functional tests look at the stool to assess digestion and the microbiome, organic compounds in the urine to assess aspects of nutritional status and microbes, and the blood to look for food reactions and nutrients. There is no hard line between what is conventional and what is functional. The biggest distinction is that functional labs are often not familiar to most conventional medical doctors. So, if you want to run them, you'll either need a functional or integrative medical doctor or an open-minded conventional medical doctor.

As you look at the following labs tests, you may think, *What should I run?* The answer to that is another question: What do you and your doctor want to know? All data is good data, and in some cases, the more data the better. But these tests are expensive and not all are easy to do. So I suggest you prioritize testing based on the health questions you'd like answered. Here are some of the tests available and the things that they can look for.

Comprehensive Digestive Stool Analysis

A comprehensive digestive stool analysis analyzes the stool for markers that help your doctor better understand your child's digestive function. Each lab is somewhat different but most look at digestion and absorption, markers of inflammation, and short-chain fatty acids, and some test for microbes.

If you want to know about the state of the gut, such as whether there is inflammation, proper chewing, sufficient digestion, adequate fat and carbohydrate absorption, healthy levels of short-chain fatty acids, and immune function, then a comprehensive digestive stool analysis can be helpful to run.

Gut Microbiome Testing

A gut microbiome test looks at the beneficial and pathogenic bacteria present and their levels. Many will look at yeast and other microbes as well. Some tests will culture and then expose the pathogens to pharmaceutical and natural agents that kill them to see if they are sensitive or resistant to the agents, so you doctor can help formulate the best strategy for eradication. Some labs use DNA identification of microbes, which is beneficial because it can be hard to culture pathogens, especially those that die when exposed to oxygen. So DNA testing can identify more microbes.

Some gut microbiome labs also include custom probiotics to help balance the microbiome. Other gut microbiome tests use these results to formulate diet recommendations. People often ask me if this is an effective way to personalize a diet. I have found that these labs are not as accurate as humans in seeing the big picture and formulating a personalized nutrition plan.

If you want to know about the balance and levels of bacteria, yeast, and other microbes in the gut, then a gut microbiome test would be beneficial.

Organic Acid Testing

Organic acids are chemical compounds found in the urine that are products of our metabolism. These organic acids can help us determine vitamin and mineral status of certain nutrients such as B_{12}, antioxidant function including glutathione and vitamin C markers, and metabolism of fatty acids, ketone markers, mitochondrial markers, and amino acid markers.

Bacterial and yeast markers of dysbiosis are also tested, sometimes as a separate add-on organic acid test. There are pros and cons to using urine or stool when testing for microbes. In the stool, you identify specific bacteria and their levels. With organic acid testing, yeast and bacteria are identified by the organic acids in the urine, which can help for microbes that are hard to culture.

Some labs also can test for oxalates in the form of oxalic acid in the urine. However, not all labs do, so if you want to know more about oxalates in your child, you'll want to take that into consideration when choosing a lab.

Organic acid testing is beneficial to get a big picture of metabolism, nutrient status, and several systems and functions in the body.

Food Sensitivity Testing

There are a number of types of food sensitivity testing. IgG testing is the most common food sensitivity testing. Some labs also test IgA levels to foods and autoimmune antibodies against different tissues. The other common and beneficial type of food sensitivity testing is cell-mediated food testing. Each of these tests for different immune system reactions and can be beneficial.

If you suspect your child is sensitive to many different foods and an elimination diet is too challenging to conduct, or you have done one and it did not yield adequate data, then a food sensitivity panel may be beneficial.

Pyroluria, Zinc, and Copper Testing

There are labs that test for nutrients and conditions affecting mental health. Tests may include kryptopyrrole urine testing for pyroluria, plasma zinc, and serum copper.

Genetics and Nutrigenetics Testing

Genetic testing provides results on genes and single nucleotide polymorphisms (SNPs), often using saliva, and many are direct to consumer. Some labs run the data and deliver it in a raw form, so it must be run through another company that can interpret this data for you. There are many companies that do both. Some of these companies simply tell you which SNPs you have, others will also provide nutrition recommendations based on the data. You'll want to feel confident about the accuracy of these recommendations.

It's important to understand the pros and cons of this type of testing. Although there are some laws in certain countries to safeguard your data and privacy, it's important that you know what you are testing and what the potential risks are. While data can help you seek solutions, some people may experience anxiety or fear, depending on what is discovered. Also, although some countries have laws to safeguard consumers from future discrimination or potential harm, it's not possible to know all of the risks that might exist for an individual now and in the future. For these reasons, it's good to do your research and feel confident in your choice before proceeding.

A benefit of genetic testing is that it provides very specific information on your child's genetic makeup, painting a picture of what may be happening in their cells on a very detailed level. There are hundreds, even thousands, of pieces of information. However, this testing can't tell us definitively what is happening. As we covered in "What Causes Autism," we don't know if these genes are expressing. Also, it gets complex, as some genes could be improving or compounding the biochemical effects of other genes. Personally, I have found genetic testing to be helpful but not a full picture by itself. I think there is still a lot to be learned about how to apply this information to clinical nutrition recommendations.

Nutrient Testing

There is no single laboratory test that will analyze all vitamins and minerals. Part of the reason for this is that there are different ways to test for the nutrient levels in your body. Some are best tested in blood, serum, plasma, hair, or urine. And others are best tested as metabolites rather than actual levels. For example, B_{12} may be normal or even high in the blood, but it is not getting into the cell and being utilized properly. Methylmalonyl-CoA (MMA) is a urine metabolite that is more sensitive at determining B_{12}

levels. MMA requires B_{12} to be converted to succinyl-coenzyme A during metabolism. High MMA levels in urine indicate there is not adequate B_{12} in the cells. There are tests for nutrients that can be beneficial. However, it's often more than one test to get the full picture of nutritional status. Nutrient testing can be helpful when you suspect a deficiency, when your child has a very limited diet, or if you want to explore common deficiencies and see if your child has any.

CONCLUSION

Nourishment is essential to all humans, especially growing children. And your child's diet and nutritional needs are as unique as they are. Therapeutic diets and nutrition are generally safe and effective for children and adults with ASD. Autism spectrum disorder is a condition affecting multiple systems, and the underlying causes and resulting symptoms are different from person to person. Creating a personalized autism nutrition plan can improve symptoms and have profound benefits.

Feeding our children is an inherent part of parenting and something we have control over right in our own kitchen. Food is medicine. It can have a powerful effect on our health, and in the words of one of my Nourishing Hope families, "Every meal is an opportunity to heal." Eating well and taking care of ourselves are lifelong strategies. It's never too late to start, and it will set your child up to reach their full potential and thrive.

Remember Matthew, the young man with autism whose story I told in the introduction? As a young boy with very little language who became an aspiring author, Matthew wanted to tell you in his own words how therapeutic nutrition changed his life.

> When it comes to nutrition, I believe that it plays a critical role in not only recovering from autism but improving life in general. It was easy being addicted to crap food; the flavors and the sugars were—and still are—certainly enticing, but it was short-term

thinking. I don't remember when I went on a diet; those memories are like puzzle pieces now lost to time. But nowadays when I eat a certain food, healthy or unhealthy, there are consequences. My mood can shift erratically. My mental health could take a dive. When I eat healthy foods—protein mostly—I feel stronger and more capable of doing things. When you eat well, you'll feel well. That's my experience with dieting. If my mom hadn't found out about the diet connection, my family and I would still be eating the standard American diet. I owe my mom a lot, and I think that I will never pay off that debt in my lifetime. However, I know I can try to reach out to others and persuade them to live the healthy lifestyle as I have. It's not easy, but nothing worth doing is easy.

I couldn't have said it better myself. Focusing on diet and nutrition is worth it. You won't regret it. Take one step and one meal at a time. Start where you can, and keep nourishing hope.

SECTION 4

Fifty Family-Friendly Recipes

A book on therapeutic diets would not be complete without recipes to support you. The following are some of my favorite recipes for children (and adults) with autism. Each recipe is tagged with diet compliance, so you can choose the right recipes for your child and family. These tags include:

- GFCFSF
- Egg-Free
- Nut-Free
- Elimination
- Low Salicylate
- Low SAG (salicylate, amine, and glutamate)
- Low Histamine
- Low Oxalate
- Low FODMAP

- *SCD/GAPS*
- *Paleo*
- *Autoimmune Paleo*
- *Ketogenic*
- *Vegan*
- *Vegetarian*

While these recipes contain ingredients and amounts that are compliant for many people on these diets, remember that multiple servings or meals can add up. Also, each person's tolerance for specific foods within a diet varies, so incorporate these meals as tolerated. I've also added notes to recipes when they can be adapted to make them diet compliant.

SOME UNIVERSAL NOTES

Choose diet-compliant cooking oils. Examples include avocado oil, extra virgin olive oil, melted coconut oil, or even lard. For low salicylate and low SAG diets, sunflower oil and rice bran oil (free of synthetic antioxidants and additives) are good choices.

For nondairy milk and nondairy butter, choose casein-free, soy-free, and other diet-compliant options. Most of these recipes were tested with salted nondairy butter. Either salted or unsalted varieties will work—simply add more salt as needed if using unsalted nondairy butter. All recipes use unsweetened plain nondairy milks. See the book extras at www .PersonalizedAutismNutritionPlan.com/extras for some of my favorite brands and products.

Choose pasture-raised meats and eggs whenever possible.

For salt, I like to use Celtic sea salt or Himalayan crystal salt with a small to medium coarseness.

The SCD/GAPS Diet recipes are intended for use with the full SCD or GAPS Diet, although some are appropriate for the introductory phases. For low oxalate diet–compliant recipes, limit the serving size to ½ cup unless otherwise specified, or if ingredients are very low oxalate and a larger serving size is acceptable.

BREAKFASTS

MAIN COURSES

VEGETABLE SIDES

BREAKFASTS

GRAIN-FREE BANANA BLUEBERRY MUFFINS

GFCFSF, SCD/GAPS, Paleo, Vegetarian

MAKES 12 MUFFINS

Ingredients

3 large very ripe bananas, mashed

3 large eggs, beaten

1 or 2 tablespoons honey (see note)

2 teaspoons gluten-free vanilla extract

2 cups blanched almond flour

½ teaspoon salt

1 teaspoon baking soda

1 tablespoon apple cider vinegar

1 cup blueberries

Instructions

1. Preheat the oven to 350°F. Line a standard muffin pan with 12 liners.
2. In a large bowl, combine the bananas, eggs, honey, and vanilla extract and stir well to combine. Stir in the almond flour and salt.
3. Place the baking soda in a small bowl. Add the apple cider vinegar and stir. As the mixture foams, quickly add it to the bowl with the banana mixture and fold it in. Fold in the blueberries.
4. Divide the batter evenly into the prepared muffin tin (a ¼-cup measure works great as a scoop!).
5. Bake for 22 to 25 minutes, until a toothpick inserted into center of a muffin comes out clean.
6. Let the muffins cool in the pan for 5 minutes, then transfer them to a wire rack to cool completely.

Note: The amount of honey (1 to 2 tablespoons) is personal preference based on how much sugar you want. I find kids like 2 tablespoons.

CHICKEN PANCAKES

GFCFSF, Nut-Free, Low Salicylate, Low SAG, Low Oxalate, Low FODMAP, SCD/GAPS, Paleo, Ketogenic

Low Histamine: Replace 3 chicken eggs with 9 quail eggs

MAKES 6 PANCAKES

Ingredients

1 chicken breast, cooked (see note)
3 large eggs
½ teaspoon salt
Diet-compliant oil, for cooking

Instructions

1. Blend the chicken breast, eggs, and salt together in a food processor until a smooth, thick batter forms.
2. Heat a large frying pan or skillet over medium heat. Melt or drizzle oil in the pan, swirling to coat, then reduce the heat to medium-low.
3. Add a dollop of the batter to the pan. Spread the batter into a 3- or 4-inch-diameter pancake ⅓ inch thick. Cook for about 5 to 6 minutes, until the pancake is firm enough to flip, then continue cooking until the inside is no longer wet, about 5 minutes more. Repeat with the remaining batter.

Note: If you are cooking the chicken breast specifically for this recipe, use a boneless, skinless breast and boil until thoroughly cooked (internal temperature reaches 165°F). If you are using a roasted chicken and don't know the precise amount of the breast, use 1⅓ cups of chopped cooked chicken.

BANANA PANCAKES

GFCFSF, Nut-Free, SCD/GAPS, Paleo, Vegetarian

Low Oxalate: Limit serving size to 2 pancakes

MAKES 12 PANCAKES

Ingredients

3 very ripe bananas
2 large eggs
½ teaspoon gluten-free vanilla extract
Pinch salt
Any diet-compliant oil, for cooking

Instructions

1. In a medium bowl, mash the bananas with a fork. Add the eggs and beat until well combined. Add the vanilla and salt and mix until combined.
2. Heat a large frying pan or skillet over medium heat. Melt or drizzle the oil in the pan, swirling to coat, then reduce the heat to medium-low.
3. Spoon enough batter into the pan to form a 3- to 4-inch pancake. Cook for about 3 minutes, until set, then flip and cook until golden brown and cooked thoroughly, about 2 minutes more. Repeat with the remaining batter.

COCONUT PANCAKES

GFCFSF, Nut-Free, Low Oxalate, SCD/GAPS, Paleo, Vegetarian

*Ketogenic: Omit the honey, and if desired, substitute
a sugar-free keto-friendly sweetener*

MAKES 12 PANCAKES

Ingredients

4 large eggs, at room temperature

¼ cup avocado oil, plus more for cooking

2 tablespoons full-fat coconut milk or other unsweetened plain
     nondairy milk

1 tablespoon honey (optional)

1 teaspoon gluten-free vanilla extract

⅓ cup coconut flour

¼ teaspoon salt

½ teaspoon baking soda

Maple syrup or diet-compliant topping of choice, for serving (see note)

Instructions

1. Beat the eggs in a large bowl. Add the oil, coconut milk, honey (if
    using), and vanilla.
2. In a separate medium bowl, combine coconut flour, salt, and
    baking soda.
3. Transfer the flour mixture to a sifter or fine-mesh strainer.
    Gradually sift the flour mixture into the egg mixture while mixing
    it with an electric mixer until smooth.
4. Heat a large frying pan or skillet over medium heat. Melt or drizzle
    oil in the pan, swirling to coat, then reduce the heat to medium-
    low. Pour the batter into the pan, making a 3- or 4-inch pancake.
    Cook on one side until firm and bubbles begin to form on top and
    pop, then flip and cook on the other side until cooked through,
    about 1 to 2 minutes more. Repeat with the remaining batter.
5. Top with maple syrup.

Note: For SCD, top the pancakes with honey that has been thinned
with a few drops of water instead of maple syrup. For ketogenic, use
a keto-friendly syrup, such as Lakanto maple syrup.

CHICKEN APPLE SAUSAGE

GFCFSF, Egg-Free, Nut-Free, Elimination, Low Salicylate, Low SAG, Low Histamine, Low Oxalate, SCD/GAPS, Paleo, Autoimmune Paleo

MAKES 6 PATTIES

Ingredients

Diet-compliant oil, for cooking

1 Golden or Red Delicious apple, peeled and finely chopped (see note)

1 pound ground chicken (see note)

½ teaspoon salt

Instructions

1. Set a large skillet over medium heat. Melt or drizzle oil in the skillet, swirling to coat. Add the apple and cook until softened, about 5 minutes. Remove the skillet from the heat and let the apple cool slightly.
2. In a large bowl, combine the chicken, cooked apple, and salt and mix until thoroughly combined. Form the mixture into 6 patties (about ⅓ inch thick).
3. Wipe out the skillet, add more oil, and warm over medium-high heat. Add the patties and cook them on both sides until the sausages are browned and the internal temperature reaches 165°F.

Note: For low salicylate, using a Golden or Red Delicious apple is very important. You could also use a pear. For other diets, any apple will work. Sweet and tart apples like Pink Lady and Granny Smith work very well. For low SAG and low histamine, the ground chicken must be freshly ground and used the same day.

MAPLE PORK SAUSAGE

GFCFSF, Egg-Free, Nut-Free, Elimination, Low Salicylate, Low Oxalate, Low FODMAP, Paleo

Ketogenic: Use a zero-sugar maple-flavored syrup, such as monk fruit syrup

SCD/GAPS: Omit maple syrup or substitute with honey

MAKES 6 PATTIES

Ingredients

1 pound ground pork
2 tablespoons maple syrup
½ teaspoon salt
Diet-compliant oil, for cooking

Instructions

1. In a large bowl, combine the pork, maple syrup, and salt and mix until thoroughly combined. Form the mixture into 6 patties (about ⅓ inch thick).
2. Set a large skillet over medium heat. Melt or drizzle oil in the skillet, swirling to coat. Add the patties and cook them on both sides, until the sausages are browned and the internal temperature reaches 165°F.

BUTTERNUT SQUASH HASH BROWNS

GFCFSF, Egg-Free, Nut-Free, Elimination, Low Salicylate, Low SAG, Low Histamine, Low Oxalate, SCD/GAPS, Paleo, Autoimmune Paleo, Vegan, Vegetarian

MAKES 6 TO 8 SERVINGS

Ingredients

1 tablespoon diet-compliant oil
2 cups peeled and grated butternut squash
Salt

Instructions

Set a large frying pan over medium heat. Melt or drizzle the oil in the pan, swirling to coat. Add ⅓ cup of butternut squash to the pan, press gently to flatten into a ⅓-inch-thick disc, and cook until browned and crispy underneath, about 5 minutes, then flip and cook on the other side until browned and crispy, about 5 minutes more. Season with salt to taste. Repeat with the remaining batter.

Note: These hash browns are great topped with poached or fried eggs or served as a side with diet-compliant sausage or scrambled eggs. They can also be made with rutabagas and other root vegetables.

RICE PORRIDGE (SLOW COOKER)

GFCFSF, Nut-Free, Vegetarian

Egg-Free, Vegan, or Elimination: Omit egg

Low Salicylate and Low SAG: Replace coconut milk with cashew milk and omit spices

Low Histamine: Omit egg or replace with 3 quail eggs, and omit vanilla if not tolerated because of fermentation

MAKES 4 SERVINGS

Ingredients

1½ cups canned full-fat coconut milk
1½ cups water
1¼ cups brown rice
1 egg, beaten (optional)
2 tablespoons maple syrup
1 teaspoon gluten-free vanilla extract
1 teaspoon ground cinnamon
½ teaspoon ground cardamom
¼ teaspoon ground nutmeg

Instructions

1. Combine all ingredients in a 5-quart slow cooker, stir ingredients, cover, and cook on low for 6 to 8 hours. Set the timer at night, and breakfast will be ready when you wake up.

MAIN COURSES

EGG-FREE CHICKEN NUGGETS

*GFCFSF, Egg-Free, Nut-Free, Elimination, Low
Histamine, Low Oxalate, Low FODMAP*

Low Salicylate: Substitute rice vinegar for white vinegar

MAKES 3 TO 4 SERVINGS

Ingredients

1 pound chicken breasts or thighs
⅔ cup gluten-free flour (see note)
½ teaspoon salt
2 teaspoons gluten-free white vinegar
½ teaspoon baking soda
⅓ cup water
Diet-compliant oil, for cooking
Diet-compliant dipping sauce of choice, for serving

Instructions

1. Cut the chicken into nugget-size pieces ½ inch thick.
2. Mix the flour and salt in a medium bowl. In a small bowl, combine the vinegar and baking soda and quickly add it to the flour mixture as it fizzes. Quickly add the water and mix everything together with a fork until combined.
3. In a large frying pan over medium heat, add a thick layer of oil (about ¹⁄₁₀ inch) and heat until hot (test by spooning in a small amount of batter; it should sizzle).
4. Dip the chicken pieces in the batter. Place the battered chicken in the pan and cook for 4 to 5 minutes, then turn them over and cook until they reach an internal temperature of 165°F, about 4 to 5 minutes more. Use internal temperature, not time, as your gauge of when they are done. Set the cooked nuggets on a paper towel–lined plate to drain any excess oil.
5. Serve the nuggets alone or with a dipping sauce. Freeze any leftovers.

Note: I use two-thirds brown rice flour and one-third potato starch or tapioca starch or a combination of both. Don't use a gluten-free baking mix with xanthan gum or other gum because it will make the batter gummy.

SUPER NUTRIENT BURGERS

GFCFSF, Egg-Free, Nut-Free, Elimination, Paleo, Ketogenic

Low Salicylate: Omit onion powder, rosemary, and pepper

Low FODMAP: Omit onion powder

SCD/GAPS: Use homemade onion powder without added starch or omit

Autoimmune Paleo: Omit onion powder and pepper

MAKES 4 PATTIES

Ingredients
2 to 3 ounces liver
1 pound ground beef
1 teaspoon onion powder
¼ teaspoon rosemary
½ teaspoon salt
¼ teaspoon white pepper (optional)

Instructions
1. Put the liver in a food processor and blend until smooth. Discard any liver that is not thoroughly blended. You should end up with about ⅓ cup of puree.
2. In a large bowl, mix the liver with the beef, onion powder, rosemary, salt, and white pepper (if using) until well combined. Form the beef mixture into 4 patties (about ½ inch thick).
3. Heat a large frying pan over medium-high heat. Place the patties in the pan and cook for 5 to 6 minutes, then flip and cook until they reach an internal temperature of 160°F to 165°F, about 5 to 6 minutes more. (Since these contain raw liver, cook them until thoroughly done.)

Note: You might have to try the recipe to believe it, but these burgers are delicious! No one will know they are eating liver. Liver is high in iron, zinc, and vitamins A, C, and B_{12}.

GROUND BEEF STUFFED ZUCCHINI (ZUCCHIN-IZZA)

GFCFSF, Egg-Free, Low Oxalate, Paleo, Ketogenic

Ketogenic: Limit serving size to 1 medium zucchini

Nut-free and SCD/GAPS: Omit the optional dairy-free cheese if it's not diet compliant

MAKES 4 SERVINGS

Ingredients

4 zucchini

2 tablespoons avocado oil

1 pound ground beef

¼ cup finely chopped onion

2 garlic cloves, finely chopped

1 tomato, finely chopped

½ teaspoon salt

1 (7-ounce) package dairy-free cheese (optional if diet compliant)

Instructions

1. Preheat the oven to 425°F.
2. Cut the very ends off the zucchini—don't cut too much because you need the zucchini to hold its boat shape when fully cut. Halve lengthwise. Use a spoon to carve into boats, scooping out the seeds.
3. Bring a large pot of water to a boil over high heat. Add the zucchini and boil for 3 to 4 minutes, depending on size and thickness, until softened and cooked about halfway through. Drain and set aside.
4. Heat a large frying pan over medium-high heat. Add the oil, swirling to coat. Add the ground beef and cook, stirring and breaking it up with a wooden spoon as it browns. When the beef is almost fully cooked, about 10 minutes, add the onion, garlic, tomato, and salt. Cook for a few more minutes, until the tomato is cooked down, the onion and garlic are fragrant, and the meat is thoroughly cooked.

5. Place the zucchini boats, cut side up, on a rimmed baking sheet. Fill each boat with some of the ground beef mixture. Sprinkle with dairy-free cheese (if using).
6. Roast the boats for 10 to 15 minutes, until the cheese is melted and/or the top of the beef is slightly browned.
7. Serve hot.

LAMB STEW (SLOW COOKER)

GFCFSF, Egg-Free, Nut-Free, Elimination

MAKES 8 TO 10 SERVINGS

Ingredients

2 pounds lamb stew cubes
2 cups beef or chicken stock
1 cup water
6 potatoes, chopped
4 carrots, chopped
2 to 3 parsnips, chopped
1 head cauliflower, chopped
2 celery ribs, finely chopped
1 small onion, finely chopped
½ to 1 bunch greens such as kale, finely chopped

Instructions

1. Combine the lamb, stock, water, potatoes, carrots, parsnips, cauliflower, celery, and onion in a slow cooker. Cover, set on high, and cook until simmering (this could take 5 or more hours), then turn to low and cook for 1 to 3 more hours, until potatoes and beef are tender. In the last 30 minutes of cooking, add the greens.
2. Serve hot.

POT ROAST

GFCFSF, Egg-Free, Nut-Free, SCD/GAPS, Paleo

Elimination Diet: Omit wine

Low Oxalate and Ketogenic: Omit carrots

Low FODMAP: Omit onion and garlic

Autoimmune Paleo: Omit wine and use diet-compliant herbs

MAKES 6 TO 8 SERVINGS

Ingredients

3 pounds chuck roast
2 teaspoons mixed dried herbs/spices (see note)
1 teaspoon sea salt
2 tablespoons diet-compliant oil
2 cups beef broth
1 large onion, quartered
3 to 4 garlic cloves, halved
Splash of red wine (optional)
4 to 5 carrots, peeled

Instructions

1. Preheat the oven to 325°F.
2. Rub the roast with the herb/spice mixture and salt.
3. Heat a large Dutch oven or a heavy-bottomed oven-safe pot over medium-high heat. Add the oil, swirling to coat. Sear each side of the roast for about 2 minutes. Add the broth, onion, garlic, and wine (if using), cover the pot with a lid or aluminum foil, and bring to a simmer on the stove.
4. Place the pot in the oven. Check every hour to ensure there is enough liquid to cover the roast about halfway, adding water if it's low.
5. After 2 hours, add the carrots and cover the pot.
6. Roast for another 1 to 1½ hours, for a total of 3 to 3½ hours of cooking time, until the beef is tender, pulling apart with a fork.
7. Serve hot.

Note: Get creative—and if your kid likes cooking, invite them to create a spice blend with you. You can use many different herbs and spices in pot roast. My favorite combo is thyme, rosemary, sage, black pepper, and paprika.

CREAMY CRUSHED GARLIC CHICKEN

GFCFSF, Egg-Free, Nut-Free, Low Oxalate, SCD/
GAPS, Paleo, Autoimmune Paleo, Ketogenic

MAKES 4 TO 6 SERVINGS

Ingredients

2 pounds boneless, skinless chicken breasts or tenders
Salt
1 tablespoon extra virgin olive oil
2 tablespoons nondairy butter (see note)
30 garlic cloves, peeled
1 cup chopped onion
1 cup full-fat coconut milk (see note)
1 cup chicken broth
1 tablespoon lemon juice

Instructions

1. If the chicken breasts are whole, halve lengthwise so they are thin. If using tenders, no slicing is necessary. Season the chicken with salt to taste.
2. Heat a large saute pan over medium-high heat. Add the oil, swirling to coat. Add the chicken and sear for 4 to 6 minutes per side, until browned (the chicken will finish cooking in the sauce). Remove the chicken from the pan and set aside.
3. Take the pan off the heat and reduce the heat to medium-low. Once the pan has cooled slightly, wipe it out, return it to the heat, and melt the nondairy butter. Add the garlic and saute for 2 minutes, until fragrant. Add the onion and cook for 3 to 5 minutes, until translucent. Add the coconut milk, chicken broth, lemon juice, and ¼ teaspoon salt. Simmer for 5 to 10 minutes, until the flavors are melded and the sauce has reduced slightly.

4. Return the chicken to the pan and simmer until the internal temperature reaches 165°F, about 5 minutes, depending on thickness.

Note: Ensure the nondairy butter is diet compliant; for example, some use cashews, which would be not allowed on a nut-free diet. For SCD/GAPS, ensure the coconut milk has no guar-gum or other non-compliant ingredients.

SALMON CAKES

GFCFSF, Nut-Free, Low Salicylate, Low Oxalate, Low FODMAP

MAKES 2 SERVINGS

Ingredients

1 (6-ounce) can salmon with bones, drained
½ cup gluten-free breadcrumbs (see note)
2 large eggs, beaten
¼ cup finely chopped fresh herbs such as chives, green onion, and/
   or parsley (optional)
1½ teaspoons avocado oil
Salt

Instructions

1. In a medium bowl, smash the salmon with a fork to break up and crush the bones. Add the breadcrumbs, eggs, and herbs (if using) and stir until everything is fully incorporated. Refrigerate the salmon mixture for 20 to 30 minutes to let it firm up slightly.
2. Form the salmon mixture into 3 to 4 patties (about ¾ inch thick).
3. Heat a large frying pan over medium heat. Add the avocado oil, swirling to coat. Cook the salmon cakes for 4 minutes on each side, or until firm and the egg has cooked. Season with salt to taste.

Note: If you don't have gluten-free breadcrumbs, you can make them by drying out a slice of gluten-free bread in the oven and crumbling it.

SQUASH MEATBALLS

GFCFSF, Nut-Free, Low Salicylate, Low Oxalate

Low SAG: Limit meat choices to beef, chicken, or other diet-complaint options

SCD/GAPS and Paleo: Omit breadcrumbs

MAKES 6 TO 8 SERVINGS

Ingredients

2 pounds ground beef, turkey, chicken, or bison (see note)
1 cup pureed cooked butternut squash
2 large eggs
1 cup gluten-free breadcrumbs (see note)
1 teaspoon salt

Instructions

1. Preheat the oven to 350°F. Line a rimmed baking sheet with parchment paper.
2. Combine all the ingredients in a large bowl until thoroughly mixed. Form the mixture into 1- to 2-inch balls and place on the prepared baking sheet.
3. Bake for about 30 minutes, or until the balls are cooked through (the internal temperature should reach 160°F for beef and bison and 165°F for chicken or turkey).

Note: For low SAG and low histamine, ground meat must be freshly ground and used immediately. *For low oxalate, ensure the breadcrumbs are made with low oxalate ingredients.*

SHEPHERD'S PIE

GFCFSF, Egg-Free, Nut-Free

Elimination: Omit cornstarch

Low FODMAP: Omit onion and garlic, and consider using onion or garlic oil to cook ground beef

MAKES 6 TO 8 SERVINGS

Ingredients

Mashed Potato Topping
3 pounds potatoes, peeled and cut into 1-inch chunks
1 cup unsweetened plain nondairy milk
2 tablespoons nondairy butter
½ teaspoon salt

Meat Filling
1 tablespoon extra virgin olive oil
1 onion, chopped
3 garlic cloves, minced
2 pounds ground beef
½ teaspoon salt
2 cups beef broth
1 cup chopped carrots
2 cups chopped kale
3 tablespoons cornstarch (optional)
½ cup cold water (optional)

Instructions

1. Preheat the oven to 400°F.
2. For the mashed potato topping: Put the potatoes in a large pot and add enough water to cover by 1 to 2 inches. Bring to a boil over high heat, then reduce the heat to medium to maintain a simmer. Simmer for 10 to 12 minutes, or until the potatoes are easily pierced with a fork. Drain well.
3. With a potato masher, mash the potatoes and mix in the nondairy milk, nondairy butter, and salt.
4. For the meat filling: While the potatoes are cooking, heat a large frying pan over medium heat. Pour in the oil, swirling to coat. Saute

the onion for a few minutes, until translucent. Add the garlic and cook, stirring occasionally, just until fragrant, about 30 seconds.

5. Add the beef and cook, crumbling and breaking the beef up with a wooden spoon, until browned, about 10 minutes. Season with the salt.
6. Pour the broth over the beef and bring it to a simmer. Add the carrots and simmer for 5 minutes, until slightly softened. Add the kale and simmer another 3 minutes, until tender.
7. If you'd like to thicken the broth, stir together the cornstarch and water until dissolved. Add it to the filling mixture and bring back to a simmer until thickened, about 2 to 3 minutes.
8. To assemble the pie, layer the filling mixture in the bottom of a large casserole dish. Dollop the mashed potatoes over the top and spread into an even layer.
9. Bake for about 20 minutes, until the potatoes are lightly browned and the filling is bubbling.

BEAN BURGERS

GFCFSF, Nut-Free, Vegetarian

SCD/GAPS: Use navy beans or another SCD/GAPS-compliant legume in place of black beans

MAKES 10 SERVINGS

Ingredients
1 cup dry black or kidney beans
1 cup sunflower seeds
4 large eggs
½ cup grated carrots
½ cup finely chopped kale
½ cup finely chopped onion
1 tablespoon finely chopped fresh parsley
1 tablespoon dried rosemary
1 tablespoon dried basil
1¼ teaspoons salt
Diet-compliant oil, for cooking

Instructions

1. Place the beans in a large bowl and add enough water to cover by about 3 inches. Let the beans soak overnight at room temperature. Drain and rinse well with water.
2. Place the beans in a large pot. Cover with 2 inches of water and boil for 20 to 25 minutes, until soft but not mushy. Add extra water if needed to keep them covered. (Do not add salt to the beans while they cook—it will make them tough.) Drain well.
3. In a food processor, grind the sunflower seeds until the consistency of nut flour, then transfer to a large bowl. In the same food processor (no need to clean between steps), process the beans until coarsely chopped.
4. Add the beans to the bowl with the sunflower seed meal. Add the eggs, carrots, kale, onion, parsley, rosemary, basil, and salt, and knead with your hands until mixed thoroughly.
5. Form the mixture into 10 patties (about ½ to ¾ inch thick).
6. Heat the oil in a large frying pan over medium heat. Working in batches, cook the burgers at least 10 minutes on each side, until they are firm, hold together, and are no longer wet inside. Lower the heat slightly if the burgers are browning too quickly.

Note: Cooked burgers can be kept for 3 to 4 days in the refrigerator. They can be eaten cold or reheated in a 350°F oven for about 10 minutes. They also freeze well.

DAIRY-FREE MAC AND CHEESE

GFCFSF, Egg-Free

Nut-Free: Use nut-free versions for nondairy butter, milk, and cheese

Low Oxalate: Use a low oxalate pasta, white rice flour instead of brown, and keep to a ½-cup serving size

MAKES 8 SERVINGS

Ingredients

1 pound gluten-free pasta (see note)
½ cup nondairy butter

¼ cup brown rice flour

1½ cups unsweetened plain nondairy milk

2 cups grated dairy-free, soy-free cheddar cheese

1 cup grated dairy-free, soy-free mozzarella cheese

½ teaspoon salt (optional)

Instructions

1. Bring a large pot of water to a boil. Cook the pasta until al dente or slightly under according to package directions. Drain well.

2. While the pasta is cooking, melt the nondairy butter in a medium saucepan over medium heat. Sprinkle in the flour and whisk until smooth. Add the nondairy milk and stir. Add the nondairy cheddar and mozzarella a little at a time until melted and stir until smooth. Taste the cheese sauce and season with the salt (if using).

3. Combine the pasta and cheese, stirring in the amount of cheese sauce to taste. Depending on how cheesy you like it, there may be extra sauce; cover any leftover cheese sauce and store in the fridge for 3 to 4 days.

Note: You may wish to make less pasta at a time if you're serving a smaller group. Personally, I prefer to make only the amount of pasta I need for one meal. Storing and reheating prepared mac and cheese will make for mushy pasta! For the next meal, make fresh pasta and gently reheat the sauce to make another batch of mac and cheese.

VEGETABLE SIDES

CONFETTI BRUSSELS SPROUTS

GFCFSF, Egg-Free, SCD/GAPS, Paleo, Ketogenic, Vegan, Vegetarian

*Nut-Free, Elimination, Low Oxalate, and
Autoimmune Paleo: Omit nuts*

Low Salicylate and Low SAG: Omit onion and nuts

MAKES 4 TO 6 SERVINGS

Ingredients

1 pound Brussels sprouts, trimmed and halved lengthwise
1 to 2 tablespoons diet-compliant oil
½ onion, chopped or sliced (optional)
½ cup chopped pecans or other nuts (optional)
¼ teaspoon salt

Instructions

1. In a food processor, pulse the Brussels sprouts into "confetti"
   (don't overprocess; the pieces should be about ½ to 1 inch in
   size). If needed, hand chop any remaining large pieces.
2. Heat a large saute pan over medium-low heat. Drizzle in the
   oil, swirling to coat. Add the onion (if using) and saute for 3 to
   4 minutes, until it is just starting to brown. Add the chopped
   Brussels sprouts, nuts (if using), and salt. Cook for 5 minutes, or
   until the Brussels sprouts and onion are soft and lightly browned.

RAINBOW SALAD

GFCFSF, Egg-Free, Nut-Free, Elimination,
Low Oxalate, Paleo, Vegetarian

SCD/GAPS: Omit jicama

Low Histamine: Omit strawberries and substitute
distilled vinegar for apple cider vingear

MAKES 6–8 SERVINGS

Ingredients

Salad
1 large jicama, peeled
1 cup sliced strawberries
1 cup sliced orange bell pepper
1 cup sliced yellow bell pepper
1 cup sliced cucumber
1 cup blueberries
1 cup thinly sliced or shaved purple cabbage

Dressing
2 tablespoons raw apple cider vinegar
2 tablespoons raw honey
6 tablespoons extra virgin olive oil

Instructions

1. For the salad: Slice the jicama into thin planks and use a star- or heart-shaped cutter to cut out fun shapes from the slices. Prepare 1 cup of jicama.
2. In a large serving bowl, arrange the fruits and vegetables in rainbow order, with the jicama shapes in the middle.
3. For the dressing: Stir together the vinegar and honey in a medium bowl until the honey is dissolved. Slowly drizzle in the oil and whisk until incorporated.
4. To serve, present the rainbow salad as arranged, then pour desired amount of dressing over the salad and toss.

CAULIFLOWER RICE

GFCFSF, Egg-Free, Nut-Free, Elimination, Low Histamine, Low Oxalate, SCD/GAPS, Paleo, Autoimmune Paleo, Ketogenic, Vegan, Vegetarian

MAKES 4 SERVINGS

Ingredients

1 head cauliflower, trimmed
1 tablespoon extra virgin olive oil
Salt

Instructions

1. Pulse the cauliflower in a food processor until it's the size of rice—a few short pulses.
2. Heat a large frying pan over medium heat. Drizzle in the oil, stirring to coat. Add the cauliflower and saute for 3 to 5 minutes, until it has softened a bit but is not mushy. Season with salt to taste.

RUTABAGA FRIES

GFCFSF, Egg-Free, Nut-Free, Elimination, Low Salicylate, Low SAG, Low Histamine, Low Oxalate, Low FODMAP, SCD/ GAPS, Paleo, Autoimmune Paleo, Vegan, Vegetarian

Ketogenic: Limit to a ½-cup serving for 4.4 grams net carbs

MAKES 4 TO 6 SERVINGS

Ingredients

3 rutabagas (see note)
2 tablespoons diet-compliant oil
1 teaspoon salt

Instructions

1. Preheat the oven to 425°F.
2. Peel the rutabagas and slice off the top end where the greens attach. Slice into planks about ¼ to ½ inch thick and 4 inches long.

3. In a large bowl, toss the raw rutabagas in the oil and salt until well coated.
4. Spread out the seasoned rutabagas into a single layer on a rimmed baking sheet. Bake for 35 to 45 minutes, until browned and caramelized, turning the fries occasionally for even browning. Be aware that they don't get fully crispy like a french fry made with potato.

Note: Carrots, sweet potatoes, other hard root vegetables, and butternut squash can be substituted for the rutabagas in this recipe. Ensure substitution is diet compliant. Cooking times may vary with other vegetables, so check the fries early and often to make sure they do not burn. You can also add other seasoning to the fries if you like, but for low salicylate and low SAG diets, stick with just salt.

CARROT CHIPS

GFCFSF, Egg-Free, Nut-Free, Elimination, Low Salicylate, Low SAG, Low Histamine, Low FODMAP, SCD/GAPS, Paleo, Autoimmune Paleo, Vegan, Vegetarian

MAKES 4 SERVINGS

Ingredients
4 large carrots
Diet-compliant oil, with high smoke point for frying (see note)
½ teaspoon salt

Instructions
1. Cut the carrots into thin discs or peel them into curls with a vegetable peeler.
2. Pour about 3 inches of oil into a small, high-sided pot (about 6 inches in diameter and 2 quarts). Heat the oil over medium-high heat until it sizzles when you drop a small bit of carrot in.
3. Working in small batches, fry the carrots until they begin to change color but are not browned around the edges; this only takes a few minutes per batch (tasting after they cool is the best way to tell if these are done).

4. Transfer the cooked carrots to a paper towel–lined plate to absorb excess oil. The chips will be a little soggy when they first come out, but they will firm up as they cool. Season the chips with salt.

Note: Use high smoke point oils when deep frying, such as grass-fed lard, refined coconut oil, and avocado oil. Diet-compliant options include lard or refined sunflower oil for low salicylate, and refined sunflower oil for low SAG. You can use butternut squash, parsnips, or beets, as well as other vegetables (if diet compliant). Parsnips are not SCD.

SAUTEED CABBAGE WITH APPLE AND BACON

GFCFSF, Egg-Free, Nut-Free, Low Oxalate, SCD/GAPS, Paleo

Low Salicylate and Low SAG: Omit bacon and onion and cook with a diet-compliant oil, such as sunflower oil

Ketogenic: Omit apples

Vegan and Vegetarian: Omit bacon and cook with preferred oil

MAKES 6 TO 10 SERVINGS

Ingredients

12 ounces bacon, chopped
1 yellow or red onion, chopped
2 garlic cloves, minced
1 medium to large green cabbage, chopped (see note)
2 apples, cored and sliced (see note)

Instructions

1. In a large skillet, cook the bacon over medium heat until crispy, about 10 to 12 minutes. Remove to a paper towel–lined plate to cool.
2. Pour out some of the bacon grease (into a container to save for later) until it thinly coats the bottom and return the skillet to the heat. Add the onion and saute for 3 to 4 minutes, until translucent. Add the garlic and cook, stirring, just until fragrant, about 30 seconds. Add the cabbage, then turn up the heat to medium-high

and saute for 5 minutes, until the cabbage begins
to brown.
3. Add the apples and cook for 3 to 4 minutes more, or until
    cabbage reaches desired tenderness. In the last minute, return
    the bacon to the pan and stir until heated through.

Note: Some cabbages are very large, so if you end up with a lot of
chopped cabbage, you may need to cook this recipe in two pans.
Sweet-tart varieties of apples, such as Pink Lady, work best in this
recipe.

CAULIFLOWER TORTILLAS

*GFCFSF, Nut-Free, Low Oxalate, SCD/
GAPS, Paleo, Ketogenic, Vegetarian*

Low Histamine: Substitute 9 quail eggs for the chicken eggs.

MAKES 6 TORTILLAS

Ingredients
1 large head cauliflower, trimmed
¼ cup water
3 large eggs
½ teaspoon salt

Instructions
1. Preheat the oven to 375°F. Line a rimmed baking sheet with
    parchment paper.
2. In a food processor, process the cauliflower into a "flour" (smaller
    pieces than cauliflower rice, but stop before you end up with a
    puree). This will yield about 3 cups of cauliflower.
3. In a large pot over low heat, combine the cauliflower and water
    and cook for 10 minutes, until tender. Remove from the heat,
    drain the water, and allow the cauliflower to cool slightly. Place
    cooked cauliflower in a kitchen towel or muslin cloth. Twist the
    ends closed and squeeze out as much water as possible.
4. In a large bowl, combine the cauliflower, eggs, and salt and mix
    well with clean hands.

5. Spoon the mixture onto the prepared baking sheet in 6 even mounds and flatten with the back of a spoon into 5-inch circles about ¼ inch thick.
6. Bake for 10 minutes, until tortillas are solidly held together and no longer appear wet. Carefully peel the tortillas away from the paper, flip, and bake 5 minutes more.
7. When you're ready to serve, heat and lightly brown the tortillas in a hot skillet. Extras can be stored in the refrigerator in an airtight bag or container until ready to eat.

BUTTERNUT SQUASH SOUP

GFCFSF, Egg-Free, Nut-Free, Elimination, Low Oxalate, SCD/GAPS, Paleo, Autoimmune Paleo

MAKES 4 SERVINGS

Ingredients

1 butternut squash
1 tablespoon extra virgin olive oil
½ cup chopped onion
1 teaspoon grated fresh ginger
1 teaspoon minced garlic
1½ cups chicken broth
1 teaspoon salt

Instructions

1. Preheat the oven to 375°F.
2. Halve the squash lengthwise and scoop out the seeds. Pierce the skin a few times with a fork.
3. Place the squash cut side down in a baking dish large enough to hold the squash and pour about ½ inch of water in the bottom. Bake for 20 to 40 minutes, until soft and easily pierced with a knife. Remove the squash from the oven and scoop out the flesh, discarding the skin.
4. While the squash is cooking, heat a large saucepan over medium heat. Drizzle in the oil, swirling to coat. Saute the onion until soft,

about 10 minutes. Add the ginger and garlic during the last few minutes of cooking.

5. Add the cooked squash, broth, and salt to the saucepan. Puree the soup until smooth, either with an immersion blender in the saucepan, or carefully transfer it to a blender (you may need to work in batches). Heat the pureed soup on medium-high heat until simmering, then serve.

KALE CHIPS

GFCFSF, Egg-Free, Nut-Free, Elimination, Low Histamine, SCD/ GAPS, Paleo, Autoimmune Paleo, Ketogenic, Vegan, Vegetarian

Low Oxalate: Use lacinato kale and limit to a ½-cup serving size

Low FODMAP: Limit to ½ cup of kale (measured when raw)

MAKES 2 TO 4 SERVINGS

Ingredients
1 bunch kale
1 tablespoon extra virgin olive oil
½ teaspoon salt

Instructions
1. After washing, thoroughly dry the kale leaves. Remove and discard the kale stems. Cut the leaves into large pieces. In a bowl, rub the kale pieces with the oil.
2. If you have an air fryer, spread the leaves in a single layer in a fry basket. Air fry at 250°F for 3 to 4 minutes, until dry, crispy, and bright green. Season with the salt. Serve.
3. If using an oven, preheat to 250°F. Spread the kale leaves on a baking sheet. Bake for 5 to 7 minutes. Flip kale leaves over, and bake for a few more minutes until dry and crispy. Watch closely and remove the kale leaves before they brown.

CANDIED GINGER SPAGHETTI SQUASH

GFCFSF, Egg-Free, Nut-Free, Low Histamine, Vegan, Vegetarian

Low FODMAP: Limit to a ½-cup serving size

MAKES 4 TO 6 SERVINGS

Ingredients

1 large spaghetti squash
⅓ cup coconut oil or nondairy butter, softened
⅓ cup brown sugar
⅓ cup maple syrup
½- to 1-inch piece fresh ginger, peeled and grated

Instructions

1. Preheat the oven to 375°F (use the convection setting if your oven has that feature). Line a rimmed baking sheet with parchment paper.
2. Halve the squash lengthwise and scrape out the seeds and pulp. Halve the pieces again to make 4 long wedges.
3. In a medium bowl, mix together the coconut oil, brown sugar, maple syrup, and ginger together until combined.
4. Spoon half of the butter-sugar mixture onto the squash and rub on all of the cut areas (everything except the skin). Arrange skin-side down on the prepared baking sheet.
5. Bake for 30 minutes, then brush on the remaining butter-sugar mixture and check your squash. If it's not starting to brown yet (and/or you do not have a convection oven), turn the oven up 400°F. Bake for 15 minutes, until the squash is browned a bit on top and the ginger is caramelized, similar to candied ginger.
6. Serve the whole squash wedges on the plate.

ZUCCHINI NOODLES

*GFCFSF, Egg-Free, Nut-Free, Elimination, Low
Histamine, Low Oxalate, SCD/GAPS, Paleo, Autoimmune
Paleo, Ketogenic, Vegan, Vegetarian*

MAKES 2 TO 4 SERVINGS

Ingredients

1 pound zucchini (2 or 3 zucchini)
Diet-compliant sauce, for cooking (optional)

Instructions

1. Use a vegetable peeler to make broad, thin noodles from the zucchini. If the zucchini are small and the seeds are very immature, you can peel all the way through. If the zucchini has more mature seeds, focus on the outside flesh, rotating the zucchini and peeling in quarter sections, then discard the center portions containing the seeds.

2. Heat a small amount of sauce or a few ounces of water in a large saute pan over medium heat. Toss the zucchini noodles in sauce or water and cook for only about 1 minute, just enough to heat the noodles through. (It's better if the noodles are slightly undercooked than overcooked so they will retain their shape and toothsome texture.)

ZUCCHINI PICKLES

GFCFSF, Egg-Free, Nut-Free, SCD/GAPS,
Paleo, Ketogenic, Vegan, Vegetarian

MAKES 12 SERVINGS

Ingredients

6 zucchini and/or summer squash, sliced into ⅛-inch disks
2 tablespoons salt
3 cups raw apple cider vinegar
1½ cups sugar
1 tablespoon mustard seeds
1 teaspoon celery seeds
¼ teaspoon ground turmeric
½ teaspoon red pepper flakes (optional)

Instructions

1. In a large bowl, cover the zucchini in cold water and add the salt. Soak for 1 hour in the refrigerator. Drain.
2. Combine the vinegar, sugar, mustard seeds, celery seeds, turmeric, and red pepper flakes in a large bowl. Stir every few minutes until the sugar is completely dissolved. (You could do this faster on the stove, but heating raw vinegar kills the beneficial bacteria.)
3. Fill very clean (or sterilized) mason jars with zucchini slices and pour the liquid mixture over the vegetables until covered. Store in the refrigerator for up to a month. (Because these are not canned, they must be stored in the refrigerator.)

Note: The amount of sugar on this recipe can be varied greatly, from ½ cup to 3 cups, depending on how sweet your child likes their pickles and how much sugar is allowed in their diet. You can also use cucumbers instead of zucchini; with cucumbers, I like to slice them thicker than zucchini so they maintain their crunch. But you can cut them as you like!

BRUSSELS SPROUT CHIPS

GFCFSF, Egg-Free, Nut-Free, Elimination, Low Salicylate, Low SAG, Low Oxalate, SCD/GAPS, Paleo, Autoimmune Paleo, Ketogenic, Vegan, Vegetarian

MAKES 4 SERVINGS

Ingredients

1 pound Brussels sprouts
1 tablespoon diet-compliant oil
½ teaspoon salt

Instructions

1. Preheat the oven to 250°F.
2. Trim the ends of the Brussels sprouts and pull off the large leaves from the outer layers; these will become your chips. (Save the remaining sprouts for another use—such as making Confetti Brussels Sprouts, page 288.)
3. Rub the leaves with the oil. Arrange the leaves in a single layer on a baking sheet, then sprinkle with the salt.
4. Bake for 8 to 10 minutes, until the leaves are slightly browned around the edges. Serve immediately.

AIR-FRIED POPCORN CAULIFLOWER

GFCFSF, Egg-Free, Nut-Free, Elimination, Low Oxalate, SCD/ GAPS, Paleo, Autoimmune Paleo, Ketogenic, Vegan, Vegetarian

Low Histamine: Use a low histamine oil instead, such as melted refined coconut oil

MAKES 2 TO 4 SERVINGS

Ingredients

1 large head cauliflower
1 tablespoon avocado oil
1 teaspoon sea salt

Instructions

1. Break the cauliflower into pieces. (I like some small crunchy bits, so I break mine up into various-size small chunks.)
2. In a large bowl, toss the cauliflower with the oil and rub to coat the pieces. Season with the salt.
3. Place in the air fryer basket. Air fry at 375°F for about 15 minutes, flipping once or twice in the basket, until all sides are browned.

LOW HISTAMINE NO-MATO SAUCE

GFCFSF, Egg-Free, Nut-Free, Elimination, Low Histamine, SCD/ GAPS, Paleo, Autoimmune Paleo, Vegan, Vegetarian

MAKES 24 OUNCES

Ingredients

1 cup chopped red beet
1 cup chopped carrots
1 cup chopped butternut squash
½ cup chopped celery
1 cup peeled and chopped zucchini
1 cup water
½ teaspoon dried basil
½ teaspoon dried oregano
½ teaspoon dried parsley
¼ teaspoon dried thyme
¼ teaspoon dried rosemary
2 teaspoons salt

Instructions

1. Fill a large pot with water and bring to a boil. Boil the beets for 20 minutes. Add the carrots, squash, and celery and boil for 20 minutes more. Add the zucchini and boil for 10 minutes, until all the vegetables are easily pierced with a fork. Drain well.
2. Transfer the vegetables to a blender. Add 1 cup of fresh water and puree until smooth.

3. Pour the puree back into the pot. Add the basil, oregano, parsley, thyme, rosemary, and salt and simmer on low for 10 minutes, until flavors have melded.

Note: If you do not need this recipe to be low histamine, garlic and onion are nice additions. Heat 1 tablespoon extra virgin olive oil in a large frying pan over medium heat. Add ½ cup chopped onion and cook, stirring occasionally, for 8 to 10 minutes until soft, then add 2 minced garlic cloves and cook for 1 minute. Puree the onion and garlic along with the boiled vegetables.

SNACKS

ROASTED PUMPKIN SEEDS

GFCFSF, Egg-Free, Nut-Free, Elimination, Low Histamine, Low Oxalate, Low FODMAP, SCD/ GAPS, Paleo, Ketogenic, Vegan, Vegetarian

Low Oxalate: Limit to a ¼-cup serving size

MAKES 16 TO 24 SERVINGS

Ingredients
3 cups shelled raw pumpkin seeds
2 tablespoons extra virgin olive oil
½ teaspoon salt

Instructions
1. Place the pumpkin seeds in a large bowl and add enough cool water to cover by 2 inches. Soak the pumpkin seeds for 8 hours. Drain and rinse the pumpkin seeds and return them to the bowl.
2. If you're using an oven to roast your seeds, preheat the oven to 200°F.
3. Drizzle the oil on the seeds and mix to coat. Sprinkle on the salt.
4. Spread out the seeds on a rimmed baking sheet or dehydrator trays. Bake for about 45 minutes, until dry and crispy. Check them every 15 minutes to make sure your oven isn't too hot. Try not

to brown them. To dehydrate, place in a dehydrator at 110°F for about 24 hours.

Note: For additional antioxidants, add spices such as ground turmeric, ginger, cinnamon, or cardamom. If added spices are desired, sprinkle them on toward the end of cooking (around the last 5 minutes) to avoid burning. This recipe is inspired by my nutrition colleague Trudy Scott, who specializes in anxiety and emphasizes foods rich in zinc.

ROASTED CHICKPEAS

GFCFSF, Egg-Free, Nut-Free, Elimination, Low Salicylate, Low SAG, Low Oxalate, Vegan, Vegetarian

Low Oxalate: Limit to a ½-cup serving size

MAKES 4 SERVINGS

Ingredients
1 (15-ounce) can chickpeas, drained and rinsed
1 tablespoon diet-compliant oil
¼ teaspoon salt

Instructions
1. Blot any excess moisture from the chickpeas with a kitchen towel.
2. Drizzle ½ to 1 tablespoon of oil over the chickpeas and mix to coat. Sprinkle with the salt and mix again.
3. Place in an air fryer basket and air fry at 350°F for about 20 minutes, until dry and crispy. Toss and mix the chickpeas halfway through cooking.

POPPED SORGHUM

GFCFSF, Egg-Free, Nut-Free, Elimination, Low Salicylate, Low SAG. Low Histamine, Low FODMAP, Vegan, Vegetarian

MAKES 1 TO 2 SERVINGS

Ingredients

2 tablespoons diet-compliant oil
1 cup whole sorghum kernels

Instructions

1. Heat the oil in a medium to large saucepan over medium-high heat. Drop a sorghum kernel into the oil to test it; if it sizzles, the oil is ready.
2. Reduce the heat to medium and add the sorghum. Swirl the pot to coat the kernels with oil and cover with a lid.
3. Continue to swirl or shake the pot as the sorghum pops. Keep going until the popping slows down to one pop every few seconds or stops. Be aware that, unlike popcorn, about one-third to one-half of the kernels will not (ever) pop. Be careful not to over-pop, or the kernels will burn.

PEAR SAUCE

GFCFSF, Egg-Free, Nut-Free, Elimination, Low Salicylate, Low SAG, Low Histamine, Low Oxalate, SCD/GAPS, Paleo, Autoimmune Paleo, Vegan, Vegetarian

Low Oxalate: Use Bartlett pears and limit serving size to ½ cup

MAKES 6 SERVINGS

Ingredients

6 pears, peeled, cored, and quartered

Instructions

1. Place the pears in a large pot with about 1 inch of water. Bring to a boil over medium-high heat, then reduce the heat to low, cover the pot, and simmer for about 25 minutes, until the pears are very soft and cook down into a sauce, stirring a few times during cooking. If the moisture level is getting low or drying out, add more water as needed.
2. If your child likes it very smooth, puree the sauce in a food processor.

PEANUT DIPPING SAUCE (FOR VEGETABLES)

GFCFSF, Egg-Free, SCD/GAPS, Vegan, Vegetarian

MAKES 2 CUPS

Ingredients

⅔ cup creamy peanut butter
¼ cup rice vinegar
¼ cup water
3 tablespoons coconut aminos
1 tablespoon honey
½ cup toasted sesame oil

Instructions

1. Place the peanut butter, rice vinegar, water, coconut aminos, and honey in a blender. Puree on high and, with the blender running, slowly drizzle in the sesame oil and blend until the sauce is emulsified and creamy.
2. Serve as a dip with diet-compliant vegetables like carrot sticks.

Note: This recipe also makes a great salad dressing when you thin the dip with more oil.

DEVILED EGGS

GFCFSF, Nut-Free, Low Oxalate, Low FODMAP,
SCD/GAPS, Paleo, Ketogenic, Vegetarian

MAKES 20 TO 24 DEVILED EGGS

Ingredients

12 large eggs
⅓ cup mayonnaise
1 teaspoon Dijon mustard
¼ teaspoon salt
Diet-compliant garnish, such as chives, chopped bacon, salmon
    eggs, or chopped olives (optional)

Instructions

1. Fill a large pot with water and bring to a boil. Remove the pot
    from the heat and carefully lower the eggs, one at a time, into the
    water. Once the last egg is in the water, set a timer for 13 minutes,
    then return the pot to the heat. Wait for the water to gently boil,
    then reduce the heat to maintain a simmer. As the eggs cook,
    gently turn and move them in the pan so that the yolks settle in
    the center.
2. At 13 minutes, take an egg out and rinse it in cool water. Working
    rapidly, peel the egg and slice it in half to make sure the yolks are
    cooked through. Cook the rest of the eggs for 1 more minute if
    necessary. When the eggs are fully cooked, cool the eggs quickly
    by transferring them to a bowl of ice water.
3. Peel the remaining eggs and halve them lengthwise.
4. Carefully scoop out the yolks and transfer them to a food
    processor with the mayo, mustard, and salt. Process until smooth
    and fully incorporated.
5. Scoop a small amount of the yolk mixture into the white halves.
    (If you want more yolk per deviled egg, discard a few whites that
    didn't peel well or broke.)
6. Add a garnish or serve them plain.

HEALTHY DESSERTS

CHOCOLATE AVOCADO PUDDING

GFCFSF, Egg-Free, Nut-Free, Paleo, Vegan, Vegetarian

MAKES 4 SERVINGS

Ingredients

2 avocados, pitted and peeled
1 cup sweetener, such as honey, maple syrup, or dates
1/3 to 1/2 cup unsweetened cocoa or carob powder

Instructions

1. Blend all ingredients in a blender or food processor until creamy.
2. Chill and serve.

DAIRY-FREE LOW SUGAR FUDGE

GFCFSF, Egg-Free, Nut-Free, Low FODMAP, Paleo, Vegan, Vegetarian
Ketogenic: Use a sugar-free chocolate, such as Lily's chocolate, or an unsweetened chocolate and add your own compliant sweetener

MAKES 12 SERVINGS

Ingredients

1 cup canned full-fat coconut milk
1½ cups soy-free, dairy-free chocolate chips (such as Enjoy Life brand)
1 teaspoon gluten-free vanilla extract
1/8 teaspoon salt

Instructions

1. Line a 6-by-8-inch or 8-inch square glass pan with parchment paper (making sure it comes up on two sides).

2. Warm the coconut milk in a medium pot over medium-low heat. Add the chocolate chips, vanilla, and salt and stir continuously with a whisk, heating slowly and making sure it does not boil or burn, until it starts to lightly steam. Watch carefully, as this only takes a few minutes. Remove from the heat.
3. Pour the mixture into the prepared pan and let set in the refrigerator for at least 2 hours. Slice into pieces.

COCONUT MACAROONS

GFCFSF, Egg-Free, SCD/GAPS, Paleo, Vegan, Vegetarian

SCD/GAPS: Use honey instead of maple syrup

MAKES 36 TO 48 MACAROONS

Ingredients

2 cups dried unsweetened finely shredded coconut
½ cup almond flour
¼ teaspoon salt
⅓ cup maple syrup
¼ cup coconut butter, softened (see note)
1 teaspoon gluten-free vanilla extract

Instructions

1. In a large bowl, combine the coconut, almond flour, and salt, mixing well.
2. Add the maple syrup, coconut butter, and vanilla and mix thoroughly with clean hands or a spoon.
3. Scoop the dough with a mini ice cream scoop (or about 1¼ tablespoons) onto dehydrator trays.
4. Place the trays in a dehydrator at 130°F for 1 hour, then turn down to 115°F and dehydrate for 12 to 15 hours more, until the macaroons are dry on the outside and inside.

Note: To make coconut butter easier to scoop from the jar, place the jar in a bowl of warm/hot water for a few minutes before measuring.

BAKED PEARS OR APPLES

GFCFSF, Egg-Free, Nut-Free, Elimination, Low Salicylate, Low SAG, Low Histamine, Low Oxalate, Paleo, Autoimmune Paleo, Vegan, Vegetarian

Low Histamine: Omit vanilla extract not tolerated because of fermentation

SCD/GAPS: Omit sugar or use honey instead

MAKES 4 SERVINGS

Ingredients

2 pears or Golden Delicious apples
½ teaspoon nondairy butter
1 tablespoon water
½ teaspoon gluten-free vanilla extract
2 tablespoons brown sugar
Salt

Instructions

1. Preheat the oven to 350°F.
2. Peel, core, and halve the pears lengthwise. Place on a 9-by-9-inch baking dish.
3. Melt the nondairy butter in a small saucepan over low heat, add vanilla and water, and whisk to combine.
4. Drizzle the mixture over the fruit and rub to coat. Sprinkle on all sides with the sugar and salt.
5. Bake for 15 minutes, then spoon the juices over the pears (add 1 tablespoon of water if there's not enough juice in the baking dish). Turn the pears to the other side and bake for 15 minutes more, or until soft.

SMOOTHIES AND BEVERAGES

BLUEBERRY CAULIFLOWER SMOOTHIE

GFCFSF, Egg-Free, Paleo, Vegan, Vegetarian

SCD/GAPS: Omit stevia

Ketogenic: Reduce blueberries to ½ cup per serving

MAKES 1 TO 2 SERVINGS

Ingredients

1¼ cups blueberries
1 cup frozen cauliflower rice
1 cup nondairy milk
½ cup water
2 tablespoons cashew butter
1 teaspoon gluten-free vanilla extract
1 teaspoon ground cardamom (optional)
5 stevia drops

Instructions

Blend all ingredients in a blender until smooth.

GREEN SMOOTHIE

GFCFSF, Egg-Free, Nut-Free, Elimination, SCD/GAPS,
Paleo, Autoimmune Paleo, Vegan, Vegetarian

MAKES 2 SERVINGS

Ingredients

1 cup frozen mango
½ cup fresh or frozen blueberries
1 ripe banana
½ avocado
5 kale leaves, destemmed (about 1 cup)
12 ounces vegetable juice (freshly pressed if possible)
2 dates (optional; see note)

Instructions

Blend all ingredients in a blender until smooth.

Note: You may want to use the dates if your berries are on the tart side.

MANGO GINGER PROBIOTIC SMOOTHIE

GFCFSF, Egg-Free, Nut-Free, SCD/GAPS, Paleo,
Autoimmune Paleo, Vegan, Vegetarian

MAKES 2 SERVINGS

Ingredients

1 cup frozen mango
1 orange, peeled
½ cup carrot juice
½ cup water
1 teaspoon grated fresh ginger
1 teaspoon grated fresh turmeric
1 tablespoon raw sauerkraut juice

Instructions

Blend the mango, orange, carrot juice, water, ginger, and turmeric in a blender until smooth, then add the sauerkraut juice and blend on low for a few seconds until just mixed in.

CHERRY APPLE CIDER VINEGAR DRINK

GFCFSF, Egg-Free, Nut-Free, Elimination, Low Oxalate, SCD/ GAPS, Paleo, Autoimmune Paleo, Vegan, Vegetarian

MAKES 2 SERVINGS

Ingredients

2 cups water (see note)
1 cup fresh or frozen pitted sweet cherries (about 16 cherries)
1 tablespoons apple cider vinegar

Instructions

Blend the water and cherries in a blender until smooth. Add the apple cider vinegar, and blend on low for a few seconds until just mixed in.

Note: You can make the beverage fizzy by blending the cherries with 1 cup of water (instead of 2 cups), then adding 1 cup of sparkling water after the apple cider vinegar.

CASHEW MILK

GFCFSF, Egg-Free, Low Salicylate, Low SAG, SCD/ GAPS, Paleo, Ketogenic, Vegan, Vegetarian

MAKES 40 OUNCES

Ingredients

1 cup raw cashews
4 cups water
1 teaspoon gluten-free vanilla extract (optional)

Instructions

1. Soak the cashews in a bowl of water that covers them by several inches for at least 2 hours or overnight.
2. Drain the cashews and rinse well.
3. In a high-powered blender, combine the soaked cashews, water, and vanilla (if using) and blend on high speed until smooth. Refrigerate and drink. You do not need to strain cashew milk.

Note: If you want this milk sweetened, you can use 1 to 2 teaspoons of raw honey for SCD/GAPS or maple syrup for low salicylate and low SAG.

SUGAR-FREE HOT COCOA

GFCFSF, Egg-Free, Nut-Free, Paleo, Ketogenic, Vegan, Vegetarian

MAKES 2 SERVINGS

Ingredients

12 ounces nondairy milk (see note)
2 tablespoons unsweetened cocoa powder
3 to 5 stevia drops (see note)

Instructions

Heat the nondairy milk in a medium pot over medium-low heat. Once it begins to warm, add the cocoa powder and whisk until smooth. Heat until hot and steaming but be careful not to let it boil. Add the stevia 1 drop at a time until desired sweetness is achieved.

Note: I like a thicker milk, like oat milk, coconut milk, or nut milk, but make sure it's gluten-free and allergen-free for your requirements. For low salicylate, use a diet-compliant milk such as cashew milk or gluten-free oat milk, and be aware that although stevia is often tolerated, its salicylate level has not been tested. You can also use other nonsugar sweeteners (liquid or powder), such as monk fruit extract, or any sweetener that is tolerated if sugar-free is not of concern.

APPENDIX A

Parent Global Impressions (PGI) Symptom Rating Scale

Please circle the severity of the following symptoms, using the following definitions.

None—no noticeable symptoms

Slight—noticeable symptoms but no significant effect on daily functioning or quality of life

Mild—mild effect on daily functioning or quality of life

Moderate—moderate effect on daily functioning or quality of life

Moderately severe—substantial effect on daily functioning or quality of life

Severe—severe effect on daily functioning or quality of life

Extremely severe—extremely severe effect on daily functioning or quality of life

1. Expressive Language/Speech	None / Slight / Mild / Moderate / Moderately Severe / Severe / Extremely Severe
2. Receptive Language/ Comprehension	None / Slight / Mild / Moderate / Moderately Severe / Severe / Extremely Severe
3. Play Skills	None / Slight / Mild / Moderate / Moderately Severe / Severe / Extremely Severe
4. Cognition/ Thinking	None / Slight / Mild / Moderate / Moderately Severe / Severe / Extremely Severe
5. Attention/Focus	None / Slight / Mild / Moderate / Moderately Severe / Severe / Extremely Severe
6. Stools/GI Problems	None / Slight / Mild / Moderate / Moderately Severe / Severe / Extremely Severe
7. Sleep	None / Slight / Mild / Moderate / Moderately Severe / Severe / Extremely Severe
8. Sociability	None / Slight / Mild / Moderate / Moderately Severe / Severe / Extremely Severe
9. Eye Contact	None / Slight / Mild / Moderate / Moderately Severe / Severe / Extremely Severe
10. Hyperactivity	None / Slight / Mild / Moderate / Moderately Severe / Severe / Extremely Severe
11. Tantrums/ Meltdowns	None / Slight / Mild / Moderate / Moderately Severe / Severe / Extremely Severe

12. Irritability/Mood	None / Slight / Mild / Moderate / Moderately Severe / Severe / Extremely Severe
13. Anxiety	None / Slight / Mild / Moderate / Moderately Severe / Severe / Extremely Severe
14. Depression	None / Slight / Mild / Moderate / Moderately Severe / Severe / Extremely Severe
15. Stimming/ Perseveration	None / Slight / Mild / Moderate / Moderately Severe / Severe / Extremely Severe
16. Sensory Sensitivity	None / Slight / Mild / Moderate / Moderately Severe / Severe / Extremely Severe
17. Aggression	None / Slight / Mild / Moderate / Moderately Severe / Severe / Extremely Severe
18. Self-Abusive	None / Slight / Mild / Moderate / Moderately Severe / Severe / Extremely Severe
19. Seizures	None / Slight / Mild / Moderate / Moderately Severe / Severe / Extremely Severe
20. Self-Limited Diet (only eat few foods)	None / Slight / Mild / Moderate / Moderately Severe / Severe / Extremely Severe
21. OVERALL Autism/ Related Symptoms	None / Slight / Mild / Moderate / Moderately Severe / Severe / Extremely Severe

APPENDIX B

Food Sources of Nutrients

Folate-Rich Foods

Liver, chicken	3.5 oz/100 g	569 mcg folate
Lentils	1 cup	358 mcg folate
Black-eyed peas, boiled	1 cup	356 mcg folate
Chickpeas, boiled	1 cup	282 mcg folate
Liver, beef	3.5 oz/100 g	258 mcg folate
Peanuts	3.5 oz/100 g	240 mcg folate
Turnip greens, raw	1 cup	194 mcg folate
Asparagus, raw	3.5 oz/100 g	191 mcg folate
Sunflower seeds, raw, hulled	½ cup	160 mcg folate
Navy beans, boiled	3.5 oz/100 g	140 mcg folate
Collard greens	1 cup	129 mcg folate
Walnuts	3.5 oz/100 g	98 mcg folate

Peanut butter	3.5 oz/100 g	97 mcg folate
Broccoli	3.5 oz/100 g	65 mcg folate
Kale, raw	3.5 oz/100 g	62 mcg folate
Brussels sprouts	3.5 oz/100 g	61 mcg folate
Nori seaweed snack	1 package/5 g	60 mcg folate
Eggs	2 eggs	35 mcg folate
Almonds	3.5 oz/100 g	35 mcg folate
Green beans	3.5 oz/100 g	33 mcg folate

B_{12}-Rich Foods

Clams	3.5 oz/100 g	98 mcg B_{12}
Liver, lamb	3.5 oz/100 g	90 mcg B_{12}
Liver, beef	3.5 oz/100 g	84 mcg B_{12}
Kidneys, lamb	3.5 oz/100 g	55 mcg B_{12}
Oysters	3.5 oz/100 g	20 mcg B_{12}
Caviar	3.5 oz/100 g	20 mcg B_{12}
Liver, chicken	3.5 oz/100 g	16 mcg B_{12}
Sardines	3.5 oz/100 g	9 mcg B_{12}
Trout	3.5 oz/100 g	7 mcg B_{12}
Salmon	3.5 oz/100 g	6 mcg B_{12}
Tuna, canned	3.5 oz/100 g	2.2 mcg B_{12}
Beef, lean ground	3.5 oz/100 g	2.1 mcg B_{12}
Eggs	2 eggs	0.8 mcg B_{12}
Chicken, ground	3.5 oz/100 g	0.5 mcg B_{12}

Vitamin B₆-Rich Foods

Pistachios	3.5 oz/100 g	1.7 mg B_6
Leeks	¼ cup	1.21 mg B_6
Sunflower seeds, raw, hulled	½ cup	1.10 mg B_6
Liver, beef	3.5 oz/100 g	1.03 mg B_6
Tuna	3.5 oz/100 g	0.98 mg B_6
Salmon	3.5 oz/100 g	0.94 mg B_6
Chicken breast	3.5 oz/100 g	0.87 mg B_6
Beef	3.5 oz/100 g	0.87 mg B_6
Walnuts	3.5 oz/100 g	0.66 mg B_6
Potatoes, russet with skin	3.5 oz/100 g	0.61 mg B_6
Buckwheat flour	3.5 oz/100 g	0.58 mg B_6
Hazelnuts	3.5 oz/100 g	0.56 mg B_6
Peppers, sweet	3.5 oz/100 g	0.29 mg B_6
Brussels sprouts	3.5 oz/100 g	0.22 mg B_6
Chickpeas, boiled	3.5 oz/100 g	0.21 mg B_6
Cauliflower	3.5 oz/100 g	0.18 mg B_6
Sweet potatoes	3.5 oz/100 g	0.16 mg B_6
Kale, raw	3.5 oz/100 g	0.15 mg B_6
Black-eyed peas, boiled	3.5 oz/100 g	0.11 mg B_6

Calcium-Rich Foods

Note: Not all calcium-containing foods are absorbed the same in the body. As discussed in step 10, oxalates in food can inhibit calcium absorption. Therefore, extremely high oxalate foods are excluded from this list. As I recommend all children follow a GFCFSF diet, I have also omitted dairy and soy.

Nondairy milk, calcium fortified	1 cup	451 mg calcium
Sardines, canned with bones	3.5 oz/100 g	382 mg calcium
Salmon, canned with bones	3.5 oz/100 g	249 mg calcium
Collard greens, raw	3.5 oz/100 g	232 mg calcium
Molasses, blackstrap	1 tablespoon	191 mg calcium
Turnip greens, raw	3.5 oz/100 g	188 mg calcium
Dandelion greens, raw	3.5 oz/100 g	187 mg calcium
Kale, raw	3.5 oz/100 g	133 mg calcium
Watercress, raw	3.5 oz/100 g	120 mg calcium
Olives, black	3.5 oz/100 g	94 mg calcium
Chickpeas, boiled	1 cup	80 mg calcium
Shrimp, cooked	3.5 oz/100 g	70 mg calcium
Dates, medjool	3.5 oz/100 g	64 mg calcium
Sunflower seeds, hulled	½ cup	48 mg calcium
Broccoli, raw	3.5 oz/100 g	47 mg calcium
Red lentils, raw	½ cup	46 mg calcium
Rutabagas, cooked	3.5 oz/100 g	45 mg calcium
Pumpkin seeds, shelled	½ cup	31 mg calcium

Magnesium-Rich Foods

Pumpkin seeds, dried and hulled	½ cup	396 mg magnesium
Sunflower seeds, dried and hulled	½ cup	227 mg magnesium
Oats, dry	½ cup	135 mg magnesium

Magnesium-Rich Foods

White beans, cooked	1 cup	135 mg magnesium
Peas, green, raw	3.5 oz/100 g	121 mg magnesium
Quinoa, cooked	1 cup	118 mg magnesium
Chickpeas, boiled	1 cup	78 mg magnesium
Millet, cooked	1 cup	76 mg magnesium
Lentils, cooked	1 cup	71 mg magnesium
Red lentils, raw	½ cup	56 mg magnesium
Flaxseed, ground	2 tablespoons	54 mg magnesium
Dates, medjool	3.5 oz/100 g	54 mg magnesium
Parsley, fresh and raw	3.5 oz/100 g	50 mg magnesium
Dark chocolate	1 oz/28 g	49 mg magnesium
Molasses, blackstrap	1 tablespoon	48 mg magnesium
Kale, raw	3.5 oz/100 g	33 mg magnesium
Collard greens, raw	3.5 oz/100 g	27 mg magnesium

Zinc-Rich Foods

Oysters, canned	3.5 oz/100 g	91 mg zinc
Crab	1 crab	6.95 mg zinc
Pumpkin seeds, dried and hulled	½ cup	5.5 mg zinc
Beef, ground	3.5 oz/100 g	4.79 mg zinc
Sunflower seeds, dried and hulled	½ cup	3.5 mg zinc
Red lentils, raw	½ cup	3.45 mg zinc
Lamb, ground	3.5 oz/100 g	3.41 mg zinc

Chickpeas, boiled	1 cup	2.51 mg zinc
Pecans, chopped	½ cup	2.26 mg zinc
Quinoa, cooked	1 cup	2.02 mg zinc
Shrimp, cooked	3.5 oz/100 g	1.64 mg zinc
Oats, dried	½ cup	1.6 mg zinc
Millet, cooked	1 cup	1.58 mg zinc
Chicken	3.5 oz/100 g	1.47 mg zinc
Wild rice, cooked	3.5 oz/100 g	1.34 mg zinc
Peas, green, raw	3.5 oz/100 g	1.24 mg zinc
White beans, cooked	1 cup	0.96 mg zinc

Other Foods Rich in Nutrients

Beta Carotene	Apricots Carrots Collard greens Kale Sweet potatoes
Betaine	Beets
Choline	Egg yolks
Iodine	Kombu flakes Nori Oysters Shrimp
Selenium	Brazil nuts
Vitamin A	Cod liver oil Egg yolks Ghee Liver

Other Foods Rich in Nutrients

Vitamin C	Acerola
	Broccoli
	Brussels sprouts
	Collard greens
	Guava
	Kale
	Oranges
	Red bell peppers
	Strawberries
	Turnip greens
Vitamin D	Cod liver oil
	Egg yolks
	Oysters
	Salmon
	Sardines
Vitamin E	Nuts
	Seeds
	Whole grains

APPENDIX C

Online Resources

Visit www.PersonalizedAutismNutritionPlan.com/extras for more handouts and more resources to guide you on your personalized nutrition journey, including:

- GFCFSF diet and meal planning worksheets
- Nourishing Hope progress tracker
- Diet journal pages
- Supplement recommendations
- Therapeutic diet resources
- Parent Global Impressions (PGI) symptom rating scale
- Contact information for the Nourishing Hope community

ENDNOTES

INTRODUCTION

1. James B. Adams et al., "Comprehensive Nutritional and Dietary Intervention for Autism Spectrum Disorder—A Randomized, Controlled 12-Month Trial," *Nutrients* 10, no. 3 (March 17, 2018): E369, https://doi.org/10.3390/nu10030369.

WHAT CAUSES AUTISM?

1. Lauren Castelbaum et al., "On the Nature of Monozygotic Twin Concordance and Discordance for Autistic Trait Severity: A Quantitative Analysis," *Behavior Genetics* 50, no. 4 (July 2020): 263–72, https://doi.org/10.1007/s10519-019-09987-2.
2. Matthew J. Maenner, "Prevalence and Characteristics of Autism Spectrum Disorder Among Children Aged 8 Years—Autism and Developmental Disabilities Monitoring Network, 11 Sites, United States, 2018," *MMWR Surveillance Summaries* 70 (2021), https://doi.org/10.15585/mmwr.ss7011a1.
3. Matthew J. Maenner et al., "Prevalence and Characteristics of Autism Spectrum Disorder Among Children Aged 8 Years—Autism and Developmental Disabilities Monitoring Network, 11 Sites, United States, 2020," *MMWR Surveillance Summaries* 72, no. 2 (March 24, 2023): 1–14, https://doi.org/10.15585/mmwr.ss7202a1.
4. Stefan N. Hansen, Diana E. Schendel, and Erik T. Parner, "Explaining the Increase in the Prevalence of Autism Spectrum Disorders: The Proportion Attributable to Changes in Reporting Practices," *JAMA Pediatrics* 169, no. 1 (January 2015): 56–62, https://doi.org/10.1001/jamapediatrics.2014.1893.

5. Martha R. Herbert, "Autism: A Brain Disorder or a Disorder That Affects the Brain?," *Clinical Neuropsychiatry* 2, no. 6 (2005): 354–79.

6. Melania Manco et al., "Cross-Sectional Investigation of Insulin Resistance in Youths with Autism Spectrum Disorder. Any Role for Reduced Brain Glucose Metabolism?," *Translational Psychiatry* 11, no. 1 (April 20, 2021): 229, https://doi.org/10.1038/s41398-021-01345-3.

7. Maria Valicenti-McDermott et al., "Frequency of Gastrointestinal Symptoms in Children with Autistic Spectrum Disorders and Association with Family History of Autoimmune Disease," *Journal of Developmental and Behavioral Pediatrics: JDBP* 27, no. 2 Suppl (April 2006): S128–136, https://doi.org/10.1097/00004703-200604002-00011.

8. Lulu W. Wang, Daniel J. Tancredi, and Dan W. Thomas, "The Prevalence of Gastrointestinal Problems in Children Across the United States with Autism Spectrum Disorders from Families with Multiple Affected Members," *Journal of Developmental and Behavioral Pediatrics: JDBP* 32, no. 5 (June 2011): 351–60, https://doi.org/10.1097/DBP.0b013e31821bd06a; James B. Adams et al., "Gastrointestinal Flora and Gastrointestinal Status in Children with Autism—Comparisons to Typical Children and Correlation with Autism Severity," *BMC Gastroenterology* 11, no. 1 (December 2011): 22, https://doi.org/10.1186/1471-230X-11-22.

9. Wang, Tancredi, and Thomas, "The Prevalence of Gastrointestinal Problems."

10. Marie Hanscom, David J. Loane, and Terez Shea-Donohue, "Brain-Gut Axis Dysfunction in the Pathogenesis of Traumatic Brain Injury," *Journal of Clinical Investigation* 131, no. 12 (June 15, 2021): e143777, https://doi.org/10.1172/JCI143777.

11. Maria De Angelis et al., "Fecal Microbiota and Metabolome of Children with Autism and Pervasive Developmental Disorder Not Otherwise Specified," *PLoS One* 8, no. 10 (October 9, 2013): e76993, https://doi.org/10.1371/journal.pone.0076993; James T. Morton et al., "Multi-Omic Analysis Along the Gut-Brain Axis Points to a Functional Architecture of Autism," preprint (*Microbiology*, February 26, 2022), https://doi.org/10.1101/2022.02.25.482050.

12. Adams et al., "Gastrointestinal Flora."

13. Sydney M. Finegold et al., "Gastrointestinal Microflora Studies in Late-Onset Autism," *Clinical Infectious Diseases: An Official Publication of the Infectious Diseases Society of America* 35, no. Suppl 1 (September 1, 2002): S6–16, https://doi.org/10.1086/341914; Khemlal Nirmalkar et al., "Bimodal Distribution of Intestinal *Candida* in Children with Autism and Its Potential Link with Worse ASD Symptoms," *Gut Microbes Reports* 1, no. 1 (December 31, 2024): 2358324, https://doi.org/10.1080/29933935.2024.2358324.

14. Amani Alharthi et al., "The Human Gut Microbiome as a Potential Factor in Autism Spectrum Disorder," *International Journal of Molecular Sciences* 23, no. 3 (January 25, 2022): 1363, https://doi.org/10.3390/ijms23031363; Rebecca S. Eshraghi et al., "Early Disruption of the Microbiome Leading to Decreased Antioxidant Capacity and Epigenetic Changes: Implications for the Rise in Autism," *Frontiers in Cellular Neuroscience* 12 (2018): 256, https://doi.org/10.3389/fncel.2018.00256.

15. Troy Vargason, Deborah L. McGuinness, and Juergen Hahn, "Gastrointestinal Symptoms and Oral Antibiotic Use in Children with Autism Spectrum Disorder: Retrospective Analysis of a Privately Insured U.S. Population," *Journal of Autism and Developmental Disorders* 49, no. 2 (February 2019): 647–59, https://doi.org/10.1007/s10803-018-3743-2.

16. Dae-Wook Kang et al., "Microbiota Transfer Therapy Alters Gut Ecosystem and Improves Gastrointestinal and Autism Symptoms: An Open-Label Study," *Microbiome* 5, no. 1 (December 2017): 10, https://doi.org/10.1186/s40168-016-0225-7.

17. Dae-Wook Kang et al., "Long-Term Benefit of Microbiota Transfer Therapy on Autism Symptoms and Gut Microbiota," *Scientific Reports* 9, no. 1 (April 9, 2019): 5821, https://doi.org/10.1038/s41598-019-42183-0.

18. Mathis Wolter et al., "Leveraging Diet to Engineer the Gut Microbiome," *Nature Reviews Gastroenterology & Hepatology* 18, no. 12 (December 2021): 885–902, https://doi.org/10.1038/s41575-021-00512-7.

19. Aleksandra Tomova et al., "The Influence of Food Intake Specificity in Children with Autism on Gut Microbiota," *International Journal of Molecular Sciences* 21, no. 8 (April 17, 2020): E2797, https://doi.org/10.3390/ijms21082797; J. Horn et al., "Role of Diet and Its Effects on the Gut Microbiome in the Pathophysiology of Mental Disorders," *Translational Psychiatry* 12, no. 1 (December 2022): 164, https://doi.org/10.1038/s41398-022-01922-0.

20. Wolter et al., "Leveraging Diet to Engineer the Gut Microbiome."

21. Nona M. Jiang et al., "The Impact of Systemic Inflammation on Neurodevelopment," *Trends in Molecular Medicine* 24, no. 9 (September 2018): 794–804, https://doi.org/10.1016/j.molmed.2018.06.008.

22. Kevin Roe, "Autism Spectrum Disorder Initiation by Inflammation-Facilitated Neurotoxin Transport," *Neurochemical Research* 47, no. 5 (May 2022): 1150–65, https://doi.org/10.1007/s11064-022-03527-x.

23. Jiang et al., "The Impact of Systemic Inflammation on Neurodevelopment."

24. Diana L. Vargas et al., "Neuroglial Activation and Neuroinflammation in the Brain of Patients with Autism," *Annals of Neurology* 57, no. 1 (January 2005): 67–81, https://doi.org/10.1002/ana.20315; Xiaohong Li et al., "Elevated Immune Response in the Brain of Autistic Patients," *Journal of Neuroimmunology* 207, no. 1–2 (February 15, 2009): 111–16, https://doi.org/10.1016/j.jneuroim.2008.12.002.

25. D. A. Rossignol and R. E. Frye, "A Review of Research Trends in Physiological Abnormalities in Autism Spectrum Disorders: Immune Dysregulation, Inflammation, Oxidative Stress, Mitochondrial Dysfunction and Environmental Toxicant Exposures," *Molecular Psychiatry* 17, no. 4 (April 2012): 389–401, https://doi.org/10.1038/mp.2011.165.

26. Maria Gevezova et al., "Inflammation and Mitochondrial Dysfunction in Autism Spectrum Disorder," *CNS & Neurological Disorders Drug Targets* 19, no. 5 (2020): 320–33, https://doi.org/10.2174/1871527319666200628 015039.

27. Sheikh Fayaz Ahmad et al., "Dysregulation of Th1, Th2, Th17, and T Regulatory Cell-Related Transcription Factor Signaling in Children with Autism," *Molecular Neurobiology* 54, no. 6 (August 2017): 4390–4400, https://doi.org /10.1007/s12035-016-9977-0; Dario Siniscalco et al., "Inflammation and Neuro-Immune Dysregulations in Autism Spectrum Disorders," *Pharmaceuticals* 11, no. 2 (June 2018), https://doi.org/10.3390/ph11020056.

28. Theoharis C. Theoharides et al., "Mast Cell Activation and Autism," *Biochimica et Biophysica Acta (BBA)—Molecular Basis of Disease* 1822, no. 1 (January 2012): 34–41, https://doi.org/10.1016/j.bbadis.2010.12.017.

29. Harumi Jyonouchi, Sining Sun, and Nanae Itokazu, "Innate Immunity Associated with Inflammatory Responses and Cytokine Production Against Common Dietary Proteins in Patients with Autism Spectrum Disorder," *Neuropsychobiology* 46, no. 2 (2002): 76–84, https://doi.org/10.1159 /000065416.

30. Maria Gevezova et al., "Inflammation and Mitochondrial Dysfunction."

31. Richard E. Frye and Daniel A. Rossignol, "Mitochondrial Dysfunction Can Connect the Diverse Medical Symptoms Associated with Autism Spectrum Disorders," *Pediatric Research* 69, no. 5 Pt 2 (May 2011): 41R–7R, https://doi .org/10.1203/PDR.0b013e318212f16b.

32. Geir Bjørklund et al., "The Role of Glutathione Redox Imbalance in Autism Spectrum Disorder: A Review," *Free Radical Biology & Medicine* 160 (November 20, 2020): 149–62, https://doi.org/10.1016/j.freeradbiomed.2020.07.017.

33. Altaf Alabdali, Laila Al-Ayadhi, and Afaf El-Ansary, "A Key Role for an Impaired Detoxification Mechanism in the Etiology and Severity of Autism Spectrum Disorders," *Behavioral and Brain Functions: BBF* 10 (April 28, 2014): 14, https://doi.org/10.1186/1744-9081-10-14.

34. Francesco De Luca, "Endocrinological Abnormalities in Autism," *Seminars in Pediatric Neurology* 35 (October 1, 2020): 100582, https://doi.org/10.1016 /j.spen.2016.04.001.

35. Melania Manco et al., "Cross-Sectional Investigation of Insulin Resistance in Youths with Autism Spectrum Disorder. Any Role for Reduced Brain Glucose Metabolism?," *Translational Psychiatry* 11, no. 1 (April 20, 2021): 229, https://doi.org/10.1038/s41398-021-01345-3.

36. Tamara Žigman et al., "Inborn Errors of Metabolism Associated with Autism Spectrum Disorders: Approaches to Intervention," *Frontiers in Neuroscience* 15 (2021): 673600, https://doi.org/10.3389/fnins.2021.673600.

37. S. Jill James et al., "Metabolic Biomarkers of Increased Oxidative Stress and Impaired Methylation Capacity in Children with Autism," *American Journal of Clinical Nutrition* 80, no. 6 (December 1, 2004): 1611–17, https://doi.org/10.1093/ajcn/80.6.1611.

38. Daniel P. Howsmon et al., "Classification and Adaptive Behavior Prediction of Children with Autism Spectrum Disorder Based upon Multivariate Data Analysis of Markers of Oxidative Stress and DNA Methylation," *PLoS Computational Biology* 13, no. 3 (March 2017): e1005385, https://doi.org/10.1371/journal.pcbi.1005385.

39. Julie S. Matthews, *Nourishing Hope for Autism: Nutrition and Diet Guide for Healing Children*, 3rd edition (San Francisco, California: Healthful Living Media, 2008).

40. Rosemary Waring and L. V. Klovrza, "Sulphur Metabolism in Autism," *Journal of Nutritional and Environmental Medicine* 10 (July 13, 2009): 25–32, https://doi.org/10.1080/13590840050000861; A. Alberti et al., "Sulphation Deficit in 'Low-Functioning' Autistic Children: A Pilot Study," *Biological Psychiatry* 46, no. 3 (August 1, 1999): 420–24, https://doi.org/10.1016/s0006-3223(98)00337-0; James B. Adams et al., "Nutritional and Metabolic Status of Children with Autism vs. Neurotypical Children, and the Association with Autism Severity," *Nutrition & Metabolism* 8, no. 1 (June 8, 2011): 34, https://doi.org/10.1186/1743-7075-8-34; Fatir Qureshi et al., "Multivariate Analysis of Metabolomic and Nutritional Profiles Among Children with Autism Spectrum Disorder," *Journal of Personalized Medicine* 12, no. 6 (June 1, 2022): 923, https://doi.org/10.3390/jpm12060923.

41. Margaret Moss and Rosemary Waring, "The Plasma Cysteine/Sulphate Ratio: A Possible Clinical Biomarker," *Journal of Nutritional & Environmental Medicine* 13, no. 4 (July 13, 2009): 215–229, https://doi.org/10.1080/13590840310001642003.

42. Anne Masi et al., "An Overview of Autism Spectrum Disorder, Heterogeneity and Treatment Options," *Neuroscience Bulletin* 33, no. 2 (April 2017): 183–93, https://doi.org/10.1007/s12264-017-0100-y.

43. Ovsanna T. Leyfer et al., "Comorbid Psychiatric Disorders in Children with Autism: Interview Development and Rates of Disorders," *Journal of Autism and Developmental Disorders* 36, no. 7 (October 2006): 849–61, https://doi.org/10.1007/s10803-006-0123-0.

44. Benjamin E. Yerys et al., "Attention Deficit/Hyperactivity Disorder Symptoms Moderate Cognition and Behavior in Children with Autism Spectrum Disorders," *Autism Research: Official Journal of the International Society for Autism Research* 2, no. 6 (December 2009): 322–33, https://doi.org/10.1002/aur.103.

PERSONALIZING NUTRITION

1. Joanna Kałużna-Czaplińska and Jagoda Jóźwik-Pruska, "Nutritional Strategies and Personalized Diet in Autism—Choice or Necessity?," *Trends in Food Science & Technology* 49 (March 1, 2016): 45–50, https://doi.org/10.1016/j.tifs.2016.01.005; Anna Mandecka and Bożena Regulska-Ilow, "The Importance of Nutritional Management and Education in the Treatment of Autism," *Annals of the National Institute of Hygiene* 73 no. 3 (2022): 247–58, https://doi.org/10.32394/rpzh.2022.0218.

STEP 1

1. Melissa M. Lane et al., "Ultra-Processed Food Consumption and Mental Health: A Systematic Review and Meta-Analysis of Observational Studies," *Nutrients* 14, no. 13 (June 21, 2022): 2568, https://doi.org/10.3390/nu14132568.

2. Subin Park et al., "Association Between Dietary Behaviors and Attention-Deficit/Hyperactivity Disorder and Learning Disabilities in School-Aged Children," *Psychiatry Research* 198, no. 3 (August 2012): 468–76, https://doi.org/10.1016/j.psychres.2012.02.012.

3. Donna McCann et al., "Food Additives and Hyperactive Behaviour in 3-Year-Old and 8/9-Year-Old Children in the Community: A Randomised, Double-Blinded, Placebo-Controlled Trial," *Lancet* 370, no. 9598 (November 3, 2007): 1560–67, https://doi.org/10.1016/S0140-6736(07)61306-3.

4. Prabasheela Bakthavachalu, S. Meenakshi Kannan, and M. Walid Qoronfleh, "Food Color and Autism: A Meta-Analysis," in *Personalized Food Intervention and Therapy for Autism Spectrum Disorder Management*, eds. M. Mohamed Essa and M. Walid Qoronfleh, vol. 24, *Advances in Neurobiology* (Cham: Springer International Publishing, 2020), 481–504, https://doi.org/10.1007/978-3-030-30402-7_15.

5. Julie S. Matthews and James B. Adams, "Ratings of the Effectiveness of 13 Therapeutic Diets for Autism Spectrum Disorder: Results of a National Survey," *Journal of Personalized Medicine* 13, no. 10 (September 29, 2023): 1448, https://doi.org/10.3390/jpm13101448.

6. Sheila M. S. Sears and Sandra J. Hewett, "Influence of Glutamate and GABA Transport on Brain Excitatory/Inhibitory Balance," *Experimental Biology and Medicine* 246, no. 9 (May 2021): 1069–83, https://doi.org/10.1177/1535370221989263.

7. Sabah Nisar et al., "Genetics of Glutamate and Its Receptors in Autism Spectrum Disorder," *Molecular Psychiatry* 27, no. 5 (May 2022): 2380–92, https://doi.org/10.1038/s41380-022-01506-w.

8. Benoit Chassaing et al., "Randomized Controlled-Feeding Study of Dietary Emulsifier Carboxymethylcellulose Reveals Detrimental Impacts on the Gut

Microbiota and Metabolome," *Gastroenterology* 162, no. 3 (March 2022): 743–56, https://doi.org/10.1053/j.gastro.2021.11.006; Katalin F. Csáki, "Synthetic Surfactant Food Additives Can Cause Intestinal Barrier Dysfunction," *Medical Hypotheses* 76, no. 5 (May 2011): 676–81, https://doi.org /10.1016/j.mehy.2011.01.030; Fatih Gültekin, "Food Additives and Microbiota," *Northern Clinics of Istanbul* 7, no. 2 (2020): 192–200, https://doi.org/10 .14744/nci.2019.92499.

9. Aaron Lerner and Torsten Matthias, "Changes in Intestinal Tight Junction Permeability Associated with Industrial Food Additives Explain the Rising Incidence of Autoimmune Disease," *Autoimmunity Reviews* 14, no. 6 (June 2015): 479–89, https://doi.org/10.1016/j.autrev.2015.01.009.

10. Gültekin, "Food Additives and Microbiota."

11. Sharon Parten Fowler et al., "Daily Early-Life Exposures to Diet Soda and Aspartame Are Associated with Autism in Males: A Case-Control Study," *Nutrients* 16, no. 5 (2023): 3772, https://doi.org/10.3390/nu15173772.

12. Hannelore Daniel et al., "Allulose in Human Diet: The Knowns and the Unknowns," *British Journal of Nutrition* 128, no. 2 (July 28, 2022): 172–78, https://doi.org/10.1017/S0007114521003172.

13. Chen Shen et al., "Evaluation of Adverse Effects/Events of Genetically Modified Food Consumption: A Systematic Review of Animal and Human Studies," *Environmental Sciences Europe* 34, no. 1 (December 2022): 8, https://doi .org/10.1186/s12302-021-00578-9.

14. Gulcin Algan Ozkok, "Genetically Modified Foods and the Probable Risks on Human Health," *International Journal of Nutrition and Food Sciences* 4, no. 3 (2015): 356, https://doi.org/10.11648/j.ijnfs.20150403.23.

15. Dennis D. Weisenburger, "A Review and Update with Perspective of Evidence That the Herbicide Glyphosate (Roundup) Is a Cause of Non-Hodgkin Lymphoma," *Clinical Lymphoma Myeloma and Leukemia* 21, no. 9 (September 2021): 621–30, https://doi.org/10.1016/j.clml.2021.04.009.

16. Qixing Mao et al., "The Ramazzini Institute 13-Week Pilot Study on Glyphosate and Roundup Administered at Human-Equivalent Dose to Sprague Dawley Rats: Effects on the Microbiome," *Environmental Health* 17, no. 1 (December 2018): 50, https://doi.org/10.1186/s12940-018-0394-x.

17. Isadora Argou-Cardozo and Fares Zeidán-Chuliá, "Clostridium Bacteria and Autism Spectrum Conditions: A Systematic Review and Hypothetical Contribution of Environmental Glyphosate Levels," *Medical Sciences* 6, no. 2 (April 4, 2018): 29, https://doi.org/10.3390/medsci6020029.

18. Carmen Costas-Ferreira, Rafael Durán, and Lilian R. F. Faro, "Toxic Effects of Glyphosate on the Nervous System: A Systematic Review," *International Journal of Molecular Sciences* 23, no. 9 (April 21, 2022): 4605, https://doi.org /10.3390/ijms23094605.

19. James R. Roberts et al., "Pesticide Exposure in Children," *Pediatrics* 130, no. 6 (December 1, 2012): e1765–88, https://doi.org/10.1542/peds.2012-2758.

20. Noemie Cresto et al., "Pesticides at Brain Borders: Impact on the Blood-Brain Barrier, Neuroinflammation, and Neurological Risk Trajectories," *Chemosphere* 324 (May 2023): 138251, https://doi.org/10.1016/j.chemosphere.2023.138251.

21. Amanda V. Bakian and James A. VanDerslice, "Pesticides and Autism," *BMJ* 364 (2019): l1149, https://doi.org/10.1136/bmj.l1149.

22. Carly Hyland et al., "Organic Diet Intervention Significantly Reduces Urinary Pesticide Levels in U.S. Children and Adults," *Environmental Research* 171 (April 2019): 568–75, https://doi.org/10.1016/j.envres.2019.01.024.

23. John Fagan et al., "Organic Diet Intervention Significantly Reduces Urinary Glyphosate Levels in U.S. Children and Adults," *Environmental Research* 189 (October 2020): 109898, https://doi.org/10.1016/j.envres.2020.109898.

24. Si Tan et al., "The Association Between Sugar-Sweetened Beverages and Milk Intake with Emotional and Behavioral Problems in Children with Autism Spectrum Disorder," *Frontiers in Nutrition* 9 (2022): 927212, https://doi.org/10.3389/fnut.2022.927212.

25. Julie S. Matthews and James B. Adams, "Ratings of the Effectiveness of 13 Therapeutic Diets for Autism Spectrum Disorder: Results of a National Survey," *Journal of Personalized Medicine* 13, no. 10 (September 29, 2023): 1448, https://doi.org/10.3390/jpm13101448.

26. Meaghan E. Glenn et al., "Dietary Intakes of Children Enrolled in US Early Child-Care Programs During Child-Care and Non-Child-Care Days," *Journal of the Academy of Nutrition and Dietetics* 122, no. 6 (June 2022): 1141–1157.e3, https://doi.org/10.1016/j.jand.2021.08.108.

27. "Get the Facts: Added Sugars," *Centers for Disease Control and Prevention* (blog), accessed August 15, 2023, https://www.cdc.gov/nutrition/data-statistics/added-sugars.html.

28. Miriam B. Vos et al., "Added Sugars and Cardiovascular Disease Risk in Children: A Scientific Statement from the American Heart Association," *Circulation* 135, no. 19 (May 9, 2017), https://doi.org/10.1161/CIR.0000000000000439.

29. "New Change4Life Campaign Encourages Parents to 'Be Food Smart,'" *GOV.UK: Public Health England* (blog), accessed August 15, 2023, https://www.gov.uk/government/news/new-change4life-campaign-encourages-parents-to-be-food-smart.

30. Lustig, Robert H., Kathleen Mulligan, Susan M. Noworolski, Viva W. Tai, Michael J. Wen, Ayca Erkin-Cakmak, Alejandro Gugliucci, and Jean-Marc Schwarz, "Isocaloric Fructose Restriction and Metabolic Improvement in Children with Obesity and Metabolic Syndrome," *Obesity* 24, no. 2 (February 2016): 453–60, https://doi.org/10.1002/oby.21371.

31. Monique Aucoin et al., "Diet and Anxiety: A Scoping Review," *Nutrients* 13, no. 12 (December 10, 2021): 4418, https://doi.org/10.3390/nu13124418.
32. Ayat Hussein B. Rashaid et al., "Heavy Metals and Trace Elements in Scalp Hair Samples of Children with Severe Autism Spectrum Disorder: A Case-Control Study on Jordanian Children," *Journal of Trace Elements in Medicine and Biology* 67 (September 1, 2021): 126790, https://doi.org/10.1016/j.jtemb.2021.126790.
33. Huamei Li et al., "Blood Mercury, Arsenic, Cadmium, and Lead in Children with Autism Spectrum Disorder," *Biological Trace Element Research* 181, no. 1 (January 1, 2018): 31–37, https://doi.org/10.1007/s12011-017-1002-6.
34. Philippe Grandjean, "Developmental Fluoride Neurotoxicity: An Updated Review," *Environmental Health* 18, no. 1 (December 2019): 110, https://doi.org/10.1186/s12940-019-0551-x.

STEP 2

1. Dominika Guzek et al., "Role of Fruit and Vegetables for the Mental Health of Children: A Systematic Review," *Roczniki Panstwowego Zakladu Higieny* 71, no. 1 (2020): 5–13, https://doi.org/10.32394/rpzh.2019.0096.
2. Kirsten Berding and Sharon M. Donovan, "Diet Can Impact Microbiota Composition in Children with Autism Spectrum Disorder," *Frontiers in Neuroscience* 12 (2018): 515, https://doi.org/10.3389/fnins.2018.00515.
3. Meaghan E. Glenn et al., "Dietary Intakes of Children Enrolled in US Early Child-Care Programs During Child-Care and Non-Child-Care Days," *Journal of the Academy of Nutrition and Dietetics* 122, no. 6 (June 2022): 1141–1157.e3, https://doi.org/10.1016/j.jand.2021.08.108.
4. Liem T. Chistol et al., "Sensory Sensitivity and Food Selectivity in Children with Autism Spectrum Disorder," *Journal of Autism and Developmental Disorders* 48, no. 2 (February 2018): 583–91, https://doi.org/10.1007/s10803-017-3340-9.
5. Xin Wang et al., "Association Between Dietary Quality and Executive Functions in School-Aged Children with Autism Spectrum Disorder," *Frontiers in Nutrition* 9 (2022): 940246, https://doi.org/10.3389/fnut.2022.940246.
6. Julie S. Matthews and James B. Adams, "Ratings of the Effectiveness of 13 Therapeutic Diets for Autism Spectrum Disorder: Results of a National Survey," *Journal of Personalized Medicine* 13, no. 10 (September 29, 2023): 1448, https://doi.org/10.3390/jpm13101448.
7. Alexander Acosta et al., "Dietary Factors Impact Developmental Trajectories in Young Autistic Children," *Journal of Autism and Developmental Disorders* (2023), https://doi.org/10.1007/s10803-023-06074-8.
8. Matthews and Adams, "Ratings of the Effectiveness of 13 Therapeutic Diets for Autism Spectrum Disorder."

9. Liane S. Roe et al., "Portion Size Can Be Used Strategically to Increase Intake of Vegetables and Fruits in Young Children over Multiple Days: A Cluster-Randomized Crossover Trial," *American Journal of Clinical Nutrition* 115, no. 1 (January 11, 2022): 272–83, https://doi.org/10.1093/ajcn/nqab321.

10. Jiaxi Yang et al., "Eating Vegetables First at Start of Meal and Food Intake Among Preschool Children in Japan," *Nutrients* 12, no. 6 (June 12, 2020): 1762, https://doi.org/10.3390/nu12061762.

11. Maria Garcia-Iborra et al., "Optimal Protein Intake in Healthy Children and Adolescents: Evaluating Current Evidence," *Nutrients* 15, no. 7 (March 30, 2023): 1683, https://doi.org/10.3390/nu15071683.

12. Rasnik K. Singh et al., "Influence of Diet on the Gut Microbiome and Implications for Human Health," *Journal of Translational Medicine* 15, no. 1 (April 8, 2017): 73, https://doi.org/10.1186/s12967-017-1175-y.

13. Iva Hojsak et al., "Benefits of Dietary Fibre for Children in Health and Disease," *Archives of Disease in Childhood* 107, no. 11 (November 2022): 973–79, https://doi.org/10.1136/archdischild-2021-323571.

14. Kay-Tee Khaw et al., "Randomised Trial of Coconut Oil, Olive Oil or Butter on Blood Lipids and Other Cardiovascular Risk Factors in Healthy Men and Women," *BMJ Open* 8, no. 3 (March 6, 2018): e020167, https://doi.org/10.1136/bmjopen-2017-020167.

15. Marcel van de Wouw et al., "Kefir Ameliorates Specific Microbiota-Gut-Brain Axis Impairments in a Mouse Model Relevant to Autism Spectrum Disorder," *Brain, Behavior, and Immunity* 97 (October 2021): 119–34, https://doi.org/10.1016/j.bbi.2021.07.004.

STEP 3

1. James B. Adams et al., "Nutritional and Metabolic Status of Children with Autism vs. Neurotypical Children, and the Association with Autism Severity," *Nutrition & Metabolism* 8, no. 1 (June 8, 2011): 34, https://doi.org/10.1186/1743-7075-8-34.

2. Saurav Nayak et al., "Assessment of Copper and Zinc Levels in Hair and Urine of Children with Attention Deficit Hyperactivity Disorder: A Case-Control Study in Eastern India," *Cureus* 13, no. 12 (December 2021): e20692, https://doi.org/10.7759/cureus.20692.

3. Geir Bjørklund et al., "The Role of Vitamins in Autism Spectrum Disorder: What Do We Know?," *Journal of Molecular Neuroscience* 67, no. 3 (March 2019): 373–87, https://doi.org/10.1007/s12031-018-1237-5.

4. Neluwa-Liyanage R. Indika et al., "The Rationale for Vitamin, Mineral, and Cofactor Treatment in the Precision Medical Care of Autism Spectrum Disorder," *Journal of Personalized Medicine* 13, no. 2 (January 29, 2023): 252, https://doi.org/10.3390/jpm13020252.

5. James B. Adams et al., "Effect of a Vitamin/Mineral Supplement on Children and Adults with Autism," *BMC Pediatrics* 11 (December 12, 2011): 111, https://doi.org/10.1186/1471-2431-11-111.

6. Heather A. Gordon et al., "Clinically Significant Symptom Reduction in Children with Attention-Deficit/Hyperactivity Disorder Treated with Micronutrients: An Open-Label Reversal Design Study," *Journal of Child and Adolescent Psychopharmacology* 25, no. 10 (December 2015): 783–98, https://doi.org/10.1089/cap.2015.0105.

7. Adams et al., "Effect of a Vitamin/Mineral Supplement"; James B. Adams et al., "Comprehensive Nutritional and Dietary Intervention for Autism Spectrum Disorder—A Randomized, Controlled 12-Month Trial," *Nutrients* 10, no. 3 (March 17, 2018): E369, https://doi.org/10.3390/nu10030369.

8. Autism Nutrition Research Center, "ANRC Autism Treatment Rater," 2022, https://apps.apple.com/us/app/anrc-autism-treatment-rater/id1616969988.

9. Si-ou Li et al., "Serum Copper and Zinc Levels in Individuals with Autism Spectrum Disorders," *Neuroreport* 25, no. 15 (October 22, 2014): 1216–20, https://doi.org/10.1097/WNR.0000000000000251.

10. Richard Stuckey, William Walsh, and Brett Lambert, "The Effectiveness of Targeted Nutrient Therapy in Treatment of Mental Illness," *Journal of the Australasian College of Nutritional and Environmental Medicine* 29, no. 3 (November 2010): 3–8.

11. Adams et al., "Nutritional and Metabolic Status of Children with Autism."

12. Umesh Padhye, "Excess Dietary Iron Is the Root Cause for Increase in Childhood Autism and Allergies," *Medical Hypotheses* 61, no. 2 (August 2003): 220–22, https://doi.org/10.1016/s0306-9877(03)00126-9.

13. Aleksandra Veselinović et al., "Neuroinflammation in Autism and Supplementation Based on Omega-3 Polyunsaturated Fatty Acids: A Narrative Review," *Medicina (Kaunas, Lithuania)* 57, no. 9 (August 28, 2021): 893, https://doi.org/10.3390/medicina57090893.

14. Danielle Swanson, Robert Block, and Shaker A. Mousa, "Omega-3 Fatty Acids EPA and DHA: Health Benefits Throughout Life," *Advances in Nutrition (Bethesda, Md.)* 3, no. 1 (January 2012): 1–7, https://doi.org/10.3945/an.111.000893.

15. Ledyane Taynara Marton et al., "Omega Fatty Acids and Inflammatory Bowel Diseases: An Overview," *International Journal of Molecular Sciences* 20, no. 19 (September 30, 2019): 4851, https://doi.org/10.3390/ijms20194851.

16. Swanson, Block, and Mousa, "Omega-3 Fatty Acids EPA and DHA."

17. Paola Bozzatello et al., "Polyunsaturated Fatty Acids: What Is Their Role in Treatment of Psychiatric Disorders?," *International Journal of Molecular Sciences* 20, no. 21 (October 23, 2019): 5257, https://doi.org/10.3390/ijms20215257.

18. Janice K. Kiecolt-Glaser et al., "Omega-3 Supplementation Lowers Inflammation and Anxiety in Medical Students: A Randomized Controlled Trial," *Brain, Behavior, and Immunity* 25, no. 8 (November 2011): 1725–34, https://doi.org/10.1016/j.bbi.2011.07.229.

19. Claudia R. Morris and Marilyn C. Agin, "Syndrome of Allergy, Apraxia, and Malabsorption: Characterization of a Neurodevelopmental Phenotype That Responds to Omega 3 and Vitamin E Supplementation," *Alternative Therapies in Health and Medicine* 15, no. 4 (2009): 34–43.

20. James B. Adams et al., "Ratings of the Effectiveness of Nutraceuticals for Autism Spectrum Disorders: Results of a National Survey," *Journal of Personalized Medicine* 11, no. 9 (August 31, 2021): 878, https://doi.org/10.3390/jpm11090878.

21. Autism Nutrition Research Center, "ANRC Autism Treatment Rater."

22. Basant K. Puri and Julian G. Martins, "Which Polyunsaturated Fatty Acids Are Active in Children with Attention-Deficit Hyperactivity Disorder Receiving PUFA Supplementation? A Fatty Acid Validated Meta-Regression Analysis of Randomized Controlled Trials," *Prostaglandins, Leukotrienes, and Essential Fatty Acids* 90, no. 5 (May 2014): 179–89, https://doi.org/10.1016/j.plefa.2014.01.004; E. Derbyshire, "Do Omega-3/6 Fatty Acids Have a Therapeutic Role in Children and Young People with ADHD?," *Journal of Lipids* 2017 (2017): 1–9, https://doi.org/10.1155/2017/6285218; Jelle D'Helft et al., "Relevance of ω-6 GLA Added to ω-3 PUFAs Supplements for ADHD: A Narrative Review," *Nutrients* 14, no. 16 (August 10, 2022): 3273, https://doi.org/10.3390/nu14163273.

23. Sarah A. Keim et al., "ω-3 and ω-6 Fatty Acid Supplementation May Reduce Autism Symptoms Based on Parent Report in Preterm Toddlers," *Journal of Nutrition* 148, no. 2 (February 1, 2018): 227–35, https://doi.org/10.1093/jn/nxx047.

24. Khaled Saad et al., "A Randomized, Placebo-Controlled Trial of Digestive Enzymes in Children with Autism Spectrum Disorders," *Clinical Psychopharmacology and Neuroscience: The Official Scientific Journal of the Korean College of Neuropsychopharmacology* 13, no. 2 (August 31, 2015): 188–93, https://doi.org/10.9758/cpn.2015.13.2.188; Mark A. Brudnak et al., "Enzyme-Based Therapy for Autism Spectrum Disorders—Is It Worth Another Look?," *Medical Hypotheses* 58, no. 5 (May 2002): 422–28, https://doi.org/10.1054/mehy.2001.1513.

25. Adams et al., "Ratings of the Effectiveness of Nutraceuticals for Autism Spectrum Disorders."

26. Rima Obeid, "The Metabolic Burden of Methyl Donor Deficiency with Focus on the Betaine Homocysteine Methyltransferase Pathway," *Nutrients* 5, no. 9 (September 9, 2013): 3481–95, https://doi.org/10.3390/nu5093481.

27. Adams et al., "Nutritional and Metabolic Status of Children with Autism."

28. Vandana Rai, "Association of Methylenetetrahydrofolate Reductase (MTHFR) Gene C677T Polymorphism with Autism: Evidence of Genetic Susceptibility," *Metabolic Brain Disease* 31, no. 4 (August 2016): 727–35, https://doi.org/10.1007/s11011-016-9815-0.

29. V. T. Ramaekers et al., "Folate Receptor Autoimmunity and Cerebral Folate Deficiency in Low-Functioning Autism with Neurological Deficits," *Neuropediatrics* 38, no. 6 (December 2007): 276–81, https://doi.org/10.1055/s-2008-1065354.

30. Edouard J. Servy et al., "MTHFR Isoform Carriers. 5-MTHF (5-Methyl Tetrahydrofolate) vs Folic Acid: A Key to Pregnancy Outcome: A Case Series," *Journal of Assisted Reproduction and Genetics* 35, no. 8 (August 2018): 1431–35, https://doi.org/10.1007/s10815-018-1225-2.

31. Karen E. Christensen et al., "High Folic Acid Consumption Leads to Pseudo-MTHFR Deficiency, Altered Lipid Metabolism, and Liver Injury in Mice," *American Journal of Clinical Nutrition* 101, no. 3 (March 2015): 646–58, https://doi.org/10.3945/ajcn.114.086603.

32. Darrell Wiens and M. DeSoto, "Is High Folic Acid Intake a Risk Factor for Autism?—A Review," *Brain Sciences* 7, no. 12 (November 10, 2017): 149, https://doi.org/10.3390/brainsci7110149.

33. Servy et al., "MTHFR Isoform Carriers."

34. Lori Lathrop Stern et al., "Conversion of 5-Formyltetrahydrofolic Acid to 5-Methyltetrahydrofolic Acid Is Unimpaired in Folate-Adequate Persons Homozygous for the C677T Mutation in the Methylenetetrahydrofolate Reductase Gene," *Journal of Nutrition* 130, no. 9 (September 1, 2000): 2238–42, https://doi.org/10.1093/jn/130.9.2238.

35. Adams et al., "Ratings of the Effectiveness of Nutraceuticals for Autism Spectrum Disorders."

36. Daniel A. Rossignol and Richard E. Frye, "The Effectiveness of Cobalamin (B$_{12}$) Treatment for Autism Spectrum Disorder: A Systematic Review and Meta-Analysis," *Journal of Personalized Medicine* 11, no. 8 (August 11, 2021): 784, https://doi.org/10.3390/jpm11080784.

37. Patricia Esteban-Figuerola et al., "Differences in Food Consumption and Nutritional Intake Between Children with Autism Spectrum Disorders and Typically Developing Children: A Meta-Analysis," *Autism: The International Journal of Research and Practice* 23, no. 5 (July 2019): 1079–95, https://doi.org/10.1177/1362361318794179.

38. Adams et al., "Ratings of the Effectiveness of Nutraceuticals for Autism Spectrum Disorders."

39. Adams et al., "Effect of a Vitamin/Mineral Supplement."

40. Adams et al., "Ratings of the Effectiveness of Nutraceuticals for Autism Spectrum Disorders."

41. Salvador Marí-Bauset et al., "Nutritional Impact of a Gluten-Free Casein-Free Diet in Children with Autism Spectrum Disorder," *Journal of Autism and Developmental Disorders* 46, no. 2 (February 2016): 673–84, https://doi .org/10.1007/s10803-015-2582-7; Adams et al., "Nutritional and Metabolic Status of Children with Autism."

42. Adams et al., "Effect of a Vitamin/Mineral Supplement."

43. Autism Nutrition Research Center, "ANRC Autism Treatment Rater."

44. Milagros G. Huerta et al., "Magnesium Deficiency Is Associated with Insulin Resistance in Obese Children," *Diabetes Care* 28, no. 5 (May 1, 2005): 1175–81, https://doi.org/10.2337/diacare.28.5.1175.

45. Richard E. Frye et al., "A Review of Traditional and Novel Treatments for Seizures in Autism Spectrum Disorder: Findings from a Systematic Review and Expert Panel," *Frontiers in Public Health* 1 (September 13, 2013): 31, https://doi.org/10.3389/fpubh.2013.00031.

46. Li et al., "Serum Copper and Zinc Levels."

47. Adams et al., "Nutritional and Metabolic Status of Children with Autism."

48. Hadeil M. Alsufiani et al., "Zinc Deficiency and Supplementation in Autism Spectrum Disorder and Phelan-McDermid Syndrome," *Journal of Neuroscience Research* 100, no. 4 (April 2022): 970–78, https://doi.org/10.1002/jnr .25019.

49. Hsun-Chin Chao et al., "Serum Trace Element Levels and Their Correlation with Picky Eating Behavior, Development, and Physical Activity in Early Childhood," *Nutrients* 13, no. 7 (July 2, 2021): 2295, https://doi.org/10.3390 /nu13072295.

50. Susan Dickerson Mayes and Hana Zickgraf, "Atypical Eating Behaviors in Children and Adolescents with Autism, ADHD, Other Disorders, and Typical Development," *Research in Autism Spectrum Disorders* 64 (August 1, 2019): 76–83, https://doi.org/10.1016/j.rasd.2019.04.002.

51. Sunit Singhi et al., "Low Plasma Zinc and Iron in Pica," *Indian Journal of Pediatrics* 70, no. 2 (February 2003): 139–43, https://doi.org/10.1007 /BF02723740.

52. Woody R. McGinnis et al., "Discerning the Mauve Factor, Part 1," *Alternative Therapies in Health and Medicine* 14, no. 2 (2008): 40–50.

53. Min Guo et al., "Vitamin A and Vitamin D Deficiencies Exacerbate Symptoms in Children with Autism Spectrum Disorders," *Nutritional Neuroscience* 22, no. 9 (September 2019): 637–47, https://doi.org/10.1080/1028415X.2017 .1423268.

54. Masako Suzuki and Meika Tomita, "Genetic Variations of Vitamin A-Absorption and Storage-Related Genes, and Their Potential Contribution to Vitamin A Deficiency Risks Among Different Ethnic Groups," *Frontiers in Nutrition* 9 (2022): 861619. https://doi.org/10.3389/fnut.2022.861619.

55. Nina S. Ma, Cynthia Thompson, and Sharon Weston, "Brief Report: Scurvy as a Manifestation of Food Selectivity in Children with Autism," *Journal of Autism and Developmental Disorders* 46, no. 4 (April 2016): 1464–70, https://doi.org/10.1007/s10803-015-2660-x.

56. Adams et al., "Nutritional and Metabolic Status of Children with Autism."

57. Jacek Baj et al., "Autism Spectrum Disorder: Trace Elements Imbalances and the Pathogenesis and Severity of Autistic Symptoms," *Neuroscience and Biobehavioral Reviews* 129 (October 2021): 117–32, https://doi.org/10.1016/j.neubiorev.2021.07.029.

58. Hongmei Wu et al., "Supplementation with Selenium Attenuates Autism-like Behaviors and Improves Oxidative Stress, Inflammation and Related Gene Expression in an Autism Disease Model," *Journal of Nutritional Biochemistry* 107 (September 2022): 109034, https://doi.org/10.1016/j.jnutbio.2022.109034.

59. John Jacob Cannell, "Vitamin D and Autism, What's New?," *Reviews in Endocrine and Metabolic Disorders* 18, no. 2 (June 2017): 183–93, https://doi.org/10.1007/s11154-017-9409-0.

60. Steven H. Zeisel, "Nutritional Genomics: Defining the Dietary Requirement and Effects of Choline," *Journal of Nutrition* 141, no. 3 (March 1, 2011): 531–34, https://doi.org/10.3945/jn.110.130369.

61. Sophie I. Hamstra et al., "Beyond Its Psychiatric Use: The Benefits of Low-Dose Lithium Supplementation," *Current Neuropharmacology* 21, no. 4 (April 2023): 891–910, https://doi.org/10.2174/1570159X20666220302151224.

62. Adams et al., "Nutritional and Metabolic Status of Children with Autism."

63. Autism Nutrition Research Center, "ANRC Autism Treatment Rater."

STEP 4

1. Susan Dickerson Mayes and Hana Zickgraf, "Atypical Eating Behaviors in Children and Adolescents with Autism, ADHD, Other Disorders, and Typical Development," *Research in Autism Spectrum Disorders* 64 (August 1, 2019): 76–83, https://doi.org/10.1016/j.rasd.2019.04.002.

2. Summer Yule et al., "Nutritional Deficiency Disease Secondary to ARFID Symptoms Associated with Autism and the Broad Autism Phenotype: A Qualitative Systematic Review of Case Reports and Case Series," *Journal of the Academy of Nutrition and Dietetics* 121, no. 3 (March 2021): 467–92, https://doi.org/10.1016/j.jand.2020.10.017.

3. Jason Allan Seng Soon Cheah et al., "Optic Neuropathy in an Autistic Child with Vitamin A Deficiency: A Case Report and Literature Review," *Cureus* 14, no. 2 (February 9, 2022): e22074, https://doi.org/10.7759/cureus.22074.

4. Yaseen Rafee, Katherine Burrell, and Crystal Cederna-Meko, "Lessons in Early Identification and Treatment from a Case of Disabling Vitamin C

Deficiency in a Child with Autism Spectrum Disorder," *International Journal of Psychiatry in Medicine* 54, no. 1 (January 2019): 64–73, https://doi.org/10.1177/0091217418791443.

5. Yule et al., "Nutritional Deficiency Disease Secondary to ARFID Symptoms."

6. Chunyan Li et al., "Study on Aberrant Eating Behaviors, Food Intolerance, and Stereotyped Behaviors in Autism Spectrum Disorder," *Frontiers in Psychiatry* 11 (November 5, 2020): 493695, https://doi.org/10.3389/fpsyt.2020.493695.

7. Xin Wang et al., "Association Between Dietary Quality and Executive Functions in School-Aged Children with Autism Spectrum Disorder," *Frontiers in Nutrition* 9 (2022): 940246, https://doi.org/10.3389/fnut.2022.940246.

8. Daniel J Tobiansky et al., "Sucrose Consumption Alters Steroid and Dopamine Signalling in the Female Rat Brain," *Journal of Endocrinology* 245, no. 2 (May 2020): 231–46, https://doi.org/10.1530/JOE-19-0386.

9. Richard J. Wurtman and Judith J. Wurtman, "Brain Serotonin, Carbohydrate-Craving, Obesity and Depression," *Obesity Research* 3, no. S4 (November 1995): 477S-480S, https://doi.org/10.1002/j.1550-8528.1995.tb00215.x.

10. Joe Alcock, Carlo C. Maley, and C. Athena Aktipis, "Is Eating Behavior Manipulated by the Gastrointestinal Microbiota? Evolutionary Pressures and Potential Mechanisms," *BioEssays* 36, no. 10 (October 2014): 940–49, https://doi.org/10.1002/bies.201400071.

11. Maria Rosaria Iovene et al., "Intestinal Dysbiosis and Yeast Isolation in Stool of Subjects with Autism Spectrum Disorders," *Mycopathologia* 182, no. 3–4 (April 2017): 349–63, https://doi.org/10.1007/s11046-016-0068-6.

12. Ahmed B. Bayoumy et al., "Gut Fermentation Syndrome: A Systematic Review of Case Reports," *United European Gastroenterology Journal* 9, no. 3 (April 2021): 332–42, https://doi.org/10.1002/ueg2.12062.

13. Pia P. Tannhauser et al., "Zinc Status and Meat Avoidance in Anorexia Nervosa," *International Journal of Adolescent Medicine and Health* 13, no. 4 (October 2001): 317–326, https://doi.org/10.1515/IJAMH.2001.13.4.317.

14. Liem T. Chistol et al., "Sensory Sensitivity and Food Selectivity in Children with Autism Spectrum Disorder," *Journal of Autism and Developmental Disorders* 48, no. 2 (February 2018): 583–91, https://doi.org/10.1007/s10803-017-3340-9.

15. Mayes and Zickgraf, "Atypical Eating Behaviors."

16. Cynthia R Johnson et al., "Parent Training for Feeding Problems in Children with Autism Spectrum Disorder: Initial Randomized Trial," *Journal of Pediatric Psychology* 44, no. 2 (March 1, 2019): 164–75, https://doi.org/10.1093/jpepsy/jsy063.

17. Timothy P. Holloway et al., "School Gardening and Health and Well-Being of School-Aged Children: A Realist Synthesis," *Nutrients* 15, no. 5 (February 27, 2023): 1190, https://doi.org/10.3390/nu15051190.

STEP 5

1. Kousaku Ohinata, Shun Agui, and Masaaki Yoshikawa, "Soymorphins, Novel μ Opioid Peptides Derived from Soy β-Conglycinin β-Subunit, Have Anxiolytic Activities," *Bioscience, Biotechnology, and Biochemistry* 71, no. 10 (October 23, 2007): 2618–21, https://doi.org/10.1271/bbb.70516.

2. Shahid Bashir and Laila AL-Ayadhi, "Alterations in Plasma Dipeptidyl Peptidase IV in Autism: A Pilot Study," *Neurology, Psychiatry and Brain Research* 20, no. 2 (June 2014): 41–44, https://doi.org/10.1016/j.npbr .2014.03.001.

3. Dag Tveiten et al., "Peptides and Exorphins in the Autism Spectrum," *Open Journal of Psychiatry* 4, no. 3 (2014): 275–87, https://doi.org/10.4236/ojpsych .2014.43034.

4. Karl L. Reichelt et al., "Probable Etiology and Possible Treatment of Childhood Autism," *Brain Dysfunction* 4 (1991): 308–19.

5. Tveiten et al., "Peptides and Exorphins in the Autism Spectrum."

6. Alessio Fasano, "All Disease Begins in the (Leaky) Gut: Role of Zonulin-Mediated Gut Permeability in the Pathogenesis of Some Chronic Inflammatory Diseases," *F1000Research* 9, F1000 Faculty Rev (January 31, 2020): 69, https://doi.org/10.12688/f1000research.20510.1.

7. Hussain Al Dera et al., "Leaky Gut Biomarkers in Casein- and Gluten-Rich Diet Fed Rat Model of Autism," *Translational Neuroscience* 12, no. 1 (January 1, 2021): 601–10, https://doi.org/10.1515/tnsci-2020-0207.

8. Alessio Fasano and Ivor Hill, "Serum Zonulin, Gut Permeability, and the Pathogenesis of Autism Spectrum Disorders: Cause, Effect, or an Epiphenomenon?," *Journal of Pediatrics* 188 (September 2017): 15–17, https://doi .org/10.1016/j.jpeds.2017.05.038.

9. Erman Esnafoglu et al., "Increased Serum Zonulin Levels as an Intestinal Permeability Marker in Autistic Subjects," *Journal of Pediatrics* 188 (September 2017): 240–44, https://doi.org/10.1016/j.jpeds.2017.04.004.

10. Laura de Magistris et al., "Antibodies Against Food Antigens in Patients with Autistic Spectrum Disorders," *BioMed Research International* (2013): 729349, https://doi.org/10.1155/2013/729349.

11. Harumi Jyonouchi et al., "Evaluation of an Association Between Gastrointestinal Symptoms and Cytokine Production Against Common Dietary Proteins in Children with Autism Spectrum Disorders," *Journal of Pediatrics* 146, no. 5 (May 2005): 605–10, https://doi.org/10.1016/j.jpeds.2005.01.027.

12. Harumi Jyonouchi, Sining Sun, and Nanae Itokazu, "Innate Immunity Associated with Inflammatory Responses and Cytokine Production Against Common Dietary Proteins in Patients with Autism Spectrum Disorder," *Neuropsychobiology* 46, no. 2 (2002): 76–84, https://doi.org/10.1159/0000 65416.

13. Robert Cade et al., "Autism and Schizophrenia: Intestinal Disorders," *Nutritional Neuroscience* 3, no. 1 (January 2000): 57–72, https://doi.org/10.1080/1028415X.2000.11747303.

14. Theoharis C. Theoharides et al., "Mast Cell Activation and Autism," *Biochimica et Biophysica Acta (BBA)—Molecular Basis of Disease* 1822, no. 1 (January 2012): 34–41, https://doi.org/10.1016/j.bbadis.2010.12.017.

15. Brent L. Williams et al., "Impaired Carbohydrate Digestion and Transport and Mucosal Dysbiosis in the Intestines of Children with Autism and Gastrointestinal Disturbances," *PloS One* 6, no. 9 (2011): e24585, https://doi.org/10.1371/journal.pone.0024585.

16. Rafail I. Kushak, Ashok Sengupta, and Harland S. Winter, "Interactions Between the Intestinal Microbiota and Epigenome in Individuals with Autism Spectrum Disorder," *Developmental Medicine and Child Neurology* 64, no. 3 (March 2022): 296–304, https://doi.org/10.1111/dmcn.15052.

17. R. E. Frye et al., "Cerebral Folate Receptor Autoantibodies in Autism Spectrum Disorder," *Molecular Psychiatry* 18, no. 3 (March 2013): 369–81, https://doi.org/10.1038/mp.2011.175.

18. Vincent T. Ramaekers et al., "A Milk-Free Diet Downregulates Folate Receptor Autoimmunity in Cerebral Folate Deficiency Syndrome," *Developmental Medicine and Child Neurology* 50, no. 5 (May 2008): 346–52, https://doi.org/10.1111/j.1469-8749.2008.02053.x.

19. Cara J. Westmark, "Soy Infant Formula and Seizures in Children with Autism: A Retrospective Study," *PloS One* 9, no. 3 (March 12, 2014): e80488, https://doi.org/10.1371/journal.pone.0080488.

20. Cara Jean Westmark, "A Hypothesis Regarding the Molecular Mechanism Underlying Dietary Soy-Induced Effects on Seizure Propensity," *Frontiers in Neurology* 5 (2014), https://doi.org/10.3389/fneur.2014.00169.

21. Paul Whiteley et al., "The ScanBrit Randomised, Controlled, Single-Blind Study of a Gluten- and Casein-Free Dietary Intervention for Children with Autism Spectrum Disorders," *Nutritional Neuroscience* 13, no. 2 (April 2010): 87–100, https://doi.org/10.1179/147683010X12611460763922.

22. Cade et al., "Autism and Schizophrenia."

23. Faezeh Ghalichi et al., "Effect of Gluten Free Diet on Gastrointestinal and Behavioral Indices for Children with Autism Spectrum Disorders: A Randomized Clinical Trial," *World Journal of Pediatrics* 12, no. 4 (November 2016): 436–42, https://doi.org/10.1007/s12519-016-0040-z.

24. James B. Adams et al., "Comprehensive Nutritional and Dietary Intervention for Autism Spectrum Disorder—A Randomized, Controlled 12-Month Trial," *Nutrients* 10, no. 3 (March 17, 2018): E369, https://doi.org/10.3390/nu10030369.

25. Julie S. Matthews and James B. Adams, "Ratings of the Effectiveness of 13 Therapeutic Diets for Autism Spectrum Disorder: Results of a National

Survey," *Journal of Personalized Medicine* 13, no. 10 (September 29, 2023): 1448, https://doi.org/10.3390/jpm13101448.

26. Salvador Marí-Bauset et al., "Nutritional Impact of a Gluten-Free Casein-Free Diet in Children with Autism Spectrum Disorder," *Journal of Autism and Developmental Disorders* 46, no. 2 (February 2016): 673–84, https://doi.org/10.1007/s10803-015-2582-7.

27. James B. Adams et al., "Nutritional and Metabolic Status of Children with Autism vs. Neurotypical Children, and the Association with Autism Severity," *Nutrition & Metabolism* 8, no. 1 (June 8, 2011): 34, https://doi.org/10.1186/1743-7075-8-34.

28. Gabriela Diaz de Barboza et al., "Oxidative Stress, Antioxidants and Intestinal Calcium Absorption," *World Journal of Gastroenterology* 23, no. 16 (April 28, 2017): 2841–53, https://doi.org/10.3748/wjg.v23.i16.2841.

29. James B. Adams et al., "Effect of a Vitamin/Mineral Supplement on Children and Adults with Autism," *BMC Pediatrics* 11 (December 12, 2011): 111, https://doi.org/10.1186/1471-2431-11-111.

30. Matthews and Adams, "Ratings of the Effectiveness of 13 Therapeutic Diets for Autism Spectrum Disorder."

STEP 6

1. Dawson Church et al., "Is Tapping on Acupuncture Points an Active Ingredient in Emotional Freedom Techniques? A Systematic Review and Meta-Analysis of Comparative Studies," *Journal of Nervous and Mental Disease* 206, no. 10 (October 2018): 783–93, https://doi.org/10.1097/NMD.0000000000000878.

2. Morgan Clond, "Emotional Freedom Techniques for Anxiety: A Systematic Review with Meta-Analysis," *Journal of Nervous & Mental Disease* 204, no. 5 (May 2016): 388–95, https://doi.org/10.1097/NMD.0000000000000483; Jerrod A. Nelms and Liana Castel, "A Systematic Review and Meta-Analysis of Randomized and Nonrandomized Trials of Clinical Emotional Freedom Techniques (EFT) for the Treatment of Depression," *EXPLORE* 12, no. 6 (November 2016): 416–26, https://doi.org/10.1016/j.explore.2016.08.001.

3. Donna Bach et al., "Clinical EFT (Emotional Freedom Techniques) Improves Multiple Physiological Markers of Health," *Journal of Evidence-Based Integrative Medicine* 24 (January 1, 2019): 2515690X1882369, https://doi.org/10.1177/2515690X18823691.

4. W. A. McCarty, "Clinical Story of a 6-Year-Old Boy's Eating Phobia: An Integrated Approach Utilizing Prenatal and Perinatal Psychology with Energy Psychology's Emotional Freedom Technique (EFT) in a Surrogate Nonlocal Application," *Journal of Prenatal & Perinatal Psychology & Health* 21, no. 2 (2006): 117–39.

STEP 7

1. A. Alberti et al., "Sulphation Deficit in 'Low-Functioning' Autistic Children: A Pilot Study," *Biological Psychiatry* 46, no. 3 (August 1, 1999): 420–24, https://doi.org/10.1016/s0006-3223(98)00337-0.

2. Marek L. Kowalski et al., "Diagnosis and Management of NSAID-Exacerbated Respiratory Disease (N-ERD)—a EAACI Position Paper," *Allergy* 74, no. 1 (January 2019): 28–39, https://doi.org/10.1111/all.13599.

3. Kunio Yui, George Imataka, and Shigemi Yoshihara, "Lipid-Based Molecules on Signaling Pathways in Autism Spectrum Disorder," *International Journal of Molecular Sciences* 23, no. 17 (August 29, 2022): 9803, https://doi.org/10.3390/ijms23179803.

4. Jayne E. Stratton et al., "Biogenic Amines in Cheese and Other Fermented Foods: A Review." *Journal of Food Protection* 54, no. 6 (June 1991): 460–70. https://doi.org/10.4315/0362-028X-54.6.460.

5. Ben F. Feingold, "Hyperkinesis and Learning Disabilities Linked to Artificial Food Flavors and Colors," *American Journal of Nursing* 75, no. 5 (1975): 797–803, https://doi.org/10.2307/3423460.

6. Saartje Hontelez et al., "Correlation Between Brain Function and ADHD Symptom Changes in Children with ADHD Following a Few-Foods Diet: An Open-Label Intervention Trial," *Scientific Reports* 11 (November 12, 2021): 22205, https://doi.org/10.1038/s41598-021-01684-7.

7. Julie S. Matthews and James B. Adams, "Ratings of the Effectiveness of 13 Therapeutic Diets for Autism Spectrum Disorder: Results of a National Survey," *Journal of Personalized Medicine* 13, no. 10 (September 29, 2023): 1448, https://doi.org/10.3390/jpm13101448.

8. James B. Adams et al., "Comprehensive Nutritional and Dietary Intervention for Autism Spectrum Disorder—A Randomized, Controlled 12-Month Trial," *Nutrients* 10, no. 3 (March 17, 2018): E369, https://doi.org/10.3390/nu10030369.

9. James B. Adams et al., "Effect of a Vitamin/Mineral Supplement on Children and Adults with Autism," *BMC Pediatrics* 11 (December 12, 2011): 111, https://doi.org/10.1186/1471-2431-11-111.

10. Autism Nutrition Research Center, "ANRC Autism Treatment Rater," 2022, https://apps.apple.com/us/app/anrc-autism-treatment-rater/id1616969988.

11. Margaret Moss and Rosemary Waring, "The Plasma Cysteine/Sulphate Ratio: A Possible Clinical Biomarker," *Journal of Nutritional & Environmental Medicine* 13, no. 4 (July 13, 2009): 215–29, https://doi.org/10.1080/13590840310001642003.

12. K. Z. Isoardi et al., "Activated Charcoal and Bicarbonate for Aspirin Toxicity: A Retrospective Series," *Journal of Medical Toxicology* 18, no. 1 (January 2022): 30–37, https://doi.org/10.1007/s13181-021-00865-0.

STEP 8

1. Hong Li et al., "Association of Food Hypersensitivity in Children with the Risk of Autism Spectrum Disorder: A Meta-Analysis," *European Journal of Pediatrics* 180, no. 4 (April 2021): 999–1008, https://doi.org/10.1007/s00431-020-03826-x.

2. Yuling Tan, Shiny Thomas, and Brian K. Lee, "Parent-Reported Prevalence of Food Allergies in Children with Autism Spectrum Disorder: National Health Interview Survey, 2011–2015," *Autism Research* 12, no. 5 (May 2019): 802–5, https://doi.org/10.1002/aur.2106.

3. Ruchi S. Gupta et al., "The Public Health Impact of Parent-Reported Childhood Food Allergies in the United States," *Pediatrics* 142, no. 6 (December 2018): e20181235, https://doi.org/10.1542/peds.2018-1235.

4. Chunyan Li et al., "Study on Aberrant Eating Behaviors, Food Intolerance, and Stereotyped Behaviors in Autism Spectrum Disorder," *Frontiers in Psychiatry* 11 (November 5, 2020): 493695, https://doi.org/10.3389/fpsyt.2020.493695.

5. Amanda Enstrom et al., "Increased IgG4 Levels in Children with Autism Disorder," *Brain, Behavior, and Immunity* 23, no. 3 (March 2009): 389–95, https://doi.org/10.1016/j.bbi.2008.12.005.

6. Milena Peruhova et al., "Specific Immunoglobulin E and G to Common Food Antigens and Increased Serum Zonulin in IBS Patients: A Single-Center Bulgarian Study," *Antibodies* 11, no. 2 (March 29, 2022): 23, https://doi.org/10.3390/antib11020023.

7. Peruhova et al., "Specific Immunoglobulin E and G."

8. Harumi Jyonouchi et al., "Evaluation of an Association Between Gastrointestinal Symptoms and Cytokine Production Against Common Dietary Proteins in Children with Autism Spectrum Disorders," *Journal of Pediatrics* 146, no. 5 (May 2005): 605–10, https://doi.org/10.1016/j.jpeds.2005.01.027; Harumi Jyonouchi et al., "Dysregulated Innate Immune Responses in Young Children with Autism Spectrum Disorders: Their Relationship to Gastrointestinal Symptoms and Dietary Intervention," *Neuropsychobiology* 51, no. 2 (2005): 77–85, https://doi.org/10.1159/000084164.

9. Li et al., "Study on Aberrant Eating Behaviors."

10. Alexander G. Singer et al., "Prevalence of Physician-Reported Food Allergy in Canadian Children," *Journal of Allergy and Clinical Immunology in Practice* 9, no. 1 (January 2021): 193–99, https://doi.org/10.1016/j.jaip.2020.07.039.

11. Peruhova et al., "Specific Immunoglobulin E and G."

12. Singer et al., "Prevalence of Physician-Reported Food Allergy in Canadian Children"; Hanna Karakuła-Juchnowicz et al., "The Role of IgG

Hypersensitivity in the Pathogenesis and Therapy of Depressive Disorders," *Nutritional Neuroscience* 20, no. 2 (February 2017): 110–18, https://doi.org/10.1179/1476830514Y.0000000158.

13. A. Vojdani et al., "Immune Response to Dietary Proteins, Gliadin and Cerebellar Peptides in Children with Autism," *Nutritional Neuroscience* 7, no. 3 (June 2004): 151–61, https://doi.org/10.1080/10284150400004155.

14. Muhammad Inam et al., "Prevalence of Sensitization to Food Allergens and Challenge Proven Food Allergy in Patients Visiting Allergy Centers in Rawalpindi and Islamabad, Pakistan," *SpringerPlus* 5, no. 1 (August 11, 2016): 1330, https://doi.org/10.1186/s40064-016-2980-0.

15. Matthews and Adams, "Ratings of the Effectiveness of 13 Therapeutic Diets for Autism Spectrum Disorder."

16. Marcin Bryła et al., "Recent Research on Fusarium Mycotoxins in Maize—A Review," *Foods (Basel, Switzerland)* 11, no. 21 (November 1, 2022): 3465, https://doi.org/10.3390/foods11213465.

17. K. J. Carpenter, "The Relationship of Pellagra to Corn and the Low Availability of Niacin in Cereals," *Experientia. Supplementum* 44 (1983): 197–222, https://doi.org/10.1007/978-3-0348-6540-1_12.

18. S. Lu et al., "[Detection and Analysis of Serum Food-Specific IgG Antibody in Beijing Area]," *Zhonghua Yu Fang Yi Xue Za Zhi [Chinese Journal of Preventive Medicine]* 55, no. 2 (February 6, 2021): 253–57, https://doi.org/10.3760/cma.j.cn112150-20201027-01309.

19. Alexandra Adorno Vita, Heather Zwickey, and Ryan Bradley, "Associations Between Food-Specific IgG Antibodies and Intestinal Permeability Biomarkers," *Frontiers in Nutrition* 9 (2022): 962093, https://doi.org/10.3389/fnut.2022.962093.

20. Vojdani et al., "Immune Response to Dietary Proteins."

21. Megan R. Sanctuary et al., "Dietary Considerations in Autism Spectrum Disorders: The Potential Role of Protein Digestion and Microbial Putrefaction in the Gut-Brain Axis," *Frontiers in Nutrition* 5 (2018): 40, https://doi.org/10.3389/fnut.2018.00040.

22. Lidy M. J. Pelsser et al., "A Randomised Controlled Trial into the Effects of Food on ADHD," *European Child & Adolescent Psychiatry* 18, no. 1 (January 2009): 12–19, https://doi.org/10.1007/s00787-008-0695-7.

23. S. Lucarelli et al., "Food Allergy and Infantile Autism," *Panminerva Medica* 37, no. 3 (September 1995): 137–41.

24. Lucyna Ostrowska et al., "Igg Food Antibody Guided Elimination-Rotation Diet Was More Effective than FODMAP Diet and Control Diet in the Treatment of Women with Mixed IBS-Results from an Open Label Study," *Journal of Clinical Medicine* 10, no. 19 (September 23, 2021): 4317, https://doi.org/10.3390/jcm10194317.

STEP 9

1. Karin de Punder and Leo Pruimboom, "The Dietary Intake of Wheat and Other Cereal Grains and Their Role in Inflammation," *Nutrients* 5, no. 3 (March 12, 2013): 771–87, https://doi.org/10.3390/nu5030771.

2. K. Horvath et al., "Gastrointestinal Abnormalities in Children with Autistic Disorder," *Journal of Pediatrics* 135, no. 5 (November 1999): 559–63, https://doi.org/10.1016/s0022-3476(99)70052-1; Brent L. Williams et al., "Impaired Carbohydrate Digestion and Transport and Mucosal Dysbiosis in the Intestines of Children with Autism and Gastrointestinal Disturbances," *PloS One* 6, no. 9 (2011): e24585, https://doi.org/10.1371/journal.pone.0024585.

3. Horvath et al., "Gastrointestinal Abnormalities in Children with Autistic Disorder"; Williams et al., "Impaired Carbohydrate Digestion."

4. S. V. Haas and M. P. Haas, "The Treatment of Celiac Disease with the Specific Carbohydrate Diet; Report on 191 Additional Cases," *American Journal of Gastroenterology* 23, no. 4 (April 1955): 344–60.

5. David L. Suskind et al., "Patients Perceive Clinical Benefit with the Specific Carbohydrate Diet for Inflammatory Bowel Disease," *Digestive Diseases and Sciences* 61, no. 11 (November 2016): 3255–60, https://doi.org/10.1007/s10620-016-4307-y.

6. Silvija Ābele et al., "Specific Carbohydrate Diet (SCD/GAPS) and Dietary Supplements for Children with Autistic Spectrum Disorder," *Proceedings of the Latvian Academy of Sciences* 75, no. 6 (2021): 417–25, https://doi.org/10.2478/prolas-2021-0062.

7. Kelly Barnhill et al., "Brief Report: Implementation of a Specific Carbohydrate Diet for a Child with Autism Spectrum Disorder and Fragile X Syndrome," *Journal of Autism and Developmental Disorders* 50, no. 5 (May 2020): 1800–1808, https://doi.org/10.1007/s10803-018-3704-9.

8. M. Barone et al., "Gut Microbiome Response to a Modern Paleolithic Diet in a Western Lifestyle Context," *PLoS One* 14, no. 8 (August 2019): e0220619, https://doi.org/10.1371/journal.pone.0220619.

9. Julia Otten et al., "Benefits of a Paleolithic Diet with and without Supervised Exercise on Fat Mass, Insulin Sensitivity, and Glycemic Control: A Randomized Controlled Trial in Individuals with Type 2 Diabetes," *Diabetes/Metabolism Research and Reviews* 33, no. 1 (January 2017), https://doi.org/10.1002/dmrr.2828.

10. Julie S. Matthews and James B. Adams, "Ratings of the Effectiveness of 13 Therapeutic Diets for Autism Spectrum Disorder: Results of a National Survey," *Journal of Personalized Medicine* 13, no. 10 (September 29, 2023): 1448, https://doi.org/10.3390/jpm13101448.

STEP 10

1. Jerzy Konstantynowicz et al., "A Potential Pathogenic Role of Oxalate in Autism," *European Journal of Paediatric Neurology* 16, no. 5 (September 2012): 485–91, https://doi.org/10.1016/j.ejpn.2011.08.004.

2. S. C. Noonan and G. P. Savage, "Oxalate Content of Foods and Its Effect on Humans," *Asia Pacific Journal of Clinical Nutrition* 8, no. 1 (March 1999): 64–74.

3. Mary Speirs, "The Utilization of the Calcium in Various Greens," *Journal of Nutrition* 17, no. 6 (June 1, 1939): 557–64, https://doi.org/10.1093/jn/17.6.557.

4. C. A. Peterson, J. A. Eurell, and J. W. Erdman, "Bone Composition and Histology of Young Growing Rats Fed Diets of Varied Calcium Bioavailability: Spinach, Nonfat Dry Milk, or Calcium Carbonate Added to Casein," *Journal of Nutrition* 122, no. 1 (January 1992): 137–44, https://doi.org/10.1093/jn/122.1.137.

5. Ross P. Holmes, Harold O. Goodman, and Dean G. Assimos, "Contribution of Dietary Oxalate to Urinary Oxalate Excretion," *Kidney International* 59, no. 1 (January 2001): 270–76, https://doi.org/10.1046/j.1523-1755.2001.00488.x.

6. Matteo Bargagli et al., "Dietary Oxalate Intake and Kidney Outcomes," *Nutrients* 12, no. 9 (September 2, 2020): 2673, https://doi.org/10.3390/nu12092673.

7. Bargagli et al., "Dietary Oxalate Intake and Kidney Outcomes."

8. Lama Nazzal et al., "Effect of Antibiotic Treatment on *Oxalobacter formigenes* Colonization of the Gut Microbiome and Urinary Oxalate Excretion," *Scientific Reports* 11, no. 1 (August 12, 2021): 16428, https://doi.org/10.1038/s41598-021-95992-7.

9. Tao Jiang et al., "Abundance, Functional, and Evolutionary Analysis of Oxalyl-Coenzyme A Decarboxylase in Human Microbiota," *Frontiers in Microbiology* 11 (April 23, 2020): 672, https://doi.org/10.3389/fmicb.2020.00672.

10. Mangesh V. Suryavanshi et al., "Hyperoxaluria Leads to Dysbiosis and Drives Selective Enrichment of Oxalate Metabolizing Bacterial Species in Recurrent Kidney Stone Endures," *Scientific Reports* 6, no. 1 (October 6, 2016): 34712, https://doi.org/10.1038/srep34712.

11. Aaron W. Miller, Colin Dale, and M. Denise Dearing, "Microbiota Diversification and Crash Induced by Dietary Oxalate in the Mammalian Herbivore *Neotoma albigula*," *mSphere* 2, no. 5 (October 25, 2017): e00428-17, https://doi.org/10.1128/mSphere.00428-17.

12. Julie Bonhomme et al., "Contribution of the Glycolytic Flux and Hypoxia Adaptation to Efficient Biofilm Formation by *Candida albicans*," *Molecular*

Microbiology 80, no. 4 (May 2011): 995–1013, https://doi.org/10.1111/j.1365 -2958.2011.07626.x.

13. Troy Vargason, Deborah L. McGuinness, and Juergen Hahn, "Gastrointestinal Symptoms and Oral Antibiotic Use in Children with Autism Spectrum Disorder: Retrospective Analysis of a Privately Insured U.S. Population," *Journal of Autism and Developmental Disorders* 49, no. 2 (February 2019): 647–59, https://doi.org/10.1007/s10803-018-3743-2.

14. Celeste Witting et al., "Pathophysiology and Treatment of Enteric Hyperoxaluria," *Clinical Journal of the American Society of Nephrology* 16, no. 3 (March 2021): 487–95, https://doi.org/10.2215/CJN.08000520.

15. John Knight et al., "Ascorbic Acid Intake and Oxalate Synthesis," *Urolithiasis* 44, no. 4 (August 2016): 289–97, https://doi.org/10.1007/s00240-016 -0868-7; R. A. Conyers, R. Bais, and A. M. Rofe, "The Relation of Clinical Catastrophes, Endogenous Oxalate Production, and Urolithiasis," *Clinical Chemistry* 36, no. 10 (October 1990): 1717–30; Chad R. Tracy and Margaret S. Pearle, "Update on the Medical Management of Stone Disease," *Current Opinion in Urology* 19, no. 2 (March 2009): 200–204, https://doi.org/10 .1097/MOU.0b013e328323a81d.

16. S. Sharma et al., "Comparative Studies on the Effect of Vitamin A, B_1 and B_6 Deficiency on Oxalate Metabolism in Male Rats," *Annals of Nutrition & Metabolism* 34, no. 2 (1990): 104–11, https://doi.org/10.1159/000177576; Madalina-Andreea Robea, Alina-Costina Luca, and Alin Ciobica, "Relationship Between Vitamin Deficiencies and Co-Occurring Symptoms in Autism Spectrum Disorder," *Medicina* 56, no. 5 (May 20, 2020): 245, https://doi.org /10.3390/medicina56050245.

17. Joseph J. Crivelli et al., "Contribution of Dietary Oxalate and Oxalate Precursors to Urinary Oxalate Excretion," *Nutrients* 13, no. 1 (December 28, 2020): 62, https://doi.org/10.3390/nu13010062.

18. Draženka Svedružić et al., "The Enzymes of Oxalate Metabolism: Unexpected Structures and Mechanisms," *Archives of Biochemistry and Biophysics* 433, no. 1 (January 2005): 176–92, https://doi.org/10.1016/j.abb.2004.08 .032.

19. Sharma et al., "Comparative Studies on the Effect of Vitamin A, B_1 and B_6 Deficiency."

20. Mikita Patel et al., "Oxalate Induces Mitochondrial Dysfunction and Disrupts Redox Homeostasis in a Human Monocyte Derived Cell Line," *Redox Biology* 15 (May 2018): 207–15, https://doi.org/10.1016/j.redox.2017.12.003.

21. Coothan Kandaswamy Veena et al., "Mitochondrial Dysfunction in an Animal Model of Hyperoxaluria: A Prophylactic Approach with Fucoidan," *European Journal of Pharmacology* 579, no. 1–3 (January 28, 2008): 330–36, https://doi.org/10.1016/j.ejphar.2007.09.044.

22. Theresa Ermer et al., "Oxalate, Inflammasome, and Progression of Kidney Disease," *Current Opinion in Nephrology and Hypertension* 25, no. 4 (July 2016): 363–71, https://doi.org/10.1097/MNH.0000000000000229.

23. John R. Lukens, Vishwa Deep Dixit, and Thirumala-Devi Kanneganti, "Inflammasome Activation in Obesity-Related Inflammatory Diseases and Autoimmunity," *Discovery Medicine* 12, no. 62 (July 2011): 65–74.

24. Bhesh Raj Sharma and Thirumala-Devi Kanneganti, "NLRP3 Inflammasome in Cancer and Metabolic Diseases," *Nature Immunology* 22, no. 5 (May 2021): 550–59, https://doi.org/10.1038/s41590-021-00886-5.

25. Federica Piancone et al., "The Role of the Inflammasome in Neurodegenerative Diseases," *Molecules* 26, no. 4 (February 11, 2021): 953, https://doi.org/10.3390/molecules26040953.

26. Carolina Pellegrini et al., "Microbiota-Gut-Brain Axis in Health and Disease: Is NLRP3 Inflammasome at the Crossroads of Microbiota-Gut-Brain Communications?," *Progress in Neurobiology* 191 (August 2020): 101806, https://doi.org/10.1016/j.pneurobio.2020.101806.

27. Lee Hsien Siang et al., "Fruits for Seizures? A Systematic Review on the Potential Anti-Convulsant Effects of Fruits and Their Phytochemicals," *Current Neuropharmacology* 20, no. 10 (2022): 1925–40, https://doi.org/10.2174/1570159X19666210913120637.

28. Konstantynowicz et al., "A Potential Pathogenic Role of Oxalate in Autism."

29. Noonan and Savage, "Oxalate Content of Foods and Its Effect on Humans."

30. Noonan and Savage, "Oxalate Content of Foods and Its Effect on Humans."

31. Ermer et al., "Oxalate, Inflammasome, and Progression of Kidney Disease."

32. Victoria Garland, Leal Herlitz, and Renu Regunathan-Shenk, "Diet-Induced Oxalate Nephropathy from Excessive Nut and Seed Consumption," *BMJ Case Reports* 13, no. 11 (November 30, 2020): e237212, https://doi.org/10.1136/bcr-2020-237212.

33. Weiwen Chai and Michael Liebman, "Effect of Different Cooking Methods on Vegetable Oxalate Content," *Journal of Agricultural and Food Chemistry* 53, no. 8 (April 20, 2005): 3027–30, https://doi.org/10.1021/jf048128d.

34. Noonan and Savage, "Oxalate Content of Foods and Its Effect on Humans."

35. Susanne Voss et al., "The Effect of Oral Administration of Calcium and Magnesium on Intestinal Oxalate Absorption in Humans," *Isotopes in Environmental and Health Studies* 40, no. 3 (September 2004): 199–205, https://doi.org/10.1080/10256010410001671609.

36. Somchai Chutipongtanate, Sakdithep Chaiyarit, and Visith Thongboonkerd, "Citrate, Not Phosphate, Can Dissolve Calcium Oxalate Monohydrate Crystals and Detach These Crystals from Renal Tubular Cells," *European Journal of Pharmacology* 689, no. 1–3 (August 2012): 219–25, https://doi.org/10.1016/j.ejphar.2012.06.012.

STEP 11

1. Ronald D. Hills et al., "Gut Microbiome: Profound Implications for Diet and Disease," *Nutrients* 11, no. 7 (July 16, 2019): 1613, https://doi.org/10.3390/nu11071613; Emanuele Rinninella et al., "Food Components and Dietary Habits: Keys for a Healthy Gut Microbiota Composition," *Nutrients* 11, no. 10 (October 7, 2019): 2393, https://doi.org/10.3390/nu11102393.

2. Carol A. Kumamoto, Mark S. Gresnigt, and Bernhard Hube, "The Gut, the Bad and the Harmless: *Candida albicans* as a Commensal and Opportunistic Pathogen in the Intestine," *Current Opinion in Microbiology* 56 (August 2020): 7–15, https://doi.org/10.1016/j.mib.2020.05.006.

3. Rinninella et al., "Food Components and Dietary Habits"; Irene L. Richardson and Steven A. Frese, "Non-Nutritive Sweeteners and Their Impacts on the Gut Microbiome and Host Physiology," *Frontiers in Nutrition* 9 (August 25, 2022): 988144, https://doi.org/10.3389/fnut.2022.988144.

4. Qixing Mao et al., "The Ramazzini Institute 13-Week Pilot Study on Glyphosate and Roundup Administered at Human-Equivalent Dose to Sprague Dawley Rats: Effects on the Microbiome," *Environmental Health* 17, no. 1 (December 2018): 50, https://doi.org/10.1186/s12940-018-0394-x.

5. Isadora Argou-Cardozo and Fares Zeidán-Chuliá, "Clostridium Bacteria and Autism Spectrum Conditions: A Systematic Review and Hypothetical Contribution of Environmental Glyphosate Levels," *Medical Sciences* 6, no. 2 (April 4, 2018): 29, https://doi.org/10.3390/medsci6020029.

6. Rasnik K. Singh et al., "Influence of Diet on the Gut Microbiome and Implications for Human Health," *Journal of Translational Medicine* 15, no. 1 (April 8, 2017): 73, https://doi.org/10.1186/s12967-017-1175-y.

7. Lawrence A. David et al., "Diet Rapidly and Reproducibly Alters the Human Gut Microbiome," *Nature* 505, no. 7484 (January 23, 2014): 559–63, https://doi.org/10.1038/nature12820.

8. Lindsey G. Albenberg and Gary D. Wu, "Diet and the Intestinal Microbiome: Associations, Functions, and Implications for Health and Disease," *Gastroenterology* 146, no. 6 (May 2014): 1564–72, https://doi.org/10.1053/j.gastro.2014.01.058.

9. Hills et al., "Gut Microbiome."

10. Kearney T. W. Gunsalus et al., "Manipulation of Host Diet to Reduce Gastrointestinal Colonization by the Opportunistic Pathogen *Candida albicans*," *mSphere* 1, no. 1 (2016): e00020-15, https://doi.org/10.1128/mSphere.00020-15.

11. M. Raithel et al., "Significance of Salicylate Intolerance in Diseases of the Lower Gastrointestinal Tract," *Journal of Physiology and Pharmacology: An Official Journal of the Polish Physiological Society* 56, Suppl 5 (September 2005): 89–102.

12. Jacqueline S. Barrett and Peter R. Gibson, "Fermentable Oligosaccharides, Disaccharides, Monosaccharides and Polyols (FODMAPs) and Nonallergic Food Intolerance: FODMAPs or Food Chemicals?," *Therapeutic Advances in Gastroenterology* 5, no. 4 (July 2012): 261–68, https://doi.org/10.1177/1756283X11436241.

13. Julie S. Matthews and James B. Adams, "Ratings of the Effectiveness of 13 Therapeutic Diets for Autism Spectrum Disorder: Results of a National Survey," *Journal of Personalized Medicine* 13, no. 10 (September 29, 2023): 1448, https://doi.org/10.3390/jpm13101448.

14. Sofia Reddel, Lorenza Putignani, and Federica Del Chierico, "The Impact of Low-FODMAPs, Gluten-Free, and Ketogenic Diets on Gut Microbiota Modulation in Pathological Conditions," *Nutrients* 11, no. 2 (February 12, 2019): 373, https://doi.org/10.3390/nu11020373.

15. Joost P. Algera et al., "Low FODMAP Diet Reduces Gastrointestinal Symptoms in Irritable Bowel Syndrome and Clinical Response Could Be Predicted by Symptom Severity: A Randomized Crossover Trial," *Clinical Nutrition* 41, no. 12 (December 2022): 2792–2800, https://doi.org/10.1016/j.clnu.2022.11.001; Jongsung Hahn, Jeongwon Choi, and Min Jung Chang, "Effect of Low FODMAPs Diet on Irritable Bowel Syndromes: A Systematic Review and Meta-Analysis of Clinical Trials," *Nutrients* 13, no. 7 (July 19, 2021): 2460, https://doi.org/10.3390/nu13072460.

16. Tanisa Patcharatrakul et al., "The Effect of Rice vs. Wheat Ingestion on Postprandial Gastroesophageal Reflux (GER) Symptoms in Patients with Overlapping GERD-Irritable Bowel Syndrome (IBS)," *Foods* 11, no. 1 (December 23, 2021): 26, https://doi.org/10.3390/foods11010026.

17. Licia Pensabene et al., "Low FODMAPs Diet for Functional Abdominal Pain Disorders in Children: Critical Review of Current Knowledge," *Jornal De Pediatria* 95, no. 6 (2019): 642–56, https://doi.org/10.1016/j.jped.2019.03.004.

18. Luisa Bittencourt de Aquino Fernandes Dias, Rafaela Alexia Kobus, and Amanda Bagolin do Nascimento, "Effectiveness of the Low-FODMAP Diet in Improving Non-Celiac Gluten Sensitivity: A Systematic Review," *British Journal of Nutrition*, November 3, 2022, 1–9, https://doi.org/10.1017/S0007114522002884.

19. J. G. Muir et al., "Gluten-Free and Low-FODMAP Sourdoughs for Patients with Coeliac Disease and Irritable Bowel Syndrome: A Clinical Perspective," *International Journal of Food Microbiology* 290 (February 2019): 237–46, https://doi.org/10.1016/j.ijfoodmicro.2018.10.016.

20. Rafail I. Kushak et al., "Intestinal Disaccharidase Activity in Patients with Autism: Effect of Age, Gender, and Intestinal Inflammation," *Autism: The International Journal of Research and Practice* 15, no. 3 (May 2011): 285–94, https://doi.org/10.1177/1362361310369142; Karoly Horvath and Jay A.

Perman, "Autistic Disorder and Gastrointestinal Disease," *Current Opinion in Pediatrics* 14, no. 5 (October 2002): 583–87, https://doi.org/10.1097/00008480-200210000-00004.

21. Brent L. Williams et al., "Impaired Carbohydrate Digestion and Transport and Mucosal Dysbiosis in the Intestines of Children with Autism and Gastrointestinal Disturbances," *PloS One* 6, no. 9 (2011): e24585, https://doi.org/10.1371/journal.pone.0024585.

22. Nalan Hakime Nogay et al., "The Effect of the Low FODMAP Diet on Gastrointestinal Symptoms, Behavioral Problems and Nutrient Intake in Children with Autism Spectrum Disorder: A Randomized Controlled Pilot Trial," *Journal of Autism and Developmental Disorders* 51, no. 8 (August 2021): 2800–2811, https://doi.org/10.1007/s10803-020-04717-8.

23. Alexander Bertuccioli et al., "Ketogenic and Low FODMAP Diet in Therapeutic Management of a Young Autistic Patient with Epilepsy and Dysmetabolism Poorly Responsive to Therapies: Clinical Response and Effects of Intestinal Microbiota," *International Journal of Molecular Sciences* 23, no. 15 (August 8, 2022): 8829, https://doi.org/10.3390/ijms23158829.

24. Egoitz Aranburu et al., "Gluten and FODMAPs Relationship with Mental Disorders: Systematic Review," *Nutrients* 13, no. 6 (May 31, 2021): 1894, https://doi.org/10.3390/nu13061894.

25. Maria Rosaria Iovene et al., "Intestinal Dysbiosis and Yeast Isolation in Stool of Subjects with Autism Spectrum Disorders," *Mycopathologia* 182, no. 3–4 (April 2017): 349–63, https://doi.org/10.1007/s11046-016-0068-6.

26. Ahmed B. Bayoumy et al., "Gut Fermentation Syndrome: A Systematic Review of Case Reports," *United European Gastroenterology Journal* 9, no. 3 (April 2021): 332–42, https://doi.org/10.1002/ueg2.12062.

27. Matthews and Adams, "Ratings of the Effectiveness of 13 Therapeutic Diets for Autism Spectrum Disorder."

28. Chunlong Mu et al., "Metabolic Framework for the Improvement of Autism Spectrum Disorders by a Modified Ketogenic Diet: A Pilot Study," *Journal of Proteome Research* 19, no. 1 (January 3, 2020): 382–90, https://doi.org/10.1021/acs.jproteome.9b00581.

29. Ryan W. Y. Lee et al., "A Modified Ketogenic Gluten-Free Diet with MCT Improves Behavior in Children with Autism Spectrum Disorder," *Physiology & Behavior* 188 (May 1, 2018): 205–11, https://doi.org/10.1016/j.physbeh.2018.02.006.

30. Omnia El-Rashidy et al., "Ketogenic Diet versus Gluten Free Casein Free Diet in Autistic Children: A Case-Control Study," *Metabolic Brain Disease* 32, no. 6 (December 1, 2017): 1935–41, https://doi.org/10.1007/s11011-017-0088-z.

31. Cristina Alicia Elizalde-Romero et al., "Solanum Fruits: Phytochemicals, Bioaccessibility and Bioavailability, and Their Relationship with Their

Health-Promoting Effects," *Frontiers in Nutrition* 8 (November 25, 2021): 790582, https://doi.org/10.3389/fnut.2021.790582.

32. Yue Zhao et al., "Phytochemical and Pharmacological Studies on *Solanum lyratum*: A Review," *Natural Products and Bioprospecting* 12, no. 1 (November 9, 2022): 39, https://doi.org/10.1007/s13659-022-00361-0.

33. Zhao et al., "Phytochemical and Pharmacological Studies."

34. Karin de Punder and Leo Pruimboom, "The Dietary Intake of Wheat and Other Cereal Grains and Their Role in Inflammation," *Nutrients* 5, no. 3 (March 12, 2013): 771–87, https://doi.org/10.3390/nu5030771.

35. N. R. Reddy and M. D. Pierson, "Reduction in Antinutritional and Toxic Components in Plant Foods by Fermentation," *Food Research International* 27, no. 3 (January 1994): 281–90, https://doi.org/10.1016/0963-9969(94)90096-5.

36. Muir et al., "Gluten-Free and Low-FODMAP Sourdoughs."

37. Warren D. Kruger and Sapna Gupta, "The Effect of Dietary Modulation of Sulfur Amino Acids on Cystathionine β Synthase–Deficient Mice," *Annals of the New York Academy of Sciences* 1363, no. 1 (January 2016): 80–90, https://doi.org/10.1111/nyas.12967; Veronica Tisato et al., "Genetics and Epigenetics of One-Carbon Metabolism Pathway in Autism Spectrum Disorder," *Genes* 12, no. 5 (May 2021): 782, https://doi.org/10.3390/genes12050782.

38. François Blachier et al., "Production of Hydrogen Sulfide by the Intestinal Microbiota and Epithelial Cells and Consequences for the Colonic and Rectal Mucosa," *American Journal of Physiology. Gastrointestinal and Liver Physiology* 320, no. 2 (January 1, 2021): G125–35, https://doi.org/10.1152/ajpgi.00261.2020.

39. Levi M. Teigen et al., "Dietary Factors in Sulfur Metabolism and Pathogenesis of Ulcerative Colitis," *Nutrients* 11, no. 4 (April 25, 2019): 931, https://doi.org/10.3390/nu11040931.

STEP 12

1. Li-Hao Cheng et al., "Psychobiotics in Mental Health, Neurodegenerative and Neurodevelopmental Disorders," *Journal of Food and Drug Analysis* 27, no. 3 (July 2019): 632–48, https://doi.org/10.1016/j.jfda.2019.01.002.

2. Emre Adıgüzel et al., "Probiotics and Prebiotics Alleviate Behavioral Deficits, Inflammatory Response, and Gut Dysbiosis in Prenatal VPA-Induced Rodent Model of Autism," *Physiology & Behavior* 256 (November 1, 2022): 113961, https://doi.org/10.1016/j.physbeh.2022.113961.

3. Autism Nutrition Research Center, "ANRC Autism Treatment Rater," 2022, https://apps.apple.com/us/app/anrc-autism-treatment-rater/id1616969988.

4. Amani Alharthi et al., "The Human Gut Microbiome as a Potential Factor in Autism Spectrum Disorder," *International Journal of Molecular Sciences*

23, no. 3 (January 25, 2022): 1363, https://doi.org/10.3390/ijms23031363; Tingting Tu and Changlin Zhao, "Treating Autism Spectrum Disorder by Intervening with Gut Microbiota," *Journal of Medical Microbiology* 70, no. 12 (December 2021), https://doi.org/10.1099/jmm.0.001469.

5. Shannon Rose et al., "Butyrate Enhances Mitochondrial Function During Oxidative Stress in Cell Lines from Boys with Autism," *Translational Psychiatry* 8, no. 1 (February 2, 2018): 42, https://doi.org/10.1038/s41398-017-0089-z.

6. C. Marques and A. Kasa, "Preliminary Report on Activity of Biocidin Against Multiple Species of Biofilms," September 30, 2013, https://anovahealth.com/content/product_pdf/Biofilm-Study-2013.pdf.

7. Melissa Van Arsdall et al., "Is There a Role for the Enteral Administration of Serum-Derived Immunoglobulins in Human Gastrointestinal Disease and Pediatric Critical Care Nutrition?," *Advances in Nutrition* 7, no. 3 (May 2016): 535–43, https://doi.org/10.3945/an.115.011924.

8. Laila Y. AL-Ayadhi and Nadra Elyass Elamin, "Camel Milk as a Potential Therapy as an Antioxidant in Autism Spectrum Disorder (ASD)," *Evidence-Based Complementary and Alternative Medicine* 2013 (2013): 1–8, https://doi.org/10.1155/2013/602834; Shahid Bashir and Laila Y. Al-Ayadhi, "Effect of Camel Milk on Thymus and Activation-Regulated Chemokine in Autistic Children: Double-Blind Study," *Pediatric Research* 75, no. 4 (April 2014): 559–63, https://doi.org/10.1038/pr.2013.248; Laila Y. Al-Ayadhi et al., "Behavioral Benefits of Camel Milk in Subjects with Autism Spectrum Disorder," *Journal of the College of Physicians and Surgeons Pakistan* 25, no. 11 (November 2015): 819–23.

9. Autism Nutrition Research Center, "ANRC Autism Treatment Rater."

10. Thomas W. Sedlak, Leslie G. Nucifora, Minori Koga, Lindsay S. Shaffer, Cecilia Higgs, Teppei Tanaka, Anna M. Wang, et al., "Sulforaphane Augments Glutathione and Influences Brain Metabolites in Human Subjects: A Clinical Pilot Study," *Molecular Neuropsychiatry* (May 2018), https://www.ncbi.nlm.nih.gov/pmc/articles/PMC5981770/.

11. Eric A. Klomparens and Yuchuan Ding, "The Neuroprotective Mechanisms and Effects of Sulforaphane," *Brain Circulation* 5, no. 2 (2019): 74, https://doi.org/10.4103/bc.bc_7_19.

12. Andrew W. Zimmerman et al., "Randomized Controlled Trial of Sulforaphane and Metabolite Discovery in Children with Autism Spectrum Disorder," *Molecular Autism* 12, no. 1 (May 25, 2021): 38, https://doi.org/10.1186/s13229-021-00447-5.

13. Kanwaljit Singh et al., "Sulforaphane Treatment of Autism Spectrum Disorder (ASD)," *Proceedings of the National Academy of Sciences* 111, no. 43 (October 28, 2014): 15550–55, https://doi.org/10.1073/pnas.1416940111.

14. Rhoda Lynch et al., "Sulforaphane from Broccoli Reduces Symptoms of Autism: A Follow-Up Case Series from a Randomized Double-Blind Study," *Global Advances in Health and Medicine* 6 (January 2017): 2164957X1773582, https://doi.org/10.1177/2164957X17735826.

15. Fatir Qureshi et al., "Multivariate Analysis of Metabolomic and Nutritional Profiles Among Children with Autism Spectrum Disorder," *Journal of Personalized Medicine* 12, no. 6 (June 1, 2022): 923, https://doi.org/10.3390/jpm12060923.

16. Geir Bjørklund et al., "The Role of Glutathione Redox Imbalance in Autism Spectrum Disorder: A Review," *Free Radical Biology & Medicine* 160 (November 20, 2020): 149–62, https://doi.org/10.1016/j.freeradbiomed.2020.07.017.

17. Janet K. Kern et al., "A Clinical Trial of Glutathione Supplementation in Autism Spectrum Disorders," *Medical Science Monitor* 17, no. 12 (2011): CR677–82, https://doi.org/10.12659/MSM.882125.

18. John P. Richie et al., "Randomized Controlled Trial of Oral Glutathione Supplementation on Body Stores of Glutathione," *European Journal of Nutrition* 54, no. 2 (March 2015): 251–63, https://doi.org/10.1007/s00394-014-0706-z; R. Sinha et al., "Oral Supplementation with Liposomal Glutathione Elevates Body Stores of Glutathione and Markers of Immune Function," *European Journal of Clinical Nutrition* 72, no. 1 (January 2018): 105–11, https://doi.org/10.1038/ejcn.2017.132.

19. Autism Nutrition Research Center, "ANRC Autism Treatment Rater."

20. Autism Nutrition Research Center, "ANRC Autism Treatment Rater."

21. Autism Nutrition Research Center, "ANRC Autism Treatment Rater."

22. Richard Stuckey, William Walsh, and Brett Lambert, "The Effectiveness of Targeted Nutrient Therapy in Treatment of Mental Illness," *Journal of the Australasian College of Nutritional and Environmental Medicine* 29, no. 3 (November 2010): 3–8.

23. Rhonda P. Patrick and Bruce N. Ames, "Vitamin D and the Omega-3 Fatty Acids Control Serotonin Synthesis and Action, Part 2: Relevance for ADHD, Bipolar Disorder, Schizophrenia, and Impulsive Behavior," *FASEB Journal: Official Publication of the Federation of American Societies for Experimental Biology* 29, no. 6 (June 2015): 2207–22, https://doi.org/10.1096/fj.14-268342.

24. Autism Nutrition Research Center, "ANRC Autism Treatment Rater."

25. Autism Nutrition Research Center, "ANRC Autism Treatment Rater."

26. Autism Nutrition Research Center, "ANRC Autism Treatment Rater."

27. Autism Nutrition Research Center, "ANRC Autism Treatment Rater."

28. D. A. Rossignol and R. E. Frye, "Mitochondrial Dysfunction in Autism Spectrum Disorders: A Systematic Review and Meta-Analysis," *Molecular Psychiatry* 17, no. 3 (March 2012): 290–314, https://doi.org/10.1038/mp.2010.136.

29. Annelies A. J. Verlaet et al., "Rationale for Dietary Antioxidant Treatment of ADHD," *Nutrients* 10, no. 4 (March 24, 2018): 405, https://doi.org/10.3390/nu10040405.

30. S. Hirayama et al., "The Effect of Phosphatidylserine Administration on Memory and Symptoms of Attention-Deficit Hyperactivity Disorder: A Randomised, Double-Blind, Placebo-Controlled Clinical Trial," *Journal of Human Nutrition and Dietetics: The Official Journal of the British Dietetic Association* 27, Suppl 2 (April 2014): 284–91, https://doi.org/10.1111/jhn.12090.

31. James B. Adams et al., "Ratings of the Effectiveness of Nutraceuticals for Autism Spectrum Disorders: Results of a National Survey," *Journal of Personalized Medicine* 11, no. 9 (August 31, 2021): 878, https://doi.org/10.3390/jpm11090878.

32. Autism Nutrition Research Center, "ANRC Autism Treatment Rater."

33. Richard E. Frye et al., "Effectiveness of Methylcobalamin and Folinic Acid Treatment on Adaptive Behavior in Children with Autistic Disorder Is Related to Glutathione Redox Status," *Autism Research and Treatment* (2013): 609705, https://doi.org/10.1155/2013/609705.

34. Guangfu Zhao et al., "Betaine in Inflammation: Mechanistic Aspects and Applications," *Frontiers in Immunology* 9 (2018): 1070, https://doi.org/10.3389/fimmu.2018.01070.

35. J. J. Strain et al., "Choline Status and Neurodevelopmental Outcomes at 5 Years of Age in the Seychelles Child Development Nutrition Study," *British Journal of Nutrition* 110, no. 2 (July 28, 2013): 330–36, https://doi.org/10.1017/S0007114512005077.

BEYOND DIET AND NUTRITION

1. Jet B. Muskens, Fleur P. Velders, and Wouter G. Staal, "Medical Comorbidities in Children and Adolescents with Autism Spectrum Disorders and Attention Deficit Hyperactivity Disorders: A Systematic Review," *European Child & Adolescent Psychiatry* 26, no. 9 (September 2017): 1093–1103, https://doi.org/10.1007/s00787-017-1020-0.

2. Theoharis C. Theoharides et al., "Mast Cell Activation and Autism," *Biochimica et Biophysica Acta (BBA)—Molecular Basis of Disease* 1822, no. 1 (January 2012): 34–41, https://doi.org/10.1016/j.bbadis.2010.12.017.

3. Margaret L. Bauman, "Medical Comorbidities in Autism: Challenges to Diagnosis and Treatment," *Neurotherapeutics: The Journal of the American Society for Experimental NeuroTherapeutics* 7, no. 3 (July 2010): 320–27, https://doi.org/10.1016/j.nurt.2010.06.001.

4. Anne Masi et al., "An Overview of Autism Spectrum Disorder, Heterogeneity and Treatment Options," *Neuroscience Bulletin* 33, no. 2 (April 2017): 183–93, https://doi.org/10.1007/s12264-017-0100-y.

5. Sydney M. Finegold et al., "Gastrointestinal Microflora Studies in Late-Onset Autism," *Clinical Infectious Diseases: An Official Publication of the Infectious Diseases Society of America* 35, no. Suppl 1 (September 1, 2002): S6–16, https://doi.org/10.1086/341914; Akhil A. Vinithakumari et al., "*Clostridioides difficile* Infection Dysregulates Brain Dopamine Metabolism," *Microbiology Spectrum* 10, no. 2 (April 27, 2022): e0007322, https://doi.org/10.1128/spectrum.00073-22; Lucía Iglesias-Vázquez et al., "Composition of Gut Microbiota in Children with Autism Spectrum Disorder: A Systematic Review and Meta-Analysis," *Nutrients* 12, no. 3 (March 17, 2020): 792, https://doi.org/10.3390/nu12030792.
6. Maria Rosaria Iovene et al., "Intestinal Dysbiosis and Yeast Isolation in Stool of Subjects with Autism Spectrum Disorders," *Mycopathologia* 182, no. 3–4 (April 2017): 349–63, https://doi.org/10.1007/s11046-016-0068-6.
7. Khemlal Nirmalkar et al., "Bimodal Distribution of Intestinal *Candida* in Children with Autism and Its Potential Link with Worse ASD Symptoms," *Gut Microbes Reports* 1, no. 1 (December 31, 2024): 2358324, https://doi.org/10.1080/29933935.2024.2358324.
8. T. C. Theoharides et al., "Atopic Diseases and Inflammation of the Brain in the Pathogenesis of Autism Spectrum Disorders," *Translational Psychiatry* 6, no. 6 (June 28, 2016): e844, https://doi.org/10.1038/tp.2016.77.
9. Samuele Cortese et al., "Association Between Autism Spectrum Disorder and Diabetes: Systematic Review and Meta-Analysis," *Neuroscience and Biobehavioral Reviews* 136 (May 2022): 104592, https://doi.org/10.1016/j.neubiorev.2022.104592.
10. Melania Manco et al., "Cross-Sectional Investigation of Insulin Resistance in Youths with Autism Spectrum Disorder. Any Role for Reduced Brain Glucose Metabolism?," *Translational Psychiatry* 11, no. 1 (April 20, 2021): 229, https://doi.org/10.1038/s41398-021-01345-3.
11. Cindy Sage and Ernesto Burgio, "Electromagnetic Fields, Pulsed Radiofrequency Radiation, and Epigenetics: How Wireless Technologies May Affect Childhood Development," *Child Development* 89, no. 1 (January 2018): 129–36, https://doi.org/10.1111/cdev.12824.
12. Martha R. Herbert and Cindy Sage, "Autism and EMF? Plausibility of a Pathophysiological Link Part II," *Pathophysiology: The Official Journal of the International Society for Pathophysiology* 20, no. 3 (June 2013): 211–34, https://doi.org/10.1016/j.pathophys.2013.08.002.
13. Liisa Hantsoo and Babette S. Zemel, "Stress Gets into the Belly: Early Life Stress and the Gut Microbiome," *Behavioural Brain Research* 414 (September 2021): 113474, https://doi.org/10.1016/j.bbr.2021.113474.

INDEX

ACKNOWLEDGMENTS

Many people contributed to the writing of this book.

To my mother and grandmother, who through their Italian heritage taught me to love cooking, enjoy eating healthy whole foods, and appreciate the value of family meals and traditions. By teaching me the skill of cooking without a recipe, you have helped me create many of the new dishes and recipes in this book. To my father, who has shown me true unconditional love, how to have faith, how to persevere in the face of adversity, and how to think for myself—I can't describe in words how grateful I am and how much I love you.

My daughter has taught me so much and has been patient and generous with her time to allow me to travel, speak, and write this book to help other children. I couldn't have done this without your love and support, not to mention your taste testing and priceless advice on making these recipes kid friendly and delicious. I love you forever and always. Thank you to my family for holding down the fort when I was traveling to conferences and allowing me the time to complete this enormous project.

Special acknowledgment goes to the pioneers in autism biomedicine and nutrition—your dedication and knowledge have made me a better practitioner.

Deep appreciation goes to my research mentors Dr. James Adams, Dr. Christy Alexon, Dr. Teresa Hart, and Susan Owens for inspiring my love of research and teaching me so much.

To my literary agents, Celeste Fine, Mia Vitale, and Sarah Passick of Park & Fine Literary and Media—thank you for your support and believing in my vision for this book. To the team at BenBella Books: Glenn Yeffeth, Leah Wilson, Madeline Grigg, Lindsay Marshall, Heather Butterfield, Victoria Carmody, Jessica Easto, Kim Broderick, Sarah Avinger, Morgan Carr, and all, thank you for allowing me the opportunity to get this important subject out into the world and for the guidance to make this book a powerful resource for so many families and individuals with autism spectrum disorder. And particular heartfelt gratitude goes out to my editor, Claire Schulz, who knows every inch of this book as well as I do and has helped me bring it to life—your skill is extraordinary.

And many thanks to my colleagues for their unwavering support and to my friends who have been there for me and encouraged me—I'm forever grateful. To Terri Hirning and the Hirning family—thanks for embracing us like your own family, for the countless hours of personal and professional advice, and your support with Nourishing Hope families. To Dr. Elisa Song—thank you for the touching foreword and years of friendship and guidance. To Trudy Scott—thanks for the years of support, from my first book more than sixteen years ago to today, and for the mastermind sessions nerding out over biochemistry and how to improve anxiety. To Drs. Kurt Woeller and Tracy Tranchitella—thank you for your hospitality, your years of expertise, and the many referrals that have translated into the principles in this book. To Annika Rockwell—I'm grateful for the years of friendship, professional support, and all I've learned from you. To Mira Dessy—thank you for taking me in when I was stranded at the airport and for your support with this book. To Jeannine Olson—thanks for the support and countless ideas on everything from my first book to this one; you are a true friend.

Thank you to all of my friends and colleagues for everything you have done for me and that I have learned from you: Dr. Madiha Saeed, Dr. Tom O'Bryan and Marzi O'Bryan, Maria Rickert Hong, Beth Lambert, Dr. Elizabeth Lipski, Dr. Maya Shetreat, Dr. Bridget Briggs, Dr. Kara Fitzgerald, Dr. Tom Moorcroft, Donna Gates, Mary Agnes Antonopoulos, Dr. Izabella Wentz and Michael Wentz, Magdalena Wszelaki, Andrea Nakayama, Jodi

Cohen, Dr. Nicole Beurkens, Polly Tommey, Betsy Hicks, Tara Hunkin, Beth Gillespie, Ari Whitten, Reed Davis, Dr. David Jockers, Dan Hanson, Marc Isaacson, Dr. Albert Mensah, Heidi Snyder, Dr. Ed Bauman, Paula Bartholomy, Dr. Nancy O'Hara, Dr. Anju Usman Singh, Dr. Elizabeth Mumper, Dr. Martha Herbert, Dr. Richard Frye, Dr. Daniel Rossignol, Dr. James Neuenschwander, Dr. William Walsh, Dr. William Shaw, Dr. Suzanne Goh, Dr. Terry Wahls, Dr. Michelle Perro, Dr. Sheila Kilbane, Dr. Heather Way, Dr. Lindsey Wells, Dr. Erica Peirson, Dana Laake, Vicki Kobliner, Maureen McDonnell, Honey Rinicella, Lori Knowles-Jimenez, Tracy Slepcevic, Peter Sullivan, J. J. Virgin, and the Mindshare team.

To my BioIndividual Nutrition Practitioners—keep nourishing hope for children and families in need and thank you for improving the BioIndividual Nutrition Institute with your contributions: Carrie Bailey, Holly Morello, Lisane Drouin, Joan Cass, Lisa Aschenbrenner, Shandy Laskey, Dr. Janice Carlin, Dr. Silvija Abele, Dr. Mary Wilde, Dr. Zendi Moldenhauer, and all students and graduates, too numerous to name.

To all parents, grandparents, aunts, uncles, and caregivers of children with autism spectrum disorder, individuals with autism, and Nourishing Hope families, thank you. I have learned so much from all of you. May you continue nourishing hope and thrive so the world may see all your gifts. Special thanks to all the families who shared their stories in this book in the hopes of helping and inspiring others.

ABOUT THE AUTHOR

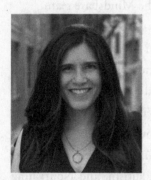

Julie Matthews is a Certified Nutrition Consultant and published researcher who received her master's degree in medical nutrition, with distinction, from Arizona State University. She has specialized in children's nutrition and complex neurological conditions, most notably autism spectrum disorder, for over twenty years. Julie sits on the Nutritional/Medical Advisory Board of the Autism Nutrition Research Center and helps children, families, and clinicians from 146 countries with her online resources, nutrition programs, and professional training courses.

Julie has educated parents and health professionals on how to use personalized nutrition and therapeutic diets to help children thrive at conferences in more than sixty-five cities over three continents including the Medical Academy of Pediatric & Special Needs (MAPS), Integrative Medicine for Mental Health (IMMH), and the American Academy of Anti-Aging Medicine (A4M). She has been featured in newspapers and blogs, and on podcasts, radio, and television including CBS. She has co-authored peer-reviewed research studies demonstrating the efficacy of nutrition and therapeutic diet intervention for ASD.

When she is not studying the latest nutrition research, supporting families, or experimenting with new recipes in her kitchen, she can be found camping with her daughter, hugging redwood trees, and gardening.